Statistical Methods for Health Care Research

Statistical Methods
for Health Care Research

Barbara Hazard Munro, Ph.D., R.N.
Associate Professor and Chairperson
Program in Nursing Research
Yale University School of Nursing
New Haven, Connecticut

Madelon A. Visintainer, Ph.D., R.N.
Associate Professor and Chairperson
Pediatric Nursing Program
Yale University School of Nursing
New Haven, Connecticut

Ellis Batten Page, Ed.D., M.A.
Professor
Educational Psychology and Research
Duke University
Durham, North Carolina

Contributing Author:
Jane Karpe Dixon, Ph.D.
Associate Professor
Program in Nursing Research
Yale University School of Nursing
New Haven, Connecticut

 J. B. Lippincott Company   Philadelphia
London   Mexico City   New York   St. Louis   São Paulo   Sydney

Acquisitions Editor: Paul Hill
Copy Editor: Ann Blum
Indexer: Barbara Farabaugh
Design Director: Tracy Baldwin
Design Coordinator: Anne O'Donnell
Designer: Katharine Nichols
Production Supervisor: J. Corey Gray
Production Editor: Rosanne Hallowell
Production Coordinator: Barney Fernandes
Compositor: Circle Graphics
Text Printer/Binder: R. R. Donnelley and Sons Company
Cover Printer: Philips Offset Co., Inc.

6 5 4 3

Library of Congress Cataloging-in-Publication Data
Munro, Barbara Hazard.
    Statistical methods for health care research.

    Bibliography: p.
    Includes index.
    1. Nursing—Research—Statistical methods.
2. Medical care—Research—Statistical methods.
I. Visintainer, Madelon A. II. Page, Ellis Batten.
III. Title. [DNLM: 1. Health Services Research—methods.
2. Statistics. WA 950 M968s]
RT81.5.M86 1986   610'.72   85–24037
ISBN 0–397–54503–7

Dedicated to
the Yale University School of Nursing
Classes of 1985, 1986, and 1987

Preface

The professional nurse or other health professional, seeking to improve practice, may wish to consult the research literature about an area of interest. Suppose one reads that hospitalized patients who received therapeutic touch

> experienced a highly significant ($p < .001$) reduction in state anxiety, according to a comparison of pre-posttest measures on A-state anxiety using a correlated t-ratio (Heidt, 1981, p. 32).

How many health professionals would understand such reporting? Certainly not as many as we would like, yet such is the language in which research is presented. If health professionals wish to use research, they must at least understand the more commonly used statistical methods. Besides terms and procedures, they must also understand the appropriate *application* of such methods to evaluate the validity of research conclusions. Thus, knowledge of statistics is important not simply for researchers, but for "consumers" of the research as well.

Our purpose is to acquaint the reader with the statistical techniques most commonly reported in the research literature of the health professions. We give examples of how such techniques are used and how results may be interpreted. Since access to computers has become fairly commonplace, it is now rare for statistics actually to be calculated by hand. For us, it is necessary to know what we can expect the computer to do and how to interpret its output. Thus, we show examples of such output throughout the book.

Calculations are presented when necessary for basic understanding of a given technique. These calculations require knowledge of only the most basic algebra, that is, how to solve an equation. Taking a square root is the most complex mathematics involved, and that is easily achieved with the use of a pocket calculator.

We hope this book opens the door of research for your understanding and enjoyment.

Acknowledgments

We would like to acknowledge the support and assistance provided by the staff members in the Program for Nursing Research at Yale University School of Nursing. They are Joan Fettes, the Administrative Assistant, and Pauline Faucher, who was the Secretary. They provided not only technical assistance with the preparation of the manuscript but understanding and encouragement as well. The students in the Yale School of Nursing graduating classes of 1985, 86, and 87 deserve very special mention. They used photocopies of the manuscript, cumbersome copies which were typed by the authors. Their comments, suggestions, and support were invaluable. In particular we would like to thank Deborah K. Mayer of the Class of 1985, who contributed excellent feedback on the first draft of the manuscript. Finally, we would like to thank Bruce Munro, husband of the first author, who assisted with the preparation of some of the figures.

Contents

SECTION 1
Understanding the Data

CHAPTER 1

Introduction to Data Analysis

Barbara Hazard Munro

OBJECTIVES FOR CHAPTER 1

After reading this chapter and completing the exercises, you should be able to

1. Discuss levels of measurement and their relationship to statistical analysis.
2. Construct a table containing absolute and relative frequencies and cumulative percents.
3. Present data by means of various graphical methods.
4. Interpret a frequency distribution created by a computer program.

LEVELS OF INQUIRY

Research studies are conducted to answer research questions and to test hypotheses. Research questions take on different forms depending on the level of inquiry. Questions at four levels of inquiry (Dickoff & James, 1968) have been posed by Diers (1979, p. 35).

1. What is this?
2. What's happening here?
3. What will happen if . . . ?
4. How can I make . . . happen?

Research questions are posed in the first two levels of inquiry, whereas hypotheses are stated for the highest two levels (levels 3 and 4). The questions or hypotheses, or both, are usually presented immediately after the review of the literature. To answer the questions or test the hypotheses, data are collected, analyzed, and interpreted.

A research study cannot be designed properly without considering the statistical techniques appropriate to answer the research questions and test the hypotheses. Conducting a study and then turning the data over to a statistician for analysis is almost guaranteed to result in useless data. The type of data that will be collected and methods of statistical analysis must be considered during the planning of the project.

LEVELS OF MEASUREMENT

In selecting measurement tools for research, it is necessary to consider the type of data the tools produce and whether or not the data are appropriate to answer the research questions. Measurement is considered the "assignment of numbers to characteristics according to some rule" (Stevens, 1951). There are various levels of measurement. We could classify subjects as older people, middle-aged people, young adults, adolescents, and children, resulting in each subject being placed in one of five categories. Or we could simply use their ages in years, resulting in a wide range of scores. The latter is a much more precise measure than classifying the subjects into a small number of categories. In the classification scheme, we would not be able to distinguish between 1 year olds and 12 year olds, since they would all fall into the category for children. In general, it is better to leave measures in their original scales, such as age in years, than to collapse the scale into groups before analysis.

Consideration of the level of measurement is important in determining the appropriate method of data analysis. Classification of measurement includes four levels, from the least precise, nominal, to the most precise, ratio.

Nominal Scale

The first and lowest scale in the hierarchy is the nominal scale. It includes *labeling* and *categories*. The numbers on baseball players' shirts are a means of labeling. No two players on the team have the same number, but the numbers do not suggest quantity of anything, that is, baseball player number 11 is not considered as having more ability than player number 2. Numbering the charts used in a study from 1 to 100 is simply a way of identifying which chart was used to obtain certain information, and in no way indicates a comparison among charts.

A second type of nominal scaling is the use of categories. More than one object may get the same number or be put into the same group, but all objects in one group are considered equal in the characteristic on which they were classified. Race, marital status, religion, and sex are categorical variables. (A variable is anything that can take on more than one value.) When using religion as a variable, all Catholics are considered equally Catholic. An individual is categorized according to the stated religion, not according to how committed he or she is to it. If amount of commitment were measured, the variable would no longer be a categorical variable. With categories, there is no attempt to quantify differences, just to group together subjects that are similar in some characteristic.

Ordinal Scale

Many measures used in behavioral research, such as measures of performance, attitude, and personality, may produce ordinal data. An ordinal scale is one in which members of a set (*e.g.*, objects, people) are ordered from most to least with respect to some characteristic. For example, a group of subjects could be lined up from shortest to tallest without any knowledge of the actual heights of the individuals. There would be no notion of equal distance between the rankings. We would not know how much taller one subject was than another, just that a given subject was taller than the person in front of him.

Another example would be asking a supervisor to rank workers from most to least capable. Again, there is no notion of equal distance between each worker. We can say that one worker is ranked as more capable than another, but not by how much.

As runners in a distance race cross the finish line, they are often given numbers indicating their positions at the finish. These numbers represent an ordinal scale. Each number tells in what place a runner finished, but not how close he or she was to the runner ahead and behind.

Interval Scale

If, in addition to being able to rank or order individuals or objects on some characteristic, the distance between the points on the scale is known, the measure is at the interval level. This means that the distance between any two adjacent points on the scale is the same as the distance between any other two adjacent points. With an interval level scale, however, no knowledge is available about the absolute magnitude of the characteristic. The Fahrenheit thermometer is an example of a tool that provides an interval scale. Zero on the Fahrenheit scale is not a "true" zero. With interval measures, we can say that there is the same distance between points one and two as between points three and four, but we cannot say that point four is twice as large as point two. Thus, it is incorrect to say that a temperature of 80° Fahrenheit is twice as hot as a temperature of 40° Fahrenheit.

Ratio Scale

The ratio scale is the most precise measurement scale; it includes all the characteristics of the lower three scales and, in addition, has a true zero. Time is a ratio measure: 10 minutes is twice as long as 5 minutes. Weight and height are also ratio measures, with 100 pounds being twice as heavy as 50 pounds, and 12 inches twice as long as 6 inches.

To compare an interval and a ratio scale, you can look at the Fahrenheit and Kelvin scales. The Kelvin is a ratio scale with a true zero, whereas the Fahrenheit is an interval scale. On the Kelvin scale, a temperature of 100° would be twice as hot as a temperature of 50°. To demonstrate that this does not hold true for the Fahrenheit scale, note that a temperature of 50° Fahrenheit is equal to 323° on the Kelvin scale, and a temperature of 100° Fahrenheit is equal to 373° Kelvin. Since 373° is not twice as large as 323°, it is obvious that 100° Fahrenheit is not twice as hot as 50° Fahrenheit.

LEVELS OF MEASUREMENT AND STATISTICAL ANALYSIS

There are those who take a very fundamentalist view on which measures of statistical analysis can be used with which levels of data. In addition to outlining the four levels of measurement, Stevens (1951) also listed which statistical techniques were appropriate for each level of data. In his opinion, it was appropriate to use the more powerful statistical tools, often called *parametrics* (*i.e.*, analysis of variance, correlation coefficients, regression, and so on) only with data that were at least at the interval level. This meant that ordinal data, which include many of the measures used in behavioral research, had to be analyzed by less powerful statistical techniques, such as the Wilcoxon Matched-Pairs Signed-Ranks test, the Mann–Whitney U Test, or Friedman's Two-Way Analysis of Variance. The Siegel book (1956) outlined nonparametric statistics that should be used with ordinal and nominal data. Researchers tended to follow the rules set down by Stevens and Siegel, and refrained from using parametric statistics with ordinal data.

Today, most researchers take a more realistic view and use parametric measures with data when they are not sure of equal intervals. They do this because it has been found to work; that is, treating ordinal data as if they were interval data has not distorted the results. As Popham and Sirotnik (1973, p. 270) report, "A number of empirical studies have demonstrated that, when parametric procedures have been employed with ordinal data, they rarely distort a relationship between variables which may be present in the data. More often than not, such parametric analysis results are nearly identical to those yielded by nonparametric procedures."

Kerlinger (1973, p. 440) reports that even though most psychological and educational scales are basically ordinal, they "approximate equality fairly well." Nunnally (1978, p. 28) agrees and says, "How seriously are such misassumptions about scale properties likely to influence the reported results of scientific experiments? In psychology at the present time, the answer in most cases is 'very little'."

Although the weaknesses of using nonparametrics have been presented in the literature for the past 30 years, the use of such techniques is frequently reported in nursing journals. Gordon Armstrong does an excellent job of describing the major points in this long-standing controversy. (His article is entitled "Parametric Statistics and Ordinal Data: A Pervasive Misconception" and can be found in the column "Methodology Corner" of *Nursing Research*, January–February, 1981. We recommend that article to readers of this book.)

The advantage of using the parametric statistics is that they are more powerful, that is, they are more likely to find a significant difference if one exists. Kerlinger

(1973, p. 441) states: "The best procedure is to treat ordinal measures as though they were interval measurements, but to be constantly alert to the possibility of *gross* inequality of intervals."

Based on these considerations, we have simplified the presentation of statistics covered in this book to the use of nonparametrics for nominal data and the use of parametrics for all other levels of data. If you are working with a very small sample or if your data seriously violate the assumption of equality of intervals, we suggest that you consult a book providing details on the nonparametric techniques, such as the Siegel book (1956).

COMPONENTS OF THE RESULTS SECTION
OF THE RESEARCH REPORT

The results section of the research report usually begins with a description of the sample. Techniques appropriate for presenting descriptive data are given in this section of the book (Chapters 1–4). Following the description of the sample, the research questions or hypotheses, or both, are presented in the order in which they were proposed. The question or hypothesis is stated, and the analysis of the data gathered to answer the question or test the hypothesis is presented. This reporting is straightforward and factual. Comments on the meaning of the results are usually presented in the discussion section. There may be a section for additional findings that were not directly related to the questions or hypotheses. The chapter ends with a brief summary of the results. Examples of appropriate presentation of statistical results using tables and narrative are presented throughout this book.

PRESENTING DESCRIPTIVE DATA

One of the purposes of statistics is to reduce data to a manageable and under-standable form. Descriptive statistics are often used to describe the characteristics of the sample under study. They are also used in factor-isolating (descriptive) studies, which seek to determine what factors are important in a given situation.

Frequency Distributions

Suppose you gave a test to a group of 50 students and the resulting scores were as listed in Table 1-1. How well did the people do on the test? It would be hard to tell from Table 1-1. One simple way to gain some order is simply to list the scores from highest to lowest and tally up how many people got each score. This technique is called a *frequency distribution*, and the result is given in Table 1-2. Although this technique has helped us to understand how the scores were distributed, it is still quite cumbersome because of the number of scores. When you have more than 10 to 20 scores, you should combine the scores into groups for presentation in tables.

Table 1-1   Scores for 50 Subjects on Test

Subject	Score	Subject	Score	Subject	Score	Subject	Score	Subject	Score
1	73	11	74	21	74	31	80	41	71
2	65	12	76	22	93	32	74	42	80
3	80	13	65	23	95	33	84	43	75
4	85	14	92	24	75	34	76	44	85
5	71	15	85	25	84	35	94	45	72
6	90	16	97	26	95	36	75	46	90
7	76	17	82	27	86	37	89	47	76
8	89	18	70	28	55	38	59	48	88
9	82	19	86	29	99	39	95	49	73
10	73	20	75	30	79	40	78	50	65

These groups are called *class intervals*. This does not mean that in analysis using these scores you would reduce them to categories. You are using categories to make the data more meaningful for the reader. For example, the ages of your subjects might be presented as grouped data in a table, but you would use each subject's age when comparing two groups on their ages. Once you group the data for presentation, some information is lost, since you only show how many subjects fell within a particular class, not the exact scores within the class. An example of class intervals using the data already presented in Table 1-1 is given in Table 1-3. For this table, the data have been grouped in a logical way according to how grades are usually assigned, that is, 90–100 are As, 80–89 are Bs, and so forth.

Although there are no absolute rules for grouping data, there are some guidelines. You would not want more than 10 to 20 class intervals, because you would not have solved the original problem of too many scores. Class intervals of equal width are preferred. In Table 1-3, this guideline was violated in interval 90–100, because

Table 1-2   Frequency Distribution of Scores for 50 Subjects

Score	Tally	f	Score	Tally	f	Score	Tally	f	Score	Tally	f	Score	Tally	f
100			90	||	2	80	|||	3	70	|	1	60		
99	|	1	89	||	2	79	|	1	69			59	|	1
98			88	|	1	78	|	1	68			58		
97	|	1	87			77			67			57		
96			86	||	2	76	||||	4	66			56		
95	|||	3	85	|||	3	75	||||	4	65	|||	3	55	|	1
94	|	1	84	||	2	74	|||	3	64			54		
93	|	1	83			73	|||	3	63			53		
92	|	1	82	||	2	72	|	1	62			52		
91			81			71	||	2	61			51		

f = frequency

**Table 1-3   Grouped Frequency Distribution
of Test Scores for 50 Subjects**

Scores	f	Relative f (%)	Cumulative Percent
50–59	2	4	4
60–69	3	6	10
70–79	20	40	50
80–89	15	30	80
90–100	10	20	100
Totals	*50*	*100%*	

that contains 11 numbers, whereas the other intervals contain 10 each. The class intervals should be *mutually exclusive* and *exhaustive*. Mutually exclusive means that any given score will fit into only one group. For example, score 95 fits into the highest group and does not fit into any other group. Exhaustive means that each score will be included in one group. If one person had scored 42 on the test, there would not be a group in which that score would fit. Thus, mutually exclusive and exhaustive means that every score fits into one and only one group.

Open-ended intervals are avoided. This means that the lowest category should not be "59 and below," because the reader would not know if there were scores that fell below 50. Open-ended intervals are avoided at both the top and the bottom of the distribution.

In Table 1-3, the width of all but one of the class intervals is equal to 10, which is an even number. This number was used because it makes sense in reporting grades, but, as will be shown in the next section of this chapter, an odd width, say 9 or 11, makes graphing of the distribution easier. When drawing some graphs, a single point, the midpoint, is used to represent the class interval. With an odd number of possible scores within a given interval, the midpoint will be a whole number rather than a decimal.

The *absolute frequency (f)* is the actual number of subjects who received a certain score or whose score fell within a particular class interval. In Table 1-3, 20 individuals scored between 70 and 79 on the test. To calculate *relative frequencies*, you convert the actual numbers to percents. Of the 50 individuals who took the test, 20 scored beteen 70 and 79, or 40% of the scores fell between 70 and 79 ($^{20}/_{50} \times 100 = 40\%$). *Cumulative percent* results from adding up each successive percent in the relative frequency column. Of those who took the test, 4% scored between 50 and 59 and another 6% scored between 60 and 69; thus, 10% of the subjects received a grade of less than 70, or 10% failed this test.

An example of the frequency distribution produced by the *Statistical Package for the Social Sciences (SPSS)* is given in Figure 1-1. These examples will appear throughout the book; for interested readers, the SPSS Procedure cards (commands) are shown, with examples of printouts. The printout in Figure 1-1 describes the

Procedure card

```
1              16
FREQUENCIES    GENERAL = MS
```

Output

MS   MARITAL STATUS

CATEGORY LABEL	CODE	ABSOLUTE FREQ	RELATIVE FREQ (PCT)	ADJUSTED FREQ (PCT)	CUM FREQ (PCT)
SINGLE	1.	10	5.7	6.0	6.0
MARRIED	2.	140	79.5	83.8	89.8
SEPARATED	3.	5	2.8	3.0	92.8
DIVORCED	4.	4	2.3	2.4	95.2
WIDOWED	5.	8	4.5	4.8	100.0
	9.	9	5.1	MISSING	100.0
TOTAL		176	100.0	100.0	

Figure 1-1 Example of output from SPSS frequency program.

marital status of 176 subjects. When the data were entered into the computer, each category of this nominal-level variable was given a code number. A single person was given a 1 on marital status; a married person, 2; and so on. Labels were added so that the printout would contain not only the code numbers but also the corresponding label. Code number 9 was given to subjects who did not answer the question about their marital status; this category is referred to as "missing data." In this case, nine individuals did not give their marital status. In addition to the parts of the frequency distribution described above, that is, absolute frequency, relative frequency (percent), and cumulative frequency (percent), note the additional column, *adjusted frequency (percent)*. In this column, the percent is adjusted for the missing data. In this sample, there are 176 subjects; 140 reported that they were married, that is, 79.5% of the total sample ($^{140}/_{176} \times 100 = 79.5\%$). However, since nine subjects (5.1%) did not give their marital status, leaving them in the calculation may distort the results. Another way to report the findings is to say that of the 167 individuals who reported their marital status, 140, or 83.8%, were married ($^{140}/_{167} \times 100 = 83.8\%$). That is the figure given under adjusted frequency. If there were no missing data, the relative and adjusted frequencies would be the same. The cumulative frequency in the SPSS output is based on the adjusted frequency, not the relative frequency ($6.0\% + 83.8\% + 3.0\%$, *etc.*).

If you presented a table containing the information in Figure 1-1 in your results section, you would only need to describe it briefly in the narrative. Tables are used to give details; it is redundant and tiresome to report them in the text. For example, you might simply write that, of those reporting their marital status, about 84% were married, 6% were single, and the rest were separated, widowed, or divorced.

Rounding Off

The following is a brief reminder about rounding off numbers:

We first must decide how many decimal places, if any, we want to round to. If the last digit in the number to be rounded off is less than 5, we round to the lower number; if it is higher than 5, we round to the higher number. For example, if we wished to round to two decimal places, 4.423 would be rounded to 4.42, and 4.426 would be rounded to 4.43. If the number to be rounded is a 5, the usual method is to round to the nearest *even* number, since that avoids any systematic bias up or down. For example, 4.425 would be rounded to 4.42, whereas 4.435 would be rounded to 4.44. If rounding to whole numbers rather than to decimals, the same rules prevail. That is,

$$8.2 = 8$$
$$8.5 = 8$$
$$8.8 = 9$$
$$9.5 = 10$$

Graphic Methods

Presenting data graphically is often useful in giving the reader a clear picture of the differences that exist. There will be greater use of these techniques in the future, since computer programs have been developed that produce sophisticated graphic representations of data. In this book, we outline the techniques most commonly used to present data collected in behavioral research.

Histogram. Histograms are probably the most commonly used graphical method. They are a type of bar graph and are used with continuous rather than categorical data, that is, usually they are used with interval and ratio-type data. When the class intervals are equal in width, the columns (or bars) are all the same width. If class intervals are unequal, corrections need to be made in the height of the columns as well as in the width to avoid misinterpretation based on the area included in the column. We present only histograms based on equal class intervals. The height of the column indicates the frequency.

Before describing histograms in more detail, we need to describe "true" class limits. In Table 1-3, we presented the class intervals as 50–59, 60–69, and so on, but suppose someone had a score of 89.5; where does that score fall? It appears that there is a gap between 89 and 90, but of course we can use our rounding-off technique to place scores in one of these categories. The notion of continuous data is that a score does not necessarily fall on discrete points (*i.e.*, on 88, 89, 90, 91, *etc.*) but may fall anywhere between, depending on how many decimal places are included. With one decimal place, there are 9 places between 89 and 90; with two decimal places, there are 99. To be continuous, the class interval 90–100 in Table 1-3 could be written as 89.5–100.5. In histograms, the"true" class intervals are usually used on the horizontal line. This is done to demonstrate that the data are continuous.

When constructing a histogram, some factors should be kept in mind:

1. Use "true" class intervals on the horizontal line.
2. If possible, have the class intervals equal.
3. With equal class intervals, all columns have the same width.
4. The vertical and horizontal axes should be about equal in length.
5. The graph should be clearly labeled with a title and labels for both axes.
6. The graph should be clear, without reference to the text.

We will create a histogram using the data from Table 1-3. Since there was no score of 100 in the data and because we would like to demonstrate a histogram with equal class intervals, we will call the highest class interval 90–99, instead of 90–100. Now, we need to add the "true" class intervals; see Table 1-4. It is important to remember that these true class intervals must be values that cannot really occur in the data. This is ensured by having these limits to the classes go to one decimal place beyond what exists in the data. If we had scores to one decimal place in our data, a score of 89.5 could fit in either the first or second category; this, of course, violates the mutually exclusive criterion. Because our data were all whole numbers, going to one decimal place was sufficient to create numbers not included in the data. If our data went to one decimal place, we would make the ends of the true class intervals go to two decimal places. The histogram created from Table 1-4 is demonstrated in Figure 1-2. Note that the frequency axis (the vertical axis) starts at zero and is approximately equal in length to the horizontal axis. The scores have been arranged so that from left to right they go from lowest to highest. Note also that both axes are labeled and that there is a caption describing the figure.

Frequency Polygon. Another commonly used graphic method is the frequency polygon. You would not use both a histogram and a frequency polygon to present

Table 1-4 Frequency Distribution with True Class Intervals

Scores	True Class Interval	f	Relative f (%)	Cumulative Percent
50–59	49.5–59.5	2	4	4
60–69	59.5–69.5	3	6	10
70–79	69.5–79.5	20	40	50
80–89	79.5–89.5	15	30	80
90–99	89.5–99.5	10	20	100
Totals		*50*	*100%*	

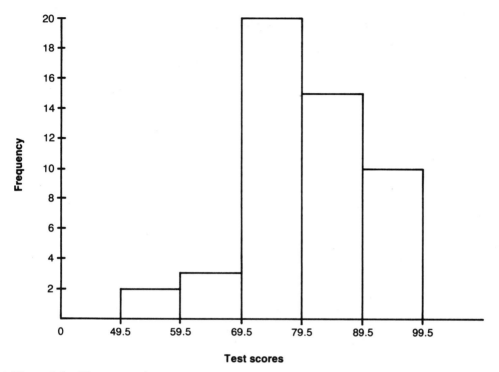

Figure 1-2 Histogram of test scores.

the data; that would be redundant. The frequency polygon is more useful if you want to place two or more distributions on the same pair of axes for the sake of making comparisons. You might, for example, want to demonstrate the difference between the scores of the experimental and control groups by displaying the scores on the same pair of axes. Although this could be done with a histogram, that technique would create more overlapping lines and the graph would not be as clear. The midpoints of the class intervals are usually used on the horizontal axis instead of the true class boundaries. In our example, the intervals are all 10 numbers wide; therefore, their midpoints must go to one decimal place. See Table 1-5 for the midpoints of the class intervals.

The vertical axis still represents the frequencies and still must start at zero. Dots represent the frequencies rather than bars, and those dots are connected by lines. The ends of the frequency polygon may be left open or closed. If the ends are closed, the polygon is connected to the horizontal axis at what would be the midpoints of the next class intervals above and below the existing intervals. Two short lines crossing the connecting lines are helpful to make clear that these are simply extensions of the polygon to the baseline. See Figure 1-3 for a polygon connected to the baseline and Figure 1-4 for one that is not.

Cumulative Percentage Polygon. The cumulative percentage polygon is used less often than the frequency polygon but is preferred when you are trying to

Table 1-5   Frequency Distributions with Midpoints of Class Intervals

Scores	Midpoints	f	Relative f (%)	Cumulative Percent
50–59	54.5	2	4	4
60–69	64.5	3	6	10
70–79	74.5	20	40	50
80–89	84.5	15	30	80
90–99	94.5	10	20	100
Totals		50	100%	

indicate the position of a given score in relation to the distribution rather than the overall form of the distribution. The results of many standardized tests are reported in this form. In a cumulative percentage polygon, the vertical axis is composed of cumulative percentages rather than frequencies. The horizontal axis is the same as in the histogram, that is, the points on the baseline are the true class intervals.

Note that the curve is plotted over the upper ends of the true class intervals, that is, the cumulative percentages for true class interval 49.5 to 59.5 is graphed over 59.5. See Figure 1-5 for a representation of the data presented in Table 1-4. To determine what percentage of scores falls below a given score, go vertically from the

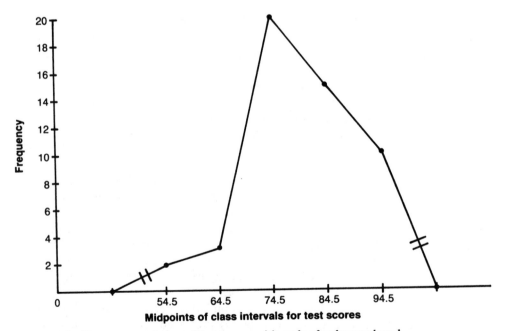

Figure 1-3   Frequency polygon of test scores with ends of polygon closed.

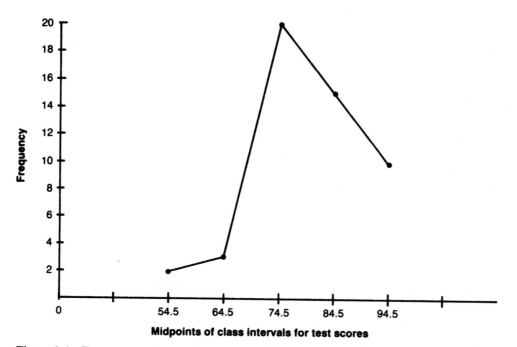

Figure 1-4   Frequency polygon of test scores with ends of polygon open.

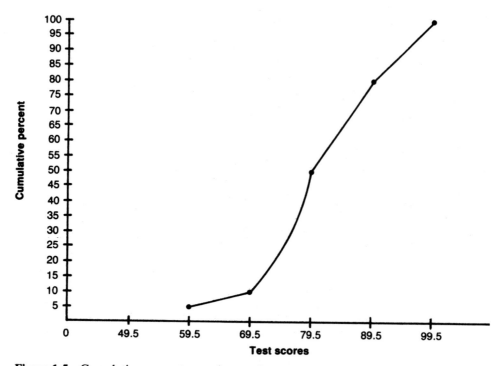

Figure 1-5   Cumulative percentage polygon of test scores.

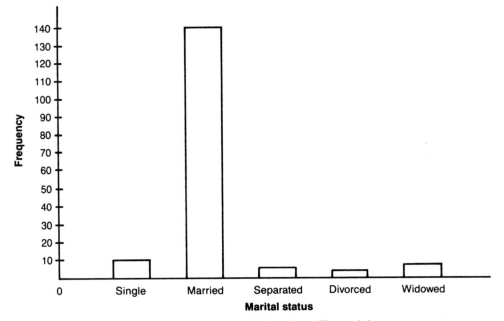

Figure 1-6   Vertical bar graph of marital status data from Figure 1-1.

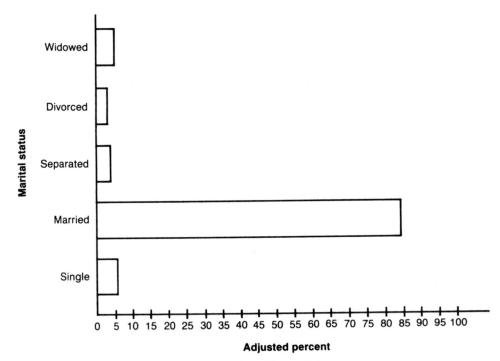

Figure 1-7   Horizontal bar graph of data from Figure 1-1.

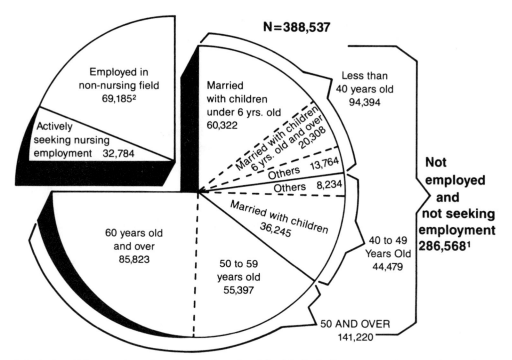

N=388,537

Employed in
non-nursing field
69,185[2]

Actively
seeking nursing
employment   32,784

Married
with children
under 6 yrs. old
60,322

Married with children
6 yrs. old and over
20,308

Others   13,764

Others   8,234

Married with children
36,245

Less than
40 years old
94,394

**Not
employed
and
not seeking
employment
286,568[1]**

60 years old
and over
85,823

50 to 59
years old
55,397

40 to 49
Years Old
44,479

50 AND OVER
141,220

[1] Includes all those not employed in nursing who did not indicate they were seeking employment or that they were employed in a field other than nursing.

[2] Excludes any who might be employed in a non-nursing field, but are actively seeking nursing employment.

Figure 1-8   Pie chart from a nursing journal. From: The registered nurse population—An overview. (DHHS Publication No. HRS-P-OD-83-1) Washington, D.C.: U.S. Department of Health & Human Services.

score to the cumulative percent line and then horizontally from that point to the vertical line. For example, start with score 69.5; go up to the cumulative percent line and then across to the vertical axis. You should come out at 10%. That means that 10% of the subjects received scores lower than 69.5. Or you could start with 79.5 and determine that half of these subjects received As and Bs and the other half received less than that.

Bar Graph. A bar graph is used with categorical data. With nominal data, the bars may be in any order that seems sensible to the researcher, but with ordinal data they should be arranged from lowest to highest. The bars may be either horizontal or vertical.

There are various ways in which bar graphs can be presented; two are given in Figures 1-6 and 1-7. In both figures, the data on marital status from Figure 1-1 are used. In Figure 1-6, a vertical bar graph was created, and the absolute frequency was used for the vertical axis. In Figure 1-7, the bars are placed horizontally and represent the adjusted percent for each category of marital status.

Pie Chart. Pie charts are not seen very often in research reports from behavioral scientists. They tend to be used by newspapers to depict such things as the federal budget. Figure 1-8 (p. 17) contains a pie chart taken from a federal report. The percentages are represented by the percent of the circle taken up by a particular category. One percent equals a slice with a central angle a $\frac{1}{100}$ of 360° or an angle of 3.6°.

Summary. Graphs are a very useful way to present data. When you are writing the data results section of your report, you should consider whether some of these methods might be useful for the presentation of your data.

EXERCISES FOR CHAPTER 1

1. For each of the following variables, specify the highest level of measurement that can be attained.

Variable	**Level of Measurement**
Sex	
Weight	
Rank in class	
Temperature: Fahrenheit scale	
Marital status	
Height	

2. Using the following data, create a *frequency distribution* with class intervals equal to 7. Include in the frequency distribution the class intervals, absolute frequency, relative frequency, and cumulative percent. Round to whole numbers.

1	22	36	23	49
8	28	40	30	8
9	24	13	25	17
15	30	16	24	20
20	31	15	31	26
27	35	7	28	21

3. Using the data in Exercise 2, draw a *histogram*, a *frequency polygon*, and a *cumulative percentage polygon*.

CHAPTER 2
Descriptive Statistics

Barbara Hazard Munro

In the first chapter, we demonstrated how data could be organized in a meaningful way. In Chapter 3, distributions will be explained in detail. In addition to understanding overall distributions, two other pieces of information assist in understanding and describing data. These are special numbers that express the "typical" score, *measures of central tendency*, and those that express the variability within the data set, *measures of dispersion*. The measures of central tendency allow us to answer questions such as, What is the average age of women seeking information from a Family Planning Clinic? Measures of dispersion allow us to answer questions such as, Among battered women, how much do the self-esteem scores vary? How much variability is there in anxiety scores for individuals 3 days after a myocardial infarction?

OBJECTIVES FOR CHAPTER 2

After reading this chapter and completing the exercises, you should be able to

1. Define both in words and in formulas measures of central tendency and dispersion.
2. Select the appropriate measures to use for a particular data set.

SAMPLES AND POPULATIONS

Because the symbols and formulas vary depending on whether one is measuring a sample or a population, the characteristics of samples and populations are reviewed here. The population includes *all* members of a defined group, and the sample is a *subset* of that population. It is important to distinguish between these. The population that is of interest to the investigator and about which he or she wishes to draw conclusions is the target population. The sample may be drawn from some other available population. For example, the researcher may be interested in knowing about *all* chemotherapy patients but will actually draw patients only from those at Yale New Haven Hospital (YNHH). In this example, the target population may be all chemotherapy patients in the United States who receive standard chemotherapy treatment. If the patients are only drawn from YNHH, however, the researcher must show that those treated at YNHH are not significantly different from those treated elsewhere, if the results are to have meaning beyond the local setting.

It is of utmost importance that the sample drawn from the population contains subjects representative of the target population. Otherwise, the researcher will not be able to generalize beyond the sample. For a more detailed description of samples and populations, the reader should consult a research text, such as Polit and Hungler's *Nursing Research—Principle and Methods* (1983).

The characteristics of populations are called *parameters,* and the characteristics of samples are called *statistics.* To distinguish between them, different sets of symbols are used. Greek letters are used to denote parameters, and Roman letters are used to denote statistics. For example, the mean, or arithmetic average, is denoted by $\overline{X}$ for the statistic and small case mu (μ) for the parameter. We have tried to keep the use of symbols in this book to a minimum. The following section includes symbols that will be used throughout the book.

SYMBOLS

The Greek letter sigma (Σ) means "the sum of." For example,

$$\sum_{i=1}^{5} X_i$$

means the summation of the X_i scores from $i = 1$ to $i = 5$, or $X_1 + X_2 + X_3 + X_4 + X_5$. If you had

$$\sum_{i=10}^{20} X_i ,$$

you would add up scores 10 through 20. See Figure 2-1 for an example. The notation

$$\sum_{i=1}^{5} X_i$$

is simplified to

$$\Sigma X$$

when all scores in the X distribution are to be added up. This is the form that we use in this book.

It is important to distinguish between ΣX, ΣX^2, and $(\Sigma X)^2$, because these symbols are frequently used in statistics (see Table 2-1). ΣX has already been

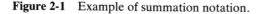

X Scores

$X_1 =$	4
$X_2 =$	4
$X_3 =$	10
$X_4 =$	5
$X_5 =$	7

$$\sum_{i=1}^{5} X_i \quad 30$$

Figure 2-1 Example of summation notation.

described as the sum of the scores in the X distribution. In our example, this is equal to 30. To calculate ΣX^2, you must first square each of the numbers in the X distribution. This results in 16, 16, 100, and so on. The sum of all these squared numbers is ΣX^2, which, in our example, is equal to 206. To calculate $(\Sigma X)^2$, you simply square the ΣX. In our example, the ΣX is 30, and squaring that number gives us 900, which is $(\Sigma X)^2$. Note particularly that $(\Sigma X)^2$ is *not* equal to ΣX^2.

MEASURES OF CENTRAL TENDENCY

Measures of central tendency are single points on the measurement scale for a given variable. Many of the variables used in the behavioral or life sciences are distributed in such a way that most scores fall in the middle, with fewer scores falling on either side, in the "tails" of the distribution. There are, however, distributions that do not assume such a "normal" distribution. Thus, we must also know the shape of the distribution and the dispersion of the scores in order to interpret the data correctly. The three most commonly reported measures of central tendency—the *mean, median,* and *mode*—are described here. These measures are used to describe the "middle" of a group of scores.

Table 2-1 Demonstration of Various Symbols

X Scores		X^2
X_1	4	16
X_2	4	16
X_3	10	100
X_4	5	25
X_5	7	49
$\Sigma X = 30$		$\Sigma X^2 = 206$
$(\Sigma X)^2 = (30)^2 = 900$		

Mean

The mean is simply the arithmetic average that we learned to calculate at some point in elementary school. You simply add up the scores and divide by the number of scores in the distribution. As previously mentioned, symbols used to designate the mean are $\overline{X}$, which stands for the mean of the sample, and μ, which stands for the mean of the population. The formula for the sample mean is written as $\overline{X} = \Sigma X / n$, where n = the number in the sample. Using the data in Table 2-1, we can calculate the mean of the X scores as $30/5 = 6$.

Characteristics of the Mean. There are three important characteristics of the mean:

1. Extreme values can distort the mean, particularly if there is a small number of subjects. For example, suppose you were trying to describe the average income of workers in a given agency and the incomes were as follows: four workers earned salaries of $18,000, $20,000, $22,000, and $24,000, and the individual responsible for managing the agency earned $75,000. The average of these salaries is $31,800, but this does not accurately describe the earnings of this group, because four of the five workers earn considerably less than $31,800, and one earns considerably more. This is an example of how one can "lie" with statistics. When average salaries are reported, always inspect the data to see what salaries are included. If a company wants to make it appear that it is paying high wages, the salaries of the administrators are averaged in with those of the workers. As will be pointed out later, the median is often a better measure of central tendency when there are data with extreme values.

2. The sum of the deviations of the scores in the distribution from the mean always equals zero. This is true because, by definition, the mean is the mathematical center of the data. Thus, half the distribution is above and half below the mean. See Table 2-2 for a demonstration of what this characteristic means. The mean is subtracted from each score $(X - \overline{X})$, and this figure is written as χ, which is the symbol for the deviation of a given score from the mean of its distribution. When the deviations $(\Sigma\chi)$ are added up, the sum is zero.

Table 2-2   Deviations Around the Mean

X	$(X - \overline{X} = \chi)$
4	$4 - 6 = -2$
4	$4 - 6 = -2$
10	$10 - 6 = 4$
5	$5 - 6 = -1$
7	$7 - 6 = 1$
$\Sigma X = 30$	$\Sigma\chi = 0$
$\overline{X} = 6$	

Table 2-3 Sums of Squares of Deviations Around Measures of Central Tendency

X	$\chi = (X - \overline{X})$	χ^2	X-median	$(X$-median$)^2$	X-mode	$(X$-mode$)^2$
4	$4-6=-2$	4	$4-5=-1$	1	$4-4=0$	0
4	$4-6=-2$	4	$4-5=-1$	1	$4-4=0$	0
10	$10-6=\ \ 4$	16	$10-5=\ \ 5$	25	$10-4=6$	36
5	$5-6=-1$	1	$5-5=\ \ 0$	0	$5-4=1$	1
7	$7-6=\ \ 1$	1	$7-5=\ \ 2$	4	$7-4=3$	9
Σ_s: 30		0	26	5	31	10	46

$\overline{X} = 6$
Median $= 5$
Mode $= 4$

3. The sum of the squares of the deviations around the mean is smaller than the sum of squares around any other value. This may not be totally clear now, but this characteristic of the mean underlies the calculation of "least squares," which is presented in later chapters. If you are trying to minimize the squared deviations in a distribution, you calculate the squared deviations from the mean. See Table 2-3 for an example. Although we have not yet described the calculation of the median or the mode, in this distribution the median equals five and the mode equals four. The sum of the squared deviations around the mean $(\Sigma\chi^2)$ equals 26; around the median, 31; and around the mode, 46. Thus, the sum of squares of the deviations around the mean is the smallest. Note also that the other deviations do not add up to zero. The sum of the deviations around the median is 5, and around the mode it is 10.

Median

The median is the midpoint in a set of ranked scores. In other words, the median is the point below which one half of the scores lie. It is, therefore, the 50th percentile. To calculate the median, you must first put the numbers in order from lowest to highest. If the number of scores is odd, the median is the middle score. If the number of scores is even, the median is halfway between the two middle scores. For example, with 4, 4, 5, 7, and 10, the median is 5. With 1, 2, 8, 9, the median is also 5; it is calculated by $(2 + 8)/2 = 5$. For other examples see Table 2-4.

Mode

The mode is used less frequently as a measure of central tendency but is the only measure applicable to categorical data. It is the most frequently occurring score in a distribution. Usually it is located at the center of the distribution, but this is not always the case. Look at Table 2-3 for an example. The score 4 occurs twice in the X

Table 2-4   Calculating the Median

Scores	Scores in Rank Order	Median
2 7 6 3	2 3 6 7	$(3+6)/2 = 4.5$
4 1 3 5 7	1 3 4 5 7	4
8 7 9 3	3 7 8 9	$(7+8)/2 = 7.5$
6 2 5 3 1	1 2 3 5 6	3

Table 2-5   Finding the Mode

Scores	Mode
5 1 7 9 3 5	5
1 3 8 7 7 3 8 7	7
1 4 5 4 6 5 8 7	4 and 5
1 3 8 2 9 5	No mode

distribution, and no other score occurs more than once. Therefore, the mode for that distribution is 4. If there are two modes, the distribution is called *bimodal*. There may be more than two modes, but that is not common. See Table 2-5 for other examples.

The mode is the only measure of central tendency that can be used with categorical data, since even for the median you must be able to rank order the data. Suppose we wanted to determine which type of wine is most popular at Yale School of Nursing. We hold a wine and cheese party, order equal quantities of red, white, and rosé wine, and the participants consume 350 glasses of white wine, 200 glasses of rosé, and 75 glasses of red wine. (The party occurs right after the statistics final!) For our next party we would, of course, buy more white wine and less red wine, because white wine was the mode.

Comparison of the Mean, Median, and Mode

Selection of a method for describing the central tendency of the data depends in part on the scale of measurement of the variable. If the data are nominal, only the mode can be used. With ordinal data, the mode or the median are often used, but if you plan to treat your ordinal data as though they were at the interval level, you may wish to use the mean when describing the center of the data. When the data represent the interval or ratio level of measurement, any of these measures of central tendency may be used.

Statistically, the mean is more stable than the median or mode and is generally considered to be the most sensitive measure of central tendency because it is the only measure that uses all the scores in the distribution in its calculation. However, as has been pointed out in the example about salaries, using all the scores has disadvantages when there are extreme scores in the distribution.

The median is helpful when you have extreme scores or when the data have been truncated, that is, cut off at one or both ends. That happens when, for example, the lowest scores are only given as 60 and below. The median may also be a good measure to use when the data are not normally distributed, that is, when you do not find most of the scores falling in the middle and a fairly even distribution on either side of the middle. If, on an examination, most of the scores fall in the highest range (90–100) and there are only a few very low scores, the data would not be normally distributed.

The mode is used mostly for qualitative data but may be interesting to report when other measures of central tendency are being reported. In reporting examination scores, one might mention the most frequently occurring score as well as the mean of the scores.

As is shown in Chapter 3, when you have a distribution that is perfectly symmetrical (*e.g.*, in a normal curve), the mean, median, and mode all fall at the same point, in the exact center of the distribution.

MEASURES OF DISPERSION

The shape of the distribution and its midpoint are two important pieces of information about our data, but something is still missing. We need to know how much variability there is. Consider two examinations in which the mean score is 80, but on one examination the scores went from a low of 50 to a high of 100, and on the other the scores went from 70 to 90. Simply reporting the means of these examinations is not enough. Four methods for describing the variability in a data set are discussed below. These methods are *range*, *interquartile range*, *standard deviation*, and *variance*.

Range

The range is the simplest method to calculate and is one that we often use. "That Sally is so smart. She got a 98 on the final, which was the highest mark on the exam! Poor Joan, she wasn't feeling well and she really bombed! She got the lowest mark on the final, a 65." We usually want to know the range of the scores. To calculate the range, simply subtract the lowest score from the highest. If we subtract Joan's score from Sally's (98 − 65 = 33), we find that the range for that examination is 33. Note that, by definition, the range is "33." In reporting results, however, you might say that the scores ranged from 65 to 98, because it seems to be more meaningful than simply saying the range was 33.

The range can be used to compare variability among distributions. For example, we said that it was not enough to report that the means for the two examinations were 80, when one went from 50 to 100 and the other from 70 to 90. We can now see that although the means were identical, the range of one was 50, and the range of the other was 20.

Interquartile Range

To understand interquartile range (IR), it is necessary to understand percentiles. (Further information on percentiles is given in Chapter 3.) Scores from standardized examinations are often reported in percentiles. The National League for Nursing Achievement scores are reported in this manner. The percentile rank for a score received on a particular test indicates what percent of the scores fall below that score. If you took a standardized test consisting of 100 questions and were told that you answered 78 of those questions correctly, you still would not know how you had done relative to others who took the test. If, in addition to knowing that you answered 78 correctly, you were told that a score of 78 represented a percentile of 94, you would know that you had done better than 94 percent of the individuals on whom the test was standardized.

When you take the Miller Analogies Test (MAT), you receive your score and an abbreviated list of percentiles arranged by field of study. For nurses, a score of 37 is at the 25th percentile, a score of 45 is at the 50th percentile, and a score of 56 is at the 75th percentile. For engineers, the percentiles change. Engineers need a score of 43 to be at the 25th percentile, 50 to be at the 50th percentile, and 56 to be at the 75th percentile. The raw scores tell you very little. Percentiles let you know how you stand among your peers.

Since the 50th percentile is at the midpoint (50% of the scores are lower), it is also the median. Percentiles are also reported in terms of quartiles. In that system, the 100 percentile points are divided into four "quarters." The 25th percentile is then called the *first quartile* (Q_1), the 50th percentile is called the *second quartile* (Q_2), the 75th percentile is the *third quartile* (Q_3), and the 100th percentile is the *fourth quartile* (Q_4).

The simple range may be unstable because of extreme values. See Table 2-6 for an example: there is one score of 2; that one score has a large effect on the range. If that score were removed, the range would only be 2 ($12 - 10$), rather than 10. The interquartile range (IR) can be used to deal with this difficulty.

Table 2-6   Instability of the Range with Extreme Values

Scores	f
2	1
10	5
11	7
12	4
Range = 12 − 2 = 10	

The IR is defined as $Q_3 - Q_1$. This gives the range of scores from the 25th to the 75th percentiles, that is, the middle 50% of the data. This is still a relatively crude measure of variability, but it provides an overview of the way in which the scores are distributed.

The *semi-interquartile range (Q)* may also be reported. This is defined as $(Q_3 - Q_1)/2$, or the average amount by which these two quartiles vary from the median (50th percentile).

To locate the 25th percentile, take the number of cases in a distribution (n) and divide by 4 (or multiply by .25), and to locate the 75th percentile, take ¾ of n (or multiply n times .75).

For example, see Table 2-7. In $X1$ there are 12 scores ($n = 12$). $Q_1 = {}^{12}\!/_4 = 3$ (or $12 \times .25 = 3$), and $Q_3 = 12 \times {}^3\!/_4 = 9$ (or $12 \times .75 = 9$). So, the first quartile is the third score from the bottom of the distribution, and the third quartile is the ninth. In this case, $Q_1 = 4$ and $Q_3 = 8$. Therefore, the interquartile range is $8 - 4 = 4$, that is, there is a four-point spread between the 25th and 75th percentiles. The semi-interquartile range is $(8 - 4)/2 = {}^4\!/_2 = 2$, and indicates that the average amount by which the 25th and 75th quartiles vary from the median is 2.

In $X2$, the percentiles are somewhat more difficult to determine because the numbers do not divide evenly. In $X2$, $n = 10$, so $Q_1 = {}^{10}\!/_4 = 2.5$, and $Q_3 = 10 \times {}^3\!/_4 = 7.5$. To locate the 2.5th score in the distribution, take the average of the second and third scores. That score $(Q_1) = (3 + 4)/2 = 3.5$. For Q_3, the 7.5th score is the average of the seventh and eighth scores in the distribution or $(8 + 9)/2 = 8.5$. The interquartile range is $8.5 - 3.5$ or 5.0, and the semi-interquartile range is

Table 2-7 Calculating Interquartile and Semi-Interquartile Ranges

	$X1$		$X2$
	10		10
	9		9
	9		9 $\leftarrow Q_3\ (8.5)$
$Q_3 \rightarrow$	8		8
	7		7
	5		5
	5		4
$Q_1 \rightarrow$	4		4 $\leftarrow Q_1\ (3.5)$
	4		3
	4		2
	3		
	2		
IR: $8 - 4 = 4$		$8.5 - 3.5 = 5$	
$Q: \dfrac{8-4}{2} = 2$		$\dfrac{8.5 - 3.5}{2} = 2.5$	

(8.5 − 3.5)/2 or 2.5. The interquartile or semi-interquartile range, or both, would be reported when the range is not representative of the distribution because of some extreme values.

Standard Deviation

The standard deviation is the most commonly reported measure of variability. Usually, if the mean is reported as the measure of central tendency, the standard deviation is reported as the measure of variability. Means and standard deviations are generally reported together, whether in the text or in tables. The standard deviation represents the average amount by which the scores vary from the central score, the mean.

Deviation. Recall from the description of the characteristics of the mean that χ stands for the deviation of a given score from the mean and is calculated as $\chi = X - \overline{X}$. $\Sigma\chi^2$ stands for the sum of the squared deviations. Also note that the small letter n stands for the number of subjects in a sample, whereas capital N stands for the number of subjects in a population. The basic formula for calculating the standard deviation varies slightly, depending on whether you are calculating the standard deviation of the population, σ, or the standard deviation of the sample, s, which is an estimation of that population parameter. Note again that Greek letters are used for measures of the population (parameters), and Roman letters for measures of the sample (statistics). Here, small case sigma, σ, is used for the parameter, and s is used for the statistic.

$$\sigma \text{ (standard deviation for population)} = \sqrt{\frac{\Sigma\chi^2}{N}}$$

$$s \text{ (standard deviation for sample)} = \sqrt{\frac{\Sigma\chi^2}{n-1}}$$

When calculating the standard deviation from sample data, you subtract 1 from the number of subjects in the sample. That, in effect, makes a correction for the fact that only certain members of the population were measured. When you calculate a statistic of a sample, you hope that you will learn from that what the associated parameter of the population is. When you measure a sample that has been drawn in such a way as to be representative of the population, you expect that the measures, such as mean and standard deviation, are close to what you would get if you had measured everyone in the population. Later, we will discuss methods by which we can say with a certain degree of confidence that a population parameter would fall between two points.

Subtracting 1 from the number of subjects in the sample gives an "unbiased" estimate of the standard deviation of the population. If 1 is not subtracted, s tends to be an underestimate of σ. Obviously, the size of the sample is most important. If the sample is very large, subtracting 1 from n makes little difference in the result, but if the sample is small, the correction can make a big difference. For example, if

$\Sigma\chi^2 = 5000$ and $n = 1000$, $\Sigma\chi^2/N = 5000/1000 = 5$ and $\Sigma\chi^2/(n-1) = 5000/999 = 5.005$. The difference between 5 and 5.005 is very small. But if $n = 10$ and $\Sigma\chi^2$ still equaled 5000, $\Sigma\chi^2/N = 5000/10 = 500$ and $\Sigma\chi^2/(n-1) = 5000/9 = 555.56$. There is a substantial difference between 500 and 555.56.

In discussing the characteristics of the mean, we demonstrated that the sum of the squares of the deviations around the mean is smaller than the sum of squares around any other value. The standard deviation is a measure of these squared deviations around the mean. It is, then, a measure of the "least squares" around the mean. All our analyses of the variance of measures are based on the notion of "least squares;" thus, it is most important to understand why the standard deviation is the "least squares solution" around the mean.

In an attempt to clarify the meaning of a standard deviation, we will first demonstrate the use of a basic formula that uses raw scores. We will then demonstrate the equivalent formula that is more commonly used to calculate standard deviations. The latter looks more complicated but is actually easier to use, because it does not require subtraction of each score from the mean.

See Table 2-8 for the figures used in the calculation of the standard deviation by the basic formula. There are five scores in X, and they add up to 30 (ΣX). The mean

Table 2-8 Standard Deviation and Variance Using Basic Formula

X	$\chi = (X - \overline{X})$ (Deviation from Mean)	χ^2
4	$4 - 6 = -2$	4
4	$4 - 6 = -2$	4
10	$10 - 6 = \ \ 4$	16
5	$5 - 6 = -1$	1
7	$7 - 6 = \ \ 1$	1
$\Sigma X = 30$	$\Sigma\chi = 0$	$\Sigma\chi^2 = 26$

Sum of Sq Deviations (handwritten annotation above χ^2 column)

$$\overline{X} = \frac{30}{5} = 6$$

$$\sigma = \sqrt{\frac{\Sigma\chi^2}{N}} = \sqrt{\frac{26}{5}} = \sqrt{5.2} = 2.28$$

$$s = \sqrt{\frac{\Sigma\chi^2}{n-1}} = \sqrt{\frac{26}{5-1}} = \sqrt{\frac{26}{4}} = \sqrt{6.5} = 2.55$$

$$\sigma^2 = \frac{\Sigma\chi^2}{N} = \frac{26}{5} = 5.2$$

$$s^2 = \frac{\Sigma\chi^2}{n-1} = \frac{26}{4} = 6.5$$

variance is st. dev. squared (handwritten annotation)

of those five scores is 6. To calculate the deviation of each score from the mean (χ), subtract the mean (6) from each score. Note that if these deviations are added up ($\Sigma\chi$), they equal 0. Each deviation is squared (χ^2), and this gives us 4, 4, 16, 1, and 1. The sum of these squared deviations ($\Sigma\chi^2$) is 26. If these scores represented the scores from all the members of a population, we would use the formula for σ. Here, the sum of the squared deviations is divided by the number of units in the population. This gives an average squared deviation. So, for this example, the average squared deviation is 5.2. To get this back into the original scale (since we have squared all the numbers), we take the square root of 5.2, which is 2.28. We now have a population in which the average score (μ) is 6, and the standard amount by which the scores vary from that middle point is 2.28. In Chapter 3, we will show more clearly what this variation about the mean is when we describe the normal curve.

The standard deviation for the sample is calculated in the same way except that when calculating the average squared deviation, the correction is made and $\Sigma\chi^2$ is divided by 1 less than the number in the sample.

We have provided these formulas to assist you in conceptualizing a standard deviation. Now, although the next formulas may appear to be more complicated, we assure you that they are easier to calculate by hand, because they do not require calculation of deviations from the mean (χ). These formulas are mathematically equivalent to the basic formulas, that is, $\Sigma\chi^2 = \Sigma X^2 - \dfrac{(\Sigma X)^2}{n}$. To demonstrate their equivalence, we will use the same scores and apply these formulas (Table 2-9). The formulas are:

$$\sigma = \sqrt{\dfrac{\Sigma X^2 - \dfrac{(\Sigma X)^2}{N}}{N}}$$

$$s = \sqrt{\dfrac{\Sigma X^2 - \dfrac{(\Sigma X)^2}{n}}{n - 1}}$$

Now, we need only to add up our scores to calculate $\Sigma X = 30$, square each score (16, 16, 100, *etc.*), and add up the sum of these squares ($\Sigma X^2 = 206$). Those figures can now be put into the formulas. For the population (σ), the denominator remains N, and for the sample (s), $n - 1$.

Variance

The variance is the average of the squared deviations. It is used in some of the statistical techniques to be described later in this book, but it is harder to interpret than the other measures of dispersion, because the numbers are not retained in their original scale. The formula is simply the one for the standard deviation without the square root sign. In the examples given, we calculated the variance on the way to

Table 2-9   Standard Deviation and Variance Using the Short Cut Formula

X	X^2
4	16
4	16
10	100
5	25
7	49
$\Sigma X = 30$	$\Sigma X^2 = 206$

$$\sigma = \sqrt{\frac{\Sigma X^2 - \frac{(\Sigma X)^2}{N}}{N}} = \sqrt{\frac{206 - \frac{(30)^2}{5}}{5}} = \sqrt{\frac{206 - \frac{(900)}{5}}{5}} = \sqrt{\frac{26}{5}} = \sqrt{5.2} = 2.28$$

$$s = \sqrt{\frac{\Sigma X^2 - \frac{(\Sigma X)^2}{n}}{n-1}} = \sqrt{\frac{206 - \frac{(30)^2}{5}}{5-1}} = \sqrt{\frac{206 - \frac{(900)}{5}}{4}} = \sqrt{\frac{26}{4}} = \sqrt{6.5} = 2.55$$

$$\sigma^2 = \frac{\Sigma X^2 - \frac{(\Sigma X)^2}{N}}{N} = \frac{206 - \frac{(30)^2}{5}}{5} = \frac{206 - \frac{(900)}{5}}{5} = \frac{26}{5} = 5.2$$

$$\sigma^2 = \frac{\Sigma X^2 - \frac{(\Sigma X)^2}{n}}{n-1} = \frac{206 - \frac{(30)^2}{5}}{5-1} = \frac{206 - \frac{(900)}{5}}{4} = \frac{26}{4} = 6.5$$

calculating the standard deviation. The population variance is denoted σ^2, and the sample is s^2. That is because the variance is the standard deviation squared. The formulas are:

$$\sigma^2 = \frac{\Sigma x^2}{N} = \frac{\Sigma X^2 - \frac{(\Sigma X)^2}{N}}{N}$$

$$s^2 = \frac{\Sigma x^2}{n-1} = \frac{\Sigma X^2 - \frac{(\Sigma X)^2}{n}}{n-1}$$

See Table 2-8 for calculation of the variances with the deviation formula. Note that the variance is equal to the squared standard deviation. The standard deviation of the population is 2.28, and the variance is $(2.28)^2$, or 5.2. For the sample, the standard deviation is 2.55, and the variance is $(2.55)^2$, or 6.5.

Table 2-9 contains the calculation of the variances with the more commonly used formula. Note that the standard deviation is equal to the square root of the variance. For example, the variance of the sample is 6.5, and the standard deviation of the sample is $\sqrt{6.5}$, or 2.55.

PROBLEMS WITH OUTLIERS

In examining the dispersion of scores around the mean, one has an opportunity to check one's data for "outliers," so that, if necessary, corrections or adjustments may be made. Outliers are specific data points distinctly further from the mean than are other data points, as in the following data set: 5, 8, 7, 215, 4. The number 215 appears to be distinctly different from the others. The appearance of an outlier may indicate that an error has been made in the data collection or coding process, and this possibility should certainly be considered. For example, the age of an 18 year old may have been entered into the computer as 81. The frequency distribution for each variable included in the analysis should be examined to be sure that no such errors have been made. An example of a frequency distribution produced by a computer program is given in the next section of this chapter.

Alternately, the appearance of an outlier may indicate an error in conceptualizing the sample or in the sampling itself, as in the earlier example, in which the income of an agency manager, who had a salary more than three times larger than that of the next highest paid worker in the agency, was averaged in as though the manager were just one more worker. Another example is the case in which the ages of six school-aged children in a play therapy group and the age of the psychiatric nurse leading the group are treated as a single set of values. Discovery of outliers, especially in demographic variables such as income or age, may lead you to realize that you have not appropriately conceptualized your sample or that sampling criteria have not been adequately set. Many situations, however, are more subtle. If, in a classroom, one child who suffers from asthma episodes has missed 57 days of school and no other child has missed more than 21 days, should this child be included by the school nurse in a study of health education? The answer is not obvious. In fact, such a question may have no right or wrong answer. But, in any case, recognizing outliers and considering their meaning and implications when they do occur is useful in any data analysis procedure.

EXAMPLE OF A COMPUTER PRINTOUT

Figure 2-2 presents a computer printout containing the statistics described in this chapter as well as some that are described in later chapters. The SPSS FREQUENCIES program was used to generate this printout. The figure contains descriptive statistics on one item from a scale that was used to measure the attitudes

Procedure Cards

```
1                 16
FREQUENCIES       GENERAL = A3
STATISTICS        ALL
```

Output

A3

CATEGORY LABEL	CODE	ABSOLUTE FREQ	RELATIVE FREQ (PCT)	ADJUSTED FREQ (PCT)	CUM FREQ (PCT)
STRONGLY AGREE	1.	26	20.2	21.5	21.5
MODERATELY AGREE	2.	26	20.2	21.5	43.0
SLIGHTLY AGREE	3.	18	14.0	14.9	57.9
SLIGHTLY DISAGREE	4.	12	9.3	9.9	67.8
MODERATELY DISAGREE	5.	12	9.3	9.9	77.7
STRONGLY DISAGREE	6.	27	20.9	22.3	100.0
	9.	8	6.2	MISSING	100.0
	TOTAL	129	100.0	100.0	

```
MEAN        3.322    STD ERR     0.170    MEDIAN      2.972
MODE        6.000    STD DEV     1.872    VARIANCE    3.504
KURTOSIS   -1.420    SKEWNESS    0.249    RANGE       5.000
MINIMUM     1.000    MAXIMUM     6.000

VALID CASES    121    MISSING CASES    8
```

Figure 2-2   Example of descriptive statistics produced by the SPSS frequencies program.

of visiting nurses and home health aides toward death and dying (Atkins & Munro, 1984). The item was, "I would not feel anxious in the presence of someone I knew was dying," and the responses ranged from strongly agree (1) to strongly disagree (6); thus, the higher the score, the more anxiety in the presence of a dying person In this sample, 21.5% of those who answered the question said they would not fe anxious (1), and an almost equal number, 22.3%, said they would be very anxi (6). The midpoint in this six-point scale was 3.5, and the overall mean for the ɡ came very close to that (3.322). The modal score was 6, that is, the reˈ "strongly disagree" was given more often than any other response (27 inⁿ strongly disagreed). The median was 2.972, somewhat less than the mɛ standard deviation and variance were 1.872 and 3.504, respectively. Th ranged from a minimum of 1 to a maximum of 6, giving a range of 5. One remember about the computer is that it will calculate statistics on any nˈ whether or not such calculations make any sense. For example, if you enter as a variable and designate Catholics to be 1; Protestants, 2; Jews, 3; and so

Table 2-10 Demographic Characteristics of Sample of 47 Male and 89 Female Respondents in Study 1

Characteristics	Male			Female		
	$\overline{X}$	SD	Range	$\overline{X}$	SD	Range
Age in years	34.96	8.93	23–67	36.31	9.92	22–62
Education in years	16.55	2.64	12–22	15.62	2.44	10–22

	Male %	Female %	Total %
Marital status			
Single, never married	59.6	38.2	45.6
Married	36.2	44.9	41.9
Divorced or separated	4.3	13.5	10.3
Widowed	0.0	3.4	2.2
Ethnic background			
Asian	6.4	13.5	11.0
Black	2.1	4.5	3.7
Caucasian	76.6	68.5	71.3
Hispanic	4.3	4.5	4.4
Native American	2.1	7.9	5.9
Other	8.5	1.1	3.7
Religious preference			
Protestant	10.6	30.3	23.5
Catholic	27.7	22.5	24.3
Jewish	12.8	6.7	8.8
Other	14.9	6.7	9.6
None	34.0	33.7	33.8

From: Norbeck, J.S., Lindsey, A.M., & Carrieri, V.L. (1983). Further development of the Norbeck social support questionnaire: Normative data and validity testing. *Nursing Research, 32*(1), 4–9.

tell the computer to calculate statistics, you will get the mean and standard deviation for the religion variable, although the numbers have no meaning.

EXAMPLE FROM PUBLISHED RESEARCH

Table 2-10 illustrates how descriptive statistics can be presented in a table. These data were collected by Norbeck, Lindsey, and Carrieri (1983) during the second phase of testing the Norbeck Social Support Questionnaire. They were describing the demographic characteristics of their sample. They present the mean, standard deviation, and range for the continuous variables and percents for the categorical variables. Males in their sample ranged in age from 23 to 67 years, with a mean age of 34.96. In terms of marital status, 59.6% of the men were single, whereas only 38.2% of the women were single. In the total sample (men and women), 45.6% were single.

SUMMARY

Using the techniques presented in this chapter and in Chapter 1, you should be able to describe your data in your research report.

EXERCISE FOR CHAPTER 2

X1	*X2*
7	10
2	12
16	9
19	6
2	22
7	17
20	9
18	6
14	15
5	9
6	
1	

For the two sets of data above, find the

	X1	*X2*
1. Mean		
2. Median		
3. Mode		
4. Range		
5. Interquartile range		
6. Semi-interquartile range		
7. Variance*		
8. Standard deviation*		

* Use formula for sample

CHAPTER 3
Distributions

Barbara Hazard Munro

In this chapter, the distribution of scores in a data set is discussed. This should provide a better understanding of the overall characteristics of a particular data set and help you to understand the relationship of a score to the entire set of data.

OBJECTIVES FOR CHAPTER 3

After reading this chapter and completing the exercises, you should be able to

1. Describe the characteristics of the normal curve.
2. Define deviations from the normal curve.
3. Calculate standard scores, percentiles, T-scores, transformed scores, and confidence intervals.

NORMAL CURVE

The *normal curve* is a theoretically perfect frequency polygon in which the mean, median, and mode all coincide in the center and which takes the form of a symmetrical bell-shaped curve (Fig. 3-1). De Moivre, a French mathematician, developed the notion of the normal curve based on his observations of games of chance. It has been found that many human traits, such as intelligence, attitudes, and personality, are distributed among the population in a fairly "normal" way. That is, if you measure a representative sample of sufficient size on something, such as an IQ test, the resulting scores will assume a distribution that is quite similar to the normal curve. Most of the scores will fall around the mean (an IQ of 100), and there will be relatively few extreme scores, such as an IQ below 55 or one above 145.

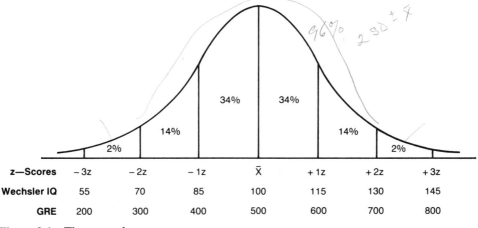

z—Scores	− 3z	− 2z	− 1z	X̄	+ 1z	+ 2z	+ 3z
Wechsler IQ	55	70	85	100	115	130	145
GRE	200	300	400	500	600	700	800

Figure 3-1   The normal curve.

The concept of the normal curve is very useful. For example, when we discuss hypothesis testing, we will talk about the probability (or the likelihood) that a given difference or relationship could have occurred by chance alone. Understanding the normal curve prepares you for understanding the concepts underlying hypothesis testing.

The baseline of the normal curve is measured off in standard deviation units. These are indicated by the small letter z in Figure 3-1. A score that is one standard deviation above the mean is symbolized by $+1z$, and $-1z$ indicates a score that is one standard deviation below the mean. For example, the Wechsler IQ test has a mean of 100 and a standard deviation of 15. Thus, one standard deviation above the mean $(+1z)$ is 115, and one standard deviation below the mean $(-1z)$ is 85.

In a normal distribution, approximately 34% of the scores fall between the mean and one standard deviation above the mean. Because the curve is symmetrical, 34% also falls between the mean and one standard deviation below the mean. So, 68% of the scores fall between $-1z$ and $+1z$. With the Wechsler IQ test, this means that 68%, or about ⅔ of the scores will fall between 85 and 115. Of the one third of the scores remaining, one sixth will fall below 85 and one sixth will be above 115.

Of the total distribution, 28% falls between one and two standard deviations from the mean. Fourteen percent falls between one and two standard deviations above the mean, and 14% falls between one and two standard deviations below the mean. Thus, 96% of the scores (14 + 34 + 34 + 14) fall between plus and minus two standard deviations from the mean. For the Wechsler IQ test, this means that 96% of the population receives scores between 70 and 130.

Most of the last 4% falls between two and three standard deviations from the mean, 2% on each side. So, 99.7% of those taking the Wechsler IQ test score between 55 and 145.

In summary,

34% of scores fall between $\overline{X}$ and $+1z$
14% of scores fall between $+1z$ and $+2z$
 2% of scores fall between $+2z$ and $+3z$

34% of scores fall between $\overline{X}$ and $-1z$
14% of scores fall between $-1z$ and $-2z$
 2% of scores fall between $-2z$ and $-3z$

or

{
68.0% of scores fall between the mean and $\pm 1z$
96.0% of scores fall between the mean and $\pm 2z$
99.7% of scores fall between the mean and $\pm 3z$

   There are two other z-scores that are quite important because we will use them when constructing confidence intervals. They are $z = \pm 1.96$ and $z = \pm 2.58$. Of the scores in a distribution, 95% fall between $\pm 1.96z$, and 99% fall between $\pm 2.58z$.
   Let's take a look at a test that many of you may be very familiar with, the Graduate Record Examination (GRE). This examination was scaled so as to have a mean of 500 and a standard deviation of 100. If 68% of the scores fall between $\pm 1z$, 68% of the scores fall between 400 and 600 ($-1z = 500 - 100 = 400$ and $+1z = 500 + 100 = 600$). Ninety-six percent of the scores fall between 300 and 700 ($-2z = 500 - (2)(100) = 300$ and $+2z = 500 + (2)(100) = 700$). Ninety-nine and seven tenths percent fall between 200 and 800 ($-3z = 500 - (3)(100) = 200$ and $+3z = 500 + (3)(100) = 800$). In the next section (percentiles), we will show more clearly what a given score means in relation to the distribution.

PERCENTILES

In the discussion of the interquartile range, we pointed out that percentiles allow us to describe a given score in relation to other scores in a distribution. A percentile tells us the relative position of a given score. It allows us to compare scores on tests that have different means and standard deviations. A percentile is calculated as

$$\frac{\text{Number of scores less than a given score}}{\text{Total number of scores}} \times 100$$

   Suppose that you received a score of 90 on a test given to a class of 50 people. Of your classmates, 40 had scores lower than 90. Your percentile rank would be

$$\frac{40}{50} \times 100 = 80.$$

You achieved a higher score than 80% of the people who took the test, which also means that almost 20% of those who took the test did better than you.

On a second test given to the same class, you also received a score of 90. Does that mean that you did equally well on the second test? No, not necessarily. You may have done the same, better, or worse. If, on the second test, you scored higher than 47 of your classmates, your percentile rank would be

$$\frac{47}{50} \times 100 = 94.$$

The 25th percentile may be referred to as the *first quartile;* the 50th, the *second quartile,* or, more commonly, the *median;* and the 75th percentile, the *third quartile.* The quartiles are points, not ranges like the interquartile range. Therefore, the third quartile is not from 50 to 75, it is just the 75th percentile. One does not usually say that a score fell within a quartile, because the quartile is only one point.

We can also determine percentile rank by using the normal curve. Again, note Figure 3-1. The IQ score of 85 exceeds the IQ score of 16% of the population, so a score of 85 is equal to a percentile rank of 16. In the same way, an IQ of 115 exceeds 84 percent of the population (50% + 34%), so an IQ of 115 has a percentile rank of 84. An IQ of 130 has a percentile rank of 98 (50% + 34% + 14%), and an IQ of 145 has a percentile rank of almost 100 (50% + 34% + 14% + 2%).

Tables have been established that make it possible to determine what proportion of the normal curve is found between various points along the baseline. They are set up as in Appendix B. To understand how to read the table, go down the first column until you come to 1.0. Note that the percent of area under the normal curve between the mean and a standard score (z-score) of 1.00 is 34.13. That is, of course, where we got the 34% that we have in Figure 3-1. Moving down the row to the right, note that the area under the curve between the mean and 1.01 is 34.38, between the mean and 1.02 is 34.61, and so on.

Suppose you have a standard score of +1.86 (we will demonstrate how to calculate the z-scores in the next section). Finding this score in the table, we see that the percent of the curve between the mean and 1.86 is 46.86. A plus z-score is above the mean, so there is 50% of the curve on the minus z side and another 46.86% between the mean and +1.86, or the percentile rank is 96.86 (50 + 46.86). If the z-score were −1.86, the score falls below the mean, and the percentile rank would be 3.14 (50 − 46.86).

In summary, to calculate a percentile when you have the standard score, you first look up the score in the table to determine what percent of the normal curve falls between the mean and the given score. Then, if the sign is positive, you add the percentage to 50. If the sign is negative, you subtract the percentage from 50.

If this seems confusing, note again the IQ scores. An IQ of 115 is +1z, and the percentile is 34.13 + 50, or 84.13. An IQ of 85 is −1z, and the percentile is 50 − 34.13, or 15.87.

In using percentiles to determine relative position, it is important to remember the following factors: (1) Because so many scores are located near the mean and so few at the ends, the distance along the baseline in terms of percentiles varies a great deal. (2) The distance between the 50th and 55th percentile is much smaller than the distance between the 90th and the 95th. What this means in practical terms is that if you raise your score on a test, there will be more impact on your percentile rank if you are near the mean than if you are near the ends of the distribution.

As an example, suppose three people retook the GRE Quantitative examination in hopes of raising their score, and thus their percentile rank (Table 3-1). All three subjects raised their score by 10 points. For subject 1, who was right at the mean, that meant an increase of 4 points in percentile rank, whereas for subject 3, who was two standard deviations above the mean to start with, the percentile rank only went up 0.5 of a point.

STANDARD SCORES

Standard scores are a way of expressing a score in terms of its relative distance from the mean. A z-score is one such standard score. As has been pointed out, the meaning of an ordinary score varies, depending on the mean and the standard deviation of the distribution from which it was drawn. In research, standard scores are used more often than percentiles. Thus far, we have used examples when the z-score was very easy to calculate. The GRE score of 600 is one standard deviation above the mean, so the z-score is $+1$. The formula used to calculate z-scores is

$$z = \frac{X - \overline{X}}{s}.$$

Remember from our discussion of standard deviation (s) that $X - \overline{X} = x$, or the deviation of a given score from the mean. For the GRE example,

$$z = \frac{600 - 500}{100} = \frac{100}{100} = 1.$$

Now let us try another example. Suppose an individual obtained a score of 48 on a test in which the mean was 35 and the standard deviation was 5. Then

$$z = \frac{48 - 35}{5} = \frac{13}{5} = 2.6.$$

Table 3-1 Relationship of Scores to Percentiles at Varying Distances from the Mean

Subject	Scores	GRE-Q	Percentile
1	1st score	500	50
	2nd score	510	54
2	1st score	600	84
	2nd score	610	86
3	1st score	700	97.7
	2nd score	710	98.2

Using the table in Appendix B, we find that 49.53% of the curve is contained between the mean and 2.6 standard deviations above the mean, so the percentile rank for this score would be 99.53 (50 + 49.53).

Suppose the national mean weight for a particular group is 120 pounds and the standard deviation is 6 pounds. An individual from the group, Mary, weighs 112 pounds. What is Mary's z-score and percentile rank?

$$z = \frac{112 - 120}{6} = \frac{-8}{6} = -1.33$$

Mary's percentile rank is 50 − 40.82, or 9.18.

If all the raw scores in a distribution are converted to z-scores, the resulting distribution will have a mean of zero and a standard deviation of one. If several distributions are converted to z-scores, the z-scores for the various measures can be compared directly. Although the new distributions have a new standard deviation and mean (1 and 0), the shape of the distribution is not altered.

Transformed Standard Scores

Because calculating z-scores results in decimals and negative numbers, some people prefer to transform them into other distributions. One distribution that has been widely used is one with a mean of 50 and a standard deviation of 10. Such *transformed standard scores* are generally referred to as *T-scores*, although some authors call them Z-scores. Some standardized test results are given in T-scores. To convert a z-score to a T-score, use the following formula.

$$T = 10z + 50.$$

For example, with a z-score of 2.5, the T-score would be

$$T = (10)(2.5) + 50$$
$$T = 25 + 50$$
$$T = 75$$

In the new distribution, the mean is 50 and the standard deviation is 10, so a score of 75 is still 2.5 standard deviations above the mean.

In the same way, other distributions can be established. This is the technique used to transform z-scores into GRE scores with a mean of 500 and a standard deviation of 100. The basic formula for transforming z-score is to multiple the z-scores times the desired standard deviation and add the desired mean.

Transformed z-scores = (new st. dev.)(z-score) + (new mean). For GRE scores, that would be $100z + 500$.

Suppose you wanted to transform your z-scores into a scale with a mean of 70 and a standard deviation of 5. Then your formula would be $5z + 70$.

Transforming scores in this way does not change the original distribution of the scores. There are circumstances, however, when a researcher may wish to change the distribution of a set of data. This might occur when you have a set of data that is not normally distributed. There are several ways to accomplish this, but it is not within the scope of this book to detail such transformations. If you need to normalize your data by making such transformations, you should consult a statistician or an advanced statistics text.

NON-NORMAL DISTRIBUTIONS

When a distribution does not have relatively equal numbers on each side of the distribution but has a large number of scores on one side, the distribution is referred to as *skewed* (see Fig. 3-2). This disproportionate hump of scores causes a "tail" to be formed at the opposite end of the distribution.

The terms *negatively* and *positively skewed* distributions are used to describe the direction in which the distribution is out of balance. The names are related to the direction of the "tail." In Figure 3-2, the positively skewed distribution has a tail extending on the right or positive side of the distribution. The opposite condition is called a negatively skewed distribution.

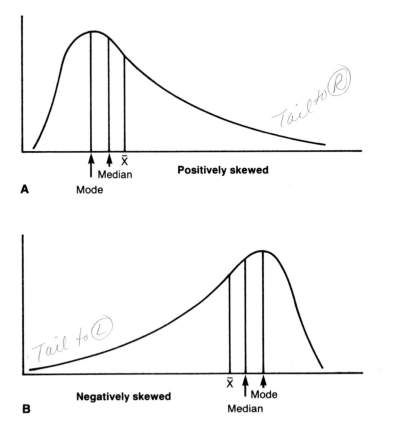

Figure 3-2 (*A* and *B*) Skewed distributions.

The amount of skewness can be described in degrees. Refer to Figure 2-2 for the way in which the SPSS program prints out the skewness of a variable. Zero indicates a symmetrical or normal distribution. A positive figure indicates a positively skewed distribution, and a negative number indicates a negatively skewed distribution.

However, even a bell-shaped curve need not be *normal*. The measure of relative peakedness or flatness of the curve is called *kurtosis*. When this is reported on your computer printouts, zero indicates a normal curve; a positive number indicates a narrow, peaked curve, also called *leptokurtic;* and a negative number indicates a flatter curve, also called *platykurtic* (remember the tail of the platypus?). The height of the curve is not the important element here; the important element is how the frequencies are distributed in the three standard deviations to either side.

If the curve varies greatly from a normal curve, you cannot use the z-scores or the percentiles in the way previously described.

CENTRAL LIMIT THEOREM

If you draw a sample from a population and calculate its mean, how close have you come to knowing the mean of the population? Statisticians have provided us with formulas that allow us to determine just how close the mean of our sample is to the mean of the population.

It has been shown that when a number of samples are drawn from a population, the *means* of these samples tend to be normally distributed, that is, when they are graphed along a baseline, they tend to form the normal curve. The larger the number of samples, the more the distribution approaches the normal curve. Also, if the average of the means of the samples is calculated (the mean of the means), this average (or mean) is very close to the actual mean of the population. Again, the larger the number of the samples, the closer this overall mean is to the population mean.

If the means form a normal distribution, we can then use the percentages under the normal curve to determine the probability statements about individual means. We would know, for example, that the probability of a given mean falling between +1 and −1 standard deviations from the mean of the population is 68%.

To calculate the standard scores necessary to determine position under the normal curve, we need to know the standard deviation of the distribution ($z = (X - \overline{X})/s$). You could calculate the s of the distribution of means by treating each mean as a raw score and applying the regular formula. This new standard deviation of the means is called the *standard error of the mean* ($S_{\overline{x}}$). The term *error* is used to indicate the fact that due to sampling error, each sample mean is likely to deviate somewhat from the true population mean.

Fortunately, statisticians have used these techniques on samples drawn from known populations and have demonstrated relationships that allow us to estimate the mean and standard deviation of a population given only the data from *one sample.* They have demonstrated that there is a constant relationship between the standard deviation of a distribution of sample means (the standard error of the mean), the standard deviation of the population from which the samples were drawn, and the size of the samples. This formula is designated as

$$\sigma_{\bar{x}} = \frac{\sigma}{\sqrt{N}}$$

Of course, we do not usually know the standard deviation of the population (σ). If we had measured the entire population, we would have no need to infer its parameters from measures taken from samples. The formula for the standard error of the mean can be written as

$$s_{\bar{x}} = \frac{s}{\sqrt{n}}$$

In that formula, $s_{\bar{x}}$ indicates that we are estimating the standard error given the standard deviation (s) of a sample of n size. It has been shown that a sample of 30 is enough to estimate the population mean with reasonable accuracy.

To summarize the central limit theorem, note that in working with samples drawn from known populations, statisticians have determined that as that sample size (n) increases:

1. The sampling distribution of the means of the samples approaches a normal distribution.
2. The mean of these means approaches the mean of the population.
3. The standard deviation of the distribution of sample means approaches

$$\frac{\sigma}{\sqrt{N}}.$$

Given the standard deviation of a sample and the size of the sample, we can estimate the standard error of the mean. For example, given a sample of 100 and a standard deviation of 20, we would estimate the standard error of the mean to be

$$s_{\bar{x}} = \frac{s}{\sqrt{n}}$$

$$s_{\bar{x}} = \frac{20}{\sqrt{100}} = \frac{20}{10} = 2$$

There are two factors that influence the standard error of the mean: the standard deviation of the sample and the sample size. Note that the sample size has a large impact on the size of the error, because the square root of n is used in the denominator. As the size of n increases, the size of the error decreases. Suppose we had the same standard deviation as just demonstrated, but a sample size of 1000 instead of 100. Now we have

$$s_{\bar{x}} = \frac{20}{\sqrt{1000}} = \frac{20}{31.62} = 0.63$$

If n is only 30, the standard error would be

$$s_{\bar{x}} = \frac{20}{\sqrt{30}} = \frac{20}{5.47} = 3.66$$

From this, we see that the larger our sample, the less error there is. If there is less error, we can estimate more precisely the parameters of the population.

If there is more variability in the sample, the standard error increases. If there is much variability, it is harder to draw a sample that is representative of the population. Given wide variability, we need larger samples. Note the effect of variability (standard deviation) on the standard error of the mean.

$$s_{\bar{x}} = \frac{5}{\sqrt{100}} = \frac{5}{10} = 0.5$$

$$s_{\bar{x}} = \frac{20}{\sqrt{100}} = \frac{20}{10} = 2$$

$$s_{\bar{x}} = \frac{40}{\sqrt{100}} = \frac{40}{10} = 4$$

CONFIDENCE INTERVALS

Since the means are normally distributed, we can use the standard deviation of the distribution of means, the standard error of the mean, to determine areas under the normal curve, and, from that, we determine how confident we are that a population mean would fall within a certain interval.

Remember from our discussion of the normal curve that we established that 95% of the distribution falls between ±1.96 standard deviations from the mean and that 99% of the distribution falls between ±2.58 standard deviations from the mean. Thus, given the characteristics of the normal curve, there is a 95% probability that a given mean will fall between ±1.96 standard deviations from the actual population mean. There is also a 99% probability that a given sample mean will fall between ±2.58 standard deviations from the actual mean. The 99% and 95% confidence intervals are those that are commonly reported in research literature.

To set the confidence intervals for the population means, we use the following formulas:

$$95\% = \overline{X} \pm 1.96\ (s_{\bar{x}})$$

$$99\% = \overline{X} \pm 2.58\ (s_{\bar{x}})$$

For example, a sample may have a mean of 100, a standard deviation of 27, and a sample size of 81. Now calculate the standard error of the mean.

$$s_{\bar{x}} = \frac{27}{\sqrt{81}} = \frac{27}{9} = 3$$

To determine the 95% confidence interval,

$$\overline{X} \pm 1.96\ (s_{\overline{x}})$$
$$100 \pm (1.96)(3)$$
$$100 \pm (5.88)$$
$$94.12 \quad \text{and} \quad 105.88$$

We could now say that the mean of our sample was 100, and we are 95% confident that the actual population mean would be between 94.12 and 105.88.

For the 99% confidence interval,

$$100 \pm (2.58)(3)$$
$$100 \pm 7.74$$
$$92.26 \quad \text{and} \quad 107.74$$

We are 99% confident that the actual population mean would fall between 92.26 and 107.74.

To demonstrate the effect of a large error on our confidence intervals, let us work through one more example.

$$\overline{X} = 100;\ n = 36;\ s = 72$$

$$s_{\overline{x}} = \frac{72}{\sqrt{36}} = \frac{72}{6} = 12$$

$$95\% = 100 \pm (1.96)(12)$$
$$100 \pm 23.52$$
$$76.48 \quad \text{and} \quad 123.52$$

$$99\% = 100 \pm (2.58)(12)$$
$$100 \pm 30.96$$
$$69.04 \quad \text{and} \quad 130.96$$

We still have a mean of 100, but the error has gone from 3 to 12. Now the confidence intervals are wide. We can say only that we are 95% confident that the actual population mean will fall between 76.48 and 123.52 and 99% confident that it will fall between 69.04 and 130.96. These figures should point out the importance of calculating the standard error of the mean and determining just how much you are able to infer about the population mean from your sample mean.

EXERCISES FOR CHAPTER 3

1. Scores on a particular test are normally distributed with a mean of 80 and a standard deviation of 20. Between what two scores would you expect:
   a. 68% of the scores to fall _____   _____
   b. 96% of the scores to fall _____   _____

2. In a negatively skewed distribution, the "tail" extends toward the _____ (right/left) or _____ (higher/lower) scores of the distribution.

3. A negative z-score indicates that the raw score is _____ (above/below) the mean.

4. When raw scores are converted to standard scores, the resulting distribution has mean equal to _____ and a standard deviation equal to _____ .

5. A distribution of scores has a mean of 70 and a standard deviation of 5. The following four scores were drawn from that distribution: 58, 65, 73, and 82.
    a. Transform the raw scores to standard scores and T-scores.
    b. Calculate the percentile for each score.
    c. Use the standard scores that you have calculated for the four scores and transform them into scores from a distribution with a mean of 100 and a standard deviation of 25.

6. You have measured 120 subjects on a particular scale. The mean is 75 and the standard deviation is 6.
    a. What is the standard error of the mean?
    b. Set up the 95% confidence interval for the mean.
    c. Set up the 99% confidence interval for the mean.

CHAPTER 4

Introduction to Inferential Statistics and Hypothesis Testing

Barbara Hazard Munro

OBJECTIVES FOR CHAPTER 4

After reading this chapter and completing the exercises, you should be able to

1. Discuss the difference between a null and a directional hypothesis.
2. Differentiate between a Type I and a Type II error.
3. Discuss the risks associated with each type of error.
4. Explain the relationship between one- and two-tailed tests and the power of a test.
5. Differentiate between parametric and nonparametric tests.
6. Explain the usefulness of the Cohen technique for determining sample size.

It was noted in Chapter 1 that research studies may be conducted either to *answer questions* or to *test hypotheses*. When you want only to describe the factors in a situation or discover whether there are relationships among those factors, you pose very general research questions. At that point, it may be difficult to state an hypothesis, because not enough is known about the situation. For example, when Elizabeth Kubler-Ross first talked to dying patients about the experience of death, she simply asked them to talk about their experiences, and she described the results.

It becomes possible to state hypotheses once the factors in a given situation and their relationships have been described. As will be demonstrated later, the use of hypotheses allows us to use more *powerful* statistical techniques, that is, techniques that are more likely to show a significant difference or relationship if one indeed exists. To state hypotheses, the researcher must make clear in the review of the literature what theoretical structure underlies the hypotheses and the deductions that led to them. From the literature review, the hypotheses should follow naturally and not be a surprise.

To answer research questions at the factor-searching or descriptive level, we may collect data at the qualitative or quantitative level, or both. Qualitative data may be reported in frequencies, as well as in verbal descriptions. Quantitative data are often presented in graphs and summarized through the use of descriptive statistics. For questions that ask about relationships, correlational techniques are often used.

At the higher levels of inquiry, hypotheses are stated about the differences between groups and about relationships among variables. We are seeking to answer, what will happen if . . . and how can I make it happen? Statistical techniques such as analysis of variance, correlation, and regression are used to test these hypotheses. In relation-searching studies, we are simply asking whether or not a relationship exists. In hypothesis testing, we are proposing a particular relationship between two or more factors and then testing to determine whether or not our proposition is supported.

In addition to looking at distinctions by level of theory, we can look at the difference between *descriptive statistics* and *inferential statistics*. Descriptive statistics are used to report what we observe in a sample, whereas inferential statistics allow us to generalize from our sample to the population. Both types of statistics are often used in the same study. In a carefully designed study from which we hope to generalize to a larger population, we may use descriptive statistics to describe our sample. But the use of a particular statistical technique by itself will not justify making inferences beyond our sample. Further, we need research design and sample selection to make such inferences. Our sample should be "representative" of the population to which we want to generalize, and we should have designed our study in such a way as to minimize the chances for error and distortion of results.

HYPOTHESIS TESTING

Given an underlying theoretical structure, a representative sample, and an appropriate research design, the researcher is able to test hypotheses. An hypothesis has been defined as "a conjectural statement of the relation between two or more variables" (Kerlinger, 1973, p. 18). We test to see whether or not the data support our hypothesis. We do not claim to "prove" that our hypothesis is true, because one study can never "prove" anything. It is always possible that some error has distorted the findings.

Statistical Significance

When talking about analyzing data, researchers talk about whether or not the results were "statistically significant." Was there a statistically significant relationship among the variables? Was there a statistically significant difference among the groups? Under the concept of statistical significance lies the notion of probability. Since the researcher usually wants to generalize beyond the sample, he or she needs to know how likely it is that the results are just a matter of chance. We use statistics to tell us how likely it is that the observed differences result from chance.

We have already presented some idea of probability when we discussed the normal curve and confidence intervals. Given the normal curve and the standard error of the mean, we can guess how close to the population the sample mean is likely to be. Commonly, people use the example of tossing coins as an example of the laws of probability. The chance of getting heads if you flip a coin once is 50%, or one out of two. It can also be shown that if you flip the coin 10 times, the chance of getting heads 10 times is 1 in 1024. These events are distributed in a manner similar to the normal curve.

Levels of Significance

The statistician determines the probability of a given result (or one more extreme) occurring by chance alone. If there is only 1 chance in 1000 that your result would occur by chance, there is only a "rare" chance that you have *not* found a real difference or relationship. Such a result would be labeled "statistically significant." Before conducting the research, the researcher decides what will be considered "rare." In most of our research, the .05 level of significance is used. This means that for a result to be statistically significant, there cannot be more than 5 chances in 100 that it would occur by chance. A .01 level means there is only one chance in 100; a .001 level, 1 in 1000, and so on. When statistics were calculated by hand, a table was usually consulted to find out whether the probability was less than .05 or less than .01. The results were then reported as greater than .05 (> 0.05), less than 0.05 ($< .05$), or less than .01 ($< .01$). As we will show you with examples from computer printouts, these new programs often give exact probabilities. When given, they should be reported. For example, if the probability was .059, it would be much more helpful to report that than just $> .05$. A probability (p) of .021 would be reported as that, rather than just $< .05$.

Null Hypothesis

The "null hypothesis" is often written H_o. It proposes that there is no difference. The null hypothesis is the basis of the statistical test. If a "significant" difference is found, the null hypothesis is *rejected*. But if no difference is found, the null hypothesis is *accepted*. In older studies, hypotheses were usually stated in null form; however, this is not done as often today. When you hypothesize, you are stating that you believe there is indeed a difference or a relationship. It is clearer if you state what differences or relationships you expect, rather than write a string of null hypotheses. It is important to understand the null hypothesis, however, because without it, there is no significance test.

Suppose you stated that there is "no significant difference" between breast- and bottle-fed babies in terms of weight gain. If you really had no idea about this issue, you would not be stating an hypothesis but would simply ask the question: Is there a difference in weight gain between breast- and bottle-fed babies? If you had rationale for an hypothesis, you might state a research hypothesis (H_1), such as: Breast-fed babies gain more weight in the first week of life than do bottle-fed babies.

Types of Error

Types of "error" are defined in terms of the null hypothesis. After analyzing the data, the researcher *accepts* the null hypothesis if there are no significant results or *rejects* the null hypothesis if there are indeed significant results. Rejecting a null hypothesis means that significant differences *have* been found. Because no study is perfect, there is always chance for error; perhaps this is one of the five chances in 100 ($p < .05$) that such an extreme result has happened by chance.

There are two potential errors that could be made. They are called *Type I* and *Type II*. Before describing these errors, the possibilities related to decisions about the null hypothesis are presented through use of the following diagram.

Null hypothesis

Decision	True	False
Accept H_0	ok	Type II
Reject H_0	Type I	ok

If we have a null hypothesis that is true and we accept that hypothesis, we have responded correctly. The incorrect response would be to reject a true null hypothesis (Type I error). If the null hypothesis is false and we reject it, we have responded correctly. The wrong response would be to accept a false null hypothesis (Type II error).

A Type I error is rejecting a *true* null hypothesis. This would occur when the data indicate a statistically significant result when, in fact, there is no difference in the population.

H_0 = no diff. betw. 2

Suppose you compared two groups taught by difference methods (A and B) on their knowledge of statistics, and the data indicated that Group A scored significantly higher than Group B. You would then reject the null hypothesis. Suppose, however, that Group A had people with higher math ability in it and that actually the method did not matter at all. Then, rejecting the null hypothesis is an error. It is called a *Type I error.*

The probability of making a Type I error is called alpha (α) and can be *decreased* by altering the level of significance. That is, you could set the *p* at .01, instead of .05. Then there is only 1 chance in 100 that the result termed "significant" could occur by chance alone. If you do that, however, you will make it more difficult to find a significant result, that is, you will decrease the *power* of the test and you will increase the risk of what is called a *Type II error*.

A Type II error is accepting a *false* null hypothesis. If the data showed no significant results, the researcher would accept the null hypothesis. If, in fact, there were significant differences, a Type II error would have been made. To avoid a Type II error, you could make the level of significance less extreme. There is a greater chance of finding significant results if you are willing to risk 10 chances in 100 that you are wrong ($p = .10$) than there is if you are willing to risk only five chances in 100 ($p = .05$). Other ways to decrease the likelihood of a Type II error are to increase the sample size, decrease sources of extraneous variation, and increase what is known as the *effect* size. The effect size is the impact made by the independent variable. For example, if Group A scored 10 points higher on the statistics final than Group B, the effect size would be 10. Of course, there is a tradeoff: decreasing the likelihood of a Type II error increases the chance of a Type I error.

If decreasing the probability of one type of error increases the probability of the other type, the question arises as to which type of error you are willing to risk. As might be expected, that depends on the study. Suppose you had a test for a particular genetic defect, and that if the defect really exists and is diagnosed early, it can be successfully treated; however, if it is not diagnosed and treated, the child will become severely retarded. On the other hand, if a child is erroneously diagnosed as having the defect and treated, no physical damage is done.

In terms of the types of errors, a Type I error would be diagnosing the defect when it does not exist. In that case, the child would be treated but not harmed by the treatment. A Type II error would be declaring the child to be normal, when he is not. In that case, irreparable damage would be done. In such a situation, it is obvious that you would make every attempt to avoid the Type II error.

On the other hand, suppose a federal study was conducted to determine whether a particular approach to pre-school preparation of underprivileged children leads to increased success in school. This approach would cost a great deal of money to implement nationwide. Those responsible for deciding whether or not to implement this approach would certainly want to be sure that a Type I error had not been made. They would not want to institute a costly new program if it did not really have any effect on success in school.

We have found that the notion of Type I and II errors is hard for some people to grasp, so we will give a few examples to allow you to determine whether or not you have grasped the concept. There are other examples in the exercises at the end of this chapter.

It is hypothesized that two groups are equal in their knowledge of statistics. Has an error been made, and, if so, what type of error, if the researcher

1. Accepts the hypothesis when the groups are really equal in statistics knowledge?
2. Rejects the hypothesis when the groups are really equal in statistics knowledge?
3. Rejects the hypothesis when the groups are really different in terms of their knowledge of statistics?
4. Accepts the hypothesis when one group has much more knowledge of statistics than the other?

These four examples summarize the possibilities surrounding these errors. First, if we are given a situation where the null hypothesis is true, that is, there is no difference, we can either accept it, making the correct decision (#1), or reject it and make an incorrect decision, or a Type I error (#2). Second, if the null hypothesis is false, we can reject it, thus making a correct decision (#3), or accept it and make an incorrect decision, or a Type II error (#4).

Power of a Test

As previously mentioned, a more *powerful* test is one that is more likely to reject a null hypothesis, that is, it is more likely to indicate a statistically significant result when such a difference exists in the population. Researchers are usually looking for significant results; they are not looking to support null hypotheses. Both the level of significance and the power of the test are important factors to consider.

One- and Two-Tailed Tests

The "tails" refer to the ends of the probability curve. When we test for statistical significance, we are asking if the difference or relationship is so extreme, so far out in the tail of the distribution, that it is unlikely to have occurred by chance alone. When we hypothesize the direction of the difference, we are indicating in which tail of the distribution we expect to find the difference.

Although there is some controversy about this, the practice among many researchers is to use a *one-tailed* test of significance when a directional hypothesis is stated and a *two-tailed* test in all other situations. The advantage of using the one-tailed test is that it is more powerful, because the value yielded by the statistical test does not have to be so large to be significant at a given level. To gain this advantage, however, you must have a sound theoretical basis for the directional hypothesis. You cannot base it on a "hunch."

Let's look at some examples to see why this is so. Since you are familiar with the normal curve, we will use that to demonstrate the difference between one- and two-tailed tests (Fig. 4-1). Recall from our discussion of confidence intervals that 95% of the distribution falls between ±1.96 standard deviations from the mean. Thus, only 5% falls beyond those two points. Two and one-half percent of the

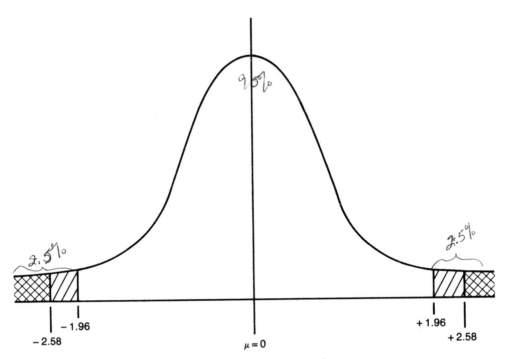

Figure 4-1   Two-tailed test of significance using the normal curve.

distribution falls below a z-score of -1.96, and 2.5% falls above $+1.96z$. To be so "rare" as to occur only 5% of the time, a z-score would have to be $-1.96z$ or less, or $+1.96z$ or greater. Note that we are using both "tails" of the distribution. Because 99% of the distribution falls between ±2.58 standard deviations from the mean of the normal curve, a score would have to be -2.58 or less, or $+2.58$ or greater, to be declared significant at the .01 level.

Figure 4-2 shows what occurs when a directional hypothesis is stated. We look at only one tail of the distribution. In this example, we will look at the positive side of the distribution. Fifty percent of the distribution falls below the mean and 45% falls between the mean and a z-score of $+1.65$ (see Appendix B). Thus, 95% $(50 + 45)$ of the distribution falls below $+1.65z$. To score in the upper 5% would require a score of $+1.65$ or greater. Given a one-tailed test of significance, you would need a score of $+1.65z$ to be significant at the .05 level, whereas with a two-tailed test, you needed a score of $\pm1.96z$. This is an example of the concept of power. With an a priori (before the fact) hypothesis, a lower z-score would be considered significant.

For the .01 level of significance and a one-tailed test, a z-score of $+2.33$ or greater is needed for significance. This is because 49% of the distribution falls between the mean and $+2.33$, and another 50% falls below the mean.

In summary, with a two-tailed test of significance, the z-score must reach

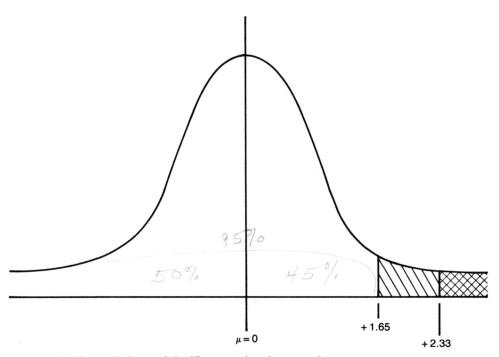

Figure 4-2   One-tailed test of significance using the normal curve.

±1.96 to be significant at the .05 level, and ±2.58 to be significant at the .01 level. With a one-tailed test, the z-score must be 1.65 for the .05 level, and 2.33 for the .01 level.

Degrees of Freedom

We have already shown the effects of degrees of freedom (df) when we discussed the denominator in the computation of the standard deviation. We pointed out that in the sample formula, the denominator is $n - 1$, thus, correcting for the possible underestimation of the population parameter. N and $n - 1$ in the denominators of the formulas for standard deviation are degrees of freedom. In describing the calculation of various statistics, we will discuss dividing by the degrees of freedom and looking up levels of significance in tables using dfs. Because this is sometimes a confusing concept, a simple example of degrees of freedom follows:

Degrees of freedom are related to the number of scores, items, or whatever in a a data set, and the idea of freedom to vary. Given three scores (1, 5, 6), we have three degrees of freedom, one for each independent item. Each score is "free to vary," that is, before collecting the data we do not know what any of these scores will be. Once we calculate the mean, however, we lose one of those dfs. This means that each of the three scores is no longer free to vary. The mean of these three scores is four. Once you know the mean and two of the three scores, you can figure out what the third score is. It is no longer free to vary. In calculating the variance or standard deviation, you are calculating how much the scores vary around the sample mean. Since the sample mean is known, one df is lost and the dfs become $n - 1$, the number of items in the set less one.

PARAMETRIC VS. NONPARAMETRIC TESTS

When we use *parametric tests* of significance, we are estimating at least one population parameter from our sample statistics. To be able to make such an estimation, we must make certain assumptions, the most important one being that the variable we have measured in the sample is normally distributed in the population to which we plan to generalize our findings. With *nonparametric tests,* there is no assumption about the distribution of the variable in the population. For that reason, nonparametric tests are often called *distribution-free.*

The main difference between these two classes of techniques is the assumptions about the population data that must be made before the parametric tests can be applied. For t-tests and analysis of variance (ANOVA), for example, it is assumed that the variable under study is normally distributed in the population and that the variance is the same at different levels of the variable. The nonparametric techniques have relatively few assumptions that must be met before they can be used.

As pointed out in Chapter 1, at one time level of measurement was considered an important element in deciding whether to use parametric or nonparametric tests. It was believed that parametric tests should be reserved for use with interval- and ratio-level data. Now, however, it has been shown that the use of parametric techniques with ordinal data rarely distorts the results. Many of the results obtained from parametric techniques are almost identical to those obtained from nonparametric techniques.

There are several advantages to the use of parametric techniques. Parametric techniques are more *powerful* and more *flexible.* They not only allow the researcher to study the effect of many independent variables on the dependent variable but also make possible the study of their interaction. Nonparametric techniques are much easier to calculate by hand, but that advantage has been eliminated by the use of computers.

We advocate the use of the parametric techniques for data at the ordinal level or higher unless the data seriously violate the assumptions of the parametric technique appropriate to the particular analysis. Small samples and serious distortions of data should lead one to explore nonparametric techniques.

SAMPLE SIZE

In planning research, the question always arises as to how large a sample one needs. With student research, the answer is often a practical one: "as many as you can get in the time allotted to collect data." There are, of course, some guidelines, such as having at least five subjects per cell in a design that will use chi square analysis. There should be fairly large numbers of subjects when one is using such techniques as multiple regression and factor analysis. Nunnally (1978) points out the difficulties in conducting such analyses with small samples. He suggests 30 subjects per independent variable in multiple regression and states that even with 10 subjects per item in a factor analysis, the chance for biased results is great. These issues will be discussed in more detail when these topics are presented.

As you may have guessed, "how many subjects?" is not a simple question to answer. This is one of those areas where "it all depends," a maddening, but true, appraisal of the situation. In planning research, we need a realistic estimate of how many subjects are needed to adequately test our hypothesis and answer our research questions. How many subjects do I need to find a significant difference? That question needs to be answered; otherwise, we may have too few subjects or, although less likely, we may waste time and effort gathering data from far more subjects than we need. One factor to be considered is how much effect the experimental condition is expected to have. If you have an experimental and control group and believe that the experimental approach will result in that group scoring 50 points higher on some measure than the control group, you will not need as many subjects in order to have that difference be statistically significant as you would if you expected the means of the two groups to differ by only five points. So, one factor to consider is how much *effect* you expect the independent variable(s) to have.

Most statistics books do not discuss how one determines appropriate sample size, nor do many research texts adequately cover this important question. One statistics book that does cover sample size in relation to the power of the statistical test is Volicer's (1981) *Advanced Statistical Methods with Nursing Research Applications*. Her presentation is derived from Cohen's (1977) approach to power analysis. A brief overview based on this method for determining sample size is presented here. For further details, see the Volicer and Cohen books.

In the Cohen approach, there are three elements required to determine sample size: effect size, significance level, and desired power. We have just given an example of what we mean by effect size, that is, the amount of impact you expect the treatment to have on the dependent variable. If two groups differ by 40 points on their mean scores, the effect size is 40. The significance level is set by the researcher; it determines the probability of making a Type I error (rejecting a *true* null hypothesis) and is called the alpha (α). The power of a test has been described as the likelihood of finding a true significant result. In other words, a power of .90 means a probability of .90 of rejecting the null hypothesis when it is indeed false. This is the opposite of making a Type II error.

Once you have selected the significance level (probably .05), determined the expected effect on the dependent variable, and determined the desired power, you can use tables in the Cohen book to determine what your sample size should be. There are separate tables for the various types of statistical tests that might be used: *t*-tests, ANOVA, multiple regression, and so on. For each test, there is a different way to calculate the estimated effect size. For example, will the means of the two

Table 4-1   Excerpts from Cohen's Tables for Determining Sample Size

One-Tailed *t*-Test (alpha = .05)

Power	Effect Size		
	.2	*.5*	*.8*
.50	136	22	9
.80	310	50	20
.90	429	69	27

Two-Tailed *t*-Test (alpha = .05)

Power	Effect Size		
	.2	*.5*	*.8*
.50	193	32	13
.80	393	64	26
.90	526	85	34

From: Cohen, J. (1977). *Statistical power analysis for the behavioral sciences.*
(Rev. ed.) New York: Academic Press.

groups vary by 10 points, 30 points, or 80 points? Obviously, we often may not have the data to calculate the estimated effect size. In such cases, Cohen suggests that we select a small, medium, or large effect size. He defines what he means by small, medium, and large for each statistical test. For the *t*-test, which compares the means of two groups, he says you should anticipate a small effect (.2) when the area of research is new, when the instruments have not been well tested, and when control is difficult. Without precise measurement tools and tight controls, you cannot expect to find a large difference or relationship. The medium effect (.5) is one that you expect will produce a noticeable difference. He gives, as an example, the difference in IQ between clerical and semiskilled workers. A large effect (.8) is expected when the groups are so different that almost half their scores do not overlap. That would be when the highest scores of one group are only at the mean of the other group.

The tables in the Cohen book list desired powers that go from .25 to .50 and then are about equally spaced between .50 and .99. Although .25 is included, it would be rare to select this level, because it means you only have one chance in four of rejecting the null hypothesis. Seeking a power of .90 to .99 would mean enormous samples. A power level of .80 is considered "good."

Let us give one example of how you might use Cohen's tables. We will use the *t*-test as an example. The purpose of the *t*-test is to determine whether or not there is a significant difference between the mean scores of two groups. If you had an experimental group and a control group, you could use the *t*-test to determine whether their scores varied. There are separate tables for one- and two-tailed tests. Suppose you hypothesized that your experimental group would score significantly higher than your control group. You would then use a one-tailed test. Next, you decide that your level of significance will be .05; that you want good power, .80; and that you expect a medium-sized effect, .5. See Table 4-1 for an abbreviated version of the appropriate Cohen table. You would need 50 subjects in each of your two groups to have a probability of .80 of finding a significant difference. If you did not hypothesize, and therefore planned to use a two-tailed test of significance, you would need 64 subjects in each of your groups.

   This brief introduction to Cohen's power analysis is to make you aware of the significance of this book, so that you will have a means for deciding more rationally how many subjects you need in your study. A great deal of effort goes into any research study, and you do not want to thwart your efforts by having an inappropriate sample size.

EXERCISES FOR CHAPTER 4

1. A researcher tests for differences between the mean scores of two groups. She sets the level of significance at 0.05. If the mean difference is so large that it would occur by chance only 1% of the time, should the researcher _____ (accept/reject) the *null hypothesis?*

2. A researcher states that there is no significant relationship between two variables and sets the level of significance at 0.01. The statistical test shows that the relationship is so small that it would occur by chance 10% of the time. The researcher should _____ (accept/reject) the hypothesis?

3. You are testing a null hypothesis at the 0.05 level. For each of the following, should you *accept* or *reject* the null hypothesis?
   a. $z = -2.00$
   b. $z = 0.19$
   c. $z = 1.98$
   d. $z = -1.50$

4. The researcher hypothesizes that one group will score significantly higher than another group. The significance level is 0.01. For each of the following results, what should the action be regarding the *directional hypothesis?*
   a. $z = 2.40$
   b. $z = -2.40$
   c. $z = 1.70$
   d. $z = 1.50$

5. When the researcher makes a prediction regarding the direction of mean differences between an experimental and control group, she should use a _____ (one-tailed/two-tailed) test of significance?

6. Which is the more powerful test?   _____ one-tailed   _____ two-tailed

7. You hypothesize that there is no significant difference between nurses and social workers in terms of weight. In each of the following, determine whether or not an error has been made, and, if so, what type of error.

   a. Social workers really weigh significantly more than nurses, and you accept the null hypothesis.
   b. Nurses really weigh more than social workers, and you reject the null hypothesis.
   c. Nurses and social workers really do weigh the same, and you accept the null hypothesis.
   d. Nurses and social workers really do weigh the same, and you reject the null hypothesis.

8. In general, will a nonparametric or parametric test, each designed to accomplish the same analytical function, more frequently reject the null hypothesis?

9. You wish to test the effects of a weight reduction program. You hypothesize that the experimental group will lose noticeably more weight than the control group, and you plan to use a t-test to test this hypothesis. What would the appropriate effect size be? Given a power of 0.80, how many subjects should you have in each group?

SECTION 2
Analyzing Relationships

CHAPTER 5
Correlation

Barbara Hazard Munro

OBJECTIVES FOR CHAPTER 5

After reading this chapter and completing the exercises, you should be able to

1. Explain when to use correlational techniques to answer research questions or test hypotheses.
2. Report a correlation coefficient in terms of its statistical significance and meaningfulness.
3. Calculate a correlation coefficient and construct a confidence interval around it.
4. Be able to read a computer printout reporting correlations.
5. Understand measures of relationship other than the Pearson Product Moment Correlation Coefficient.
6. Know when it is appropriate to use multiple correlation, partial correlation, and semi-partial correlation.

Correlational techniques are used to study relationships. They may be used in relation-searching, that is, exploratory studies in which one intent is to determine whether or not relationships exist, and in association-testing studies in which we test a hypothesis about a particular relationship.

Numan, Barklind, and Lubin (1981) sought to determine whether there was a relationship between depression and morbidity (number of months of hospitalization) among chronic dialysis patients. They reported that such a relationship did exist ($r = .25$, $p < .05$). Would you agree that a correlation of .25 gives evidence of such a relationship? It is a significant relationship, but does significance tell you how much meaning the relationship has? One aim of this chapter is to help you answer such questions.

In a study of coping behaviors following surgery, Ziemer (1983) used correlation coefficients to test the hypotheses that two kinds of coping (physiological and psychological) would be *inversely* related to the development of symptoms; that is, individuals with more coping strategies would develop fewer symptoms. As it happened, neither of the hypotheses was supported.

The term correlation is used in everyday language. We hear people state that something is correlated with something else. Here we are speaking about a relation that can be measured mathematically, in that we can calculate a number representing how strong a relation is. But a correlation, showing that two variables are related, does *not* mean that one variable *caused* the other. It is a mistake to infer causation from correlation alone. For example, more people die in hospitals than any place else. Does that mean that hospitals cause deaths? There is a relation between the number of police cars at an accident and the amount of damage done to the vehicles and people involved. Do police cars *cause* the damage? The point is, there may be a relationship, but there may also be other factors affecting the variables under study.

TYPE OF DATA REQUIRED

The Pearson Product Moment Correlation Coefficient (r) is the most usual method by which the relation between two variables is quantified and is the focus of this chapter. A brief description of other formulas, most of which have been derived from the Pearson r, will be given. To calculate r, there must be at least two measures on each subject. It is often assumed that both of these measures must be at the interval level. In most cases, however, valid results may also be obtained with ordinal data. Moreover, as will be seen, we can code categorical variables for use with r and with regression equations. Mathematically, then, it is possible to use any level of data when calculating r, but there are factors to consider other than the level of the data when deciding whether or not a correlation coefficient is appropriate.

ASSUMPTIONS

Although we can calculate correlations with data at all levels, there are certain assumptions if we are to generalize beyond the sample statistic, that is, if one is to make inferences about the population itself. First, of course, the sample must be representative of the population to which the inference will be made. Second, the variables that are being correlated, say X and Y, must each have a normal distribution, that is, the distribution of their scores must approximate the normal curve. Third, for every value of X, the distribution of Y scores must have approximately equal variability. This is called the *assumption of homoscedasticity*. Fourth, the relationship between X and Y must be linear, that is, when the two scores for each individual are graphed, they should tend to form a straight line. Of course, the points will not all fall on this line, but they should be scattered closely around it. The technique for graphing the relationship between two variables is demonstrated in

the next section of this chapter. In Figure 5-1, *A* and *B* demonstrate linear relationships, and *D* a curvilinear relationship. A technique for measuring curvilinear
relationships is presented later in this chapter.

CORRELATION COEFFICIENT

As has been pointed out, the correlation coefficient *r* allows us to state mathematically what relationship exists between two variables. It also tells us the *type* of
relationship that exists, that is, whether the relationship is *positive* or *negative*. The
relationship between job satisfaction and job turnover has been shown to be negative (we say that an *inverse* relationship exists between them). These terms mean
that as one variable increases, the other decreases. People with higher job satisfaction have lower rates of job turnover, and vice versa. Similarly, those with higher

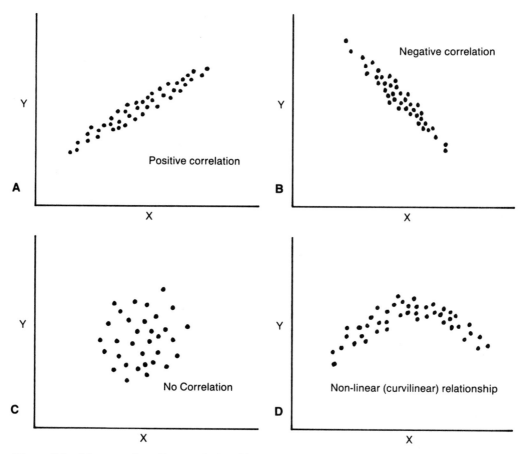

Figure 5-1   Linear and nonlinear relationships.

college grades have lower dropout rates. There is a positive relationship between GRE scores and graduate grades, that is, those with higher GRE scores usually have higher grades.

If you were to look at scores on two variables, as in Table 5-1, you might observe that those who scored high on one measure tended to score high on the other, and those who did poorly on one measure did poorly on the other. It is common to use X to designate the independent variable and Y for the dependent variable; we will use these designations throughout the book. In this example, however, it is not necessary to think of one as independent and the other as dependent. The two sets of scores might represent a quiz and an examination given to students in some class, with no notion of one causing the other.

In addition to "eyeballing" these figures, you might graph the data to see what they look like. Such a graph is called a *scatter diagram* (Fig. 5-2). To draw such a graph, you plot the pair of scores for each subject. For subject 1, the X-score was 2, so you move to 2 on the horizontal scale where the X scores are plotted. The Y-score was one, so you move straight up from the 2 on the horizontal axis to the spot opposite the 1 on the vertical axis, where the Y scores are plotted. The dot that represents subject 1's scores is labeled in the graph. In the same way, all other scores are plotted. In this example, the scores extend diagonally from the lower left to the upper right corner of the graph. Such a configuration indicates a positive relationship between the two scores: low scores on X tend to go with low scores on Y, and vice versa. If there were a negative relationship, high scores on one variable going with low scores on the other, the dots on the graph would go from the upper left to the lower right. When no relationship exists, the dots are scattered into a central cluster, like a target (see Fig. 5-1). Although the graph indicates a positive relationship between the two variables, it does not tell us just how strong the relationship is. To make such a determination, we need to calculate a correlation coefficient, r.

The correlation coefficient may range from $+1.00$ through 0.00 to -1.00. A $+1.00$ indicates a perfect positive relationship, 0.00 indicates no relationship, and

Table 5-1   Subjects' Scores on Two Measures

Subjects	X	Y
1	2	1
2	5	6
3	7	9
4	3	2
5	10	8
6	1	3
7	9	10
8	4	3
9	8	9
10	6	7

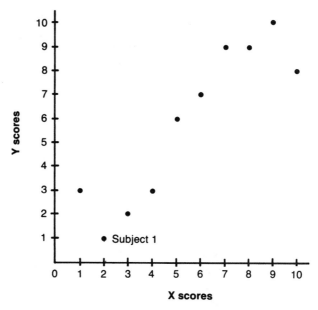

Figure 5-2   Graph of scores from Table 5-1.

−1.00 indicates a perfect negative relationship. Such relationships will now be demonstrated. To aid in explaining the concept of correlation, a formula that makes use of standard scores (z-scores) will be used. In explaining standard deviation, a formula based on deviations from the mean,

$$ s = \sqrt{\frac{\Sigma x^2}{n-1}}, $$

was used first, because that is what the measure is all about. Then another formula that was mathematically equivalent and easier to calculate was shown. The same technique is being used here. In using the formula with z-scores, we will see that r is the average of the cross-products of the z-scores ($r = (\Sigma zXzY)/n$). (Hopefully, that will be clear when we have taken you through this process.) Later in this chapter, the "computational" formula for r will be introduced. It is commonly used, easier to calculate than the z-score formula, but not as simple conceptually.

A perfect positive relationship, +1.00, is demonstrated in Table 5-2. The five subjects took a quiz, X, on which the scores ranged from 6 to 10 and an examination, Y, on which the scores ranged from 82 to 98. You can see that the subjects have the same *rank* on both measures. Subject 1 had the lowest score on both tests, subject 2 had the next lowest scores on both, and so on.

Since the means and standard deviations of the two tests are different, we cannot directly compare the scores from the two tests. Note that in Table 5-2, we have indicated the mean of the X scores by $\overline{X}$, and the mean of the Y scores by $\overline{Y}$. we will continue to use this symbolism throughout the book. To compare the scores

Table 5-2 A Perfect Positive Relationship Between Two Variables

Subjects	X	χ	Y	y	zX	zY	$zXzY$
1	6	−2	82	−8	−1.42	−1.42	2.0
2	7	−1	86	−4	−0.71	−0.71	0.5
3	8	0	90	0	0.00	0.00	0.0
4	9	1	94	4	0.71	0.71	0.5
5	10	2	98	8	1.42	1.42	2.0

$\overline{X} = 8, \sigma = 1.41$ $\qquad \Sigma zXzY = 5.00$

$\overline{Y} = 90, \sigma = 5.66$ $\qquad r = \dfrac{\Sigma zXzY}{n} = \dfrac{5.00}{5} = 1$

of the two tests directly, we can transform them so that both distributions have the same mean and standard deviation. In this example, all the scores are transformed to z-scores with a mean of zero and a standard deviation of one. The formula for converting a score to a z-score is $z = (X - \overline{X})/s$, or χ/s, where χ indicates the deviation of a score for its mean. In Table 5-2, the deviation scores for the X distribution are labeled χ and those from the Y distribution are labeled y.

To calculate the z-score for each of the original scores, we divide the χ scores by the standard deviation for X, and the y scores by the standard deviation for Y. For subject 1, the raw score on the quiz X was two points below the mean, so that $\chi = -2$. Dividing this by the standard deviation for the X scores ($\sigma = 1.41$), we find that the z-score on the quiz is -1.42 $(-2/1.41)$. For the score on the examination (Y), we see that the subject was 8 points below the mean; this also equals a z-score of -1.42 $(-8/5.66 = -1.42)$. Now, we can compare the z-scores for X and Y and see that each subject received matching z-scores for the two tests. By definition, that is a perfect positive correlation; now we must see how to calculate it.

The correlation is the mean of the cross-product of the z-scores for each subject. This is a measure of how much each pair of scores varies together. The cross-products are labeled as $zXzY$ in the table. For subject 2, the cross-product is calculated as -0.071 $(zX) \times -0.071$ (zY) and is 0.50. To take the average of the cross-products, you add them and divide by the number of cross-products. Thus, the formula for r is $(\Sigma zXzY)/n$. The sum of the cross-products $((\Sigma zXzY)/n)$ is 5.00; dividing that by 5 (the number of cross-products) results in an r equal to 1.00. The scores are plotted in Figure 5-3. When the dots are joined, they form a straight line, which indicates a perfect relationship.

To demonstrate a perfect negative correlation, we simply reversed the scores on the Y variable (Table 5-3). Subject 1 still gets the lowest score on X but now also gets the highest score on Y. Carrying out the same procedure, we find that the sum of the cross-products is -5.00; thus, $r = -5.00/5$, or -1.00, a perfect negative correlation. Figure 5-4 shows the graph of these scores.

In Table 5-4, the Y scores are scrambled in such a way that there is no relationship between the X and Y scores. These scores are plotted in Figure 5-5.

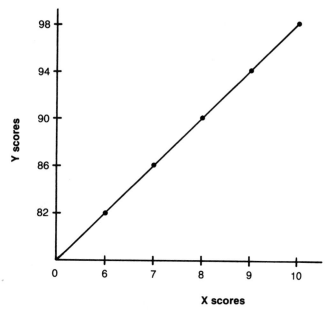

Figure 5-3 Graph of scores from Table 5-2.

Table 5-3 A Perfect Negative Correlation Between Two Variables

Subjects	X	χ	Y	y	zX	zY	zXzY
1	6	−2	98	8	−1.42	1.42	−2.0
2	7	−1	94	4	−0.71	0.71	−0.5
3	8	0	90	0	0.00	0.00	0.0
4	9	1	86	−4	0.71	−0.71	−0.5
5	10	2	82	−8	1.42	−1.42	−2.0

$\overline{X} = 8, \sigma = 1.41$

$\overline{Y} = 90, \sigma = 5.66$

$$\Sigma zXzY = -5.00$$

$$r = \frac{\Sigma zXzY}{n} = \frac{-5.00}{5} = -1.00$$

Strength of Correlation Coefficient

How large should r be in order for it to be useful? As is often the case, the answer is, "it depends." Alternate forms of a test should be measuring the same thing, so the correlation between them should be high. With tests (such as GREs) whose results are used in important decision making, the correlations between two forms of the same test must be very high, about 0.95. On the other hand, when we are studying the relationships among various aspects of human behavior, we may be quite happy with a correlation of 0.50. Some "descriptors" that can be attached to rs of varying strengths are listed below. It should be noted that the *direction* of the relationship

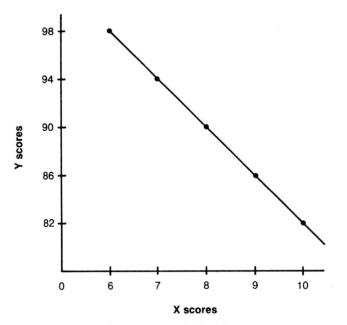

Figure 5-4   Graph of scores in Table 5-3.

does not affect the *strength* of the relationship. A correlation of −0.90 is just as high, or just as "strong," as an *r* of +0.90. The following categories include + and − *r*s:

0.00–0.25   little, if any
0.26–0.49   low
0.50–0.69   moderate
0.70–0.89   high
0.90–1.00   very high

Significance of the Correlation

If you want to generalize the *r* that you calculate from the sample to the correlation of these two variables in the population, you must determine the level of probability of *r*, that is, what is the probability that this *r* occurred by chance alone. You may use either a one- or two-tailed test for significance, depending on whether or not you hypothesized about the relationship. When you use the packaged statistical programs for the computer, the exact probability of *r* is given, 0.032 or whatever. When you calculate *r* by hand, you can consult a table such as that in Appendix C. The level of statistical significance is greatly affected by the size of the sample, *n*. It makes sense that if *r* is based on a sample of 1000, there is a much greater likelihood that it represents the *r* of the population than if *r* was based on a sample of 10. With

Table 5-4   A Demonstration of No Relationship Between Two Variables

Subjects	X	χ	Y	y	zX	zY	$zXzY$
1	6	−2	94	4	−1.42	0.71	−1.0
2	7	−1	82	−8	−0.71	−1.42	1.0
3	8	0	90	0	0.00	0.00	0.0
4	9	1	98	8	0.71	1.42	1.0
5	10	2	86	−4	1.42	−0.71	−1.0

$\overline{X} = 8, \sigma = 1.41$

$\overline{Y} = 90, \sigma = 5.66$

$\Sigma zXzY = 0.00$

$$r = \frac{\Sigma zXzY}{n} = \frac{0.00}{5} = 0.00$$

Figure 5-5   Graph of scores in Table 5-4.

a two-tailed test and a sample of 100, an *r* of 0.20 is statistically significant at the 0.05 level, but if you have a sample of 10, the correlation must be 0.632 or larger to be significant. You should note that, given large samples, *r*s that are described as demonstrating "little, if any" relationship are statistically significant. To reiterate, the statistical significance implies that the *r* did not occur by chance, that the relationship actually is greater than zero. However, a "highly significant" correlation may in fact be quite small. For that reason, many people also speak about the *meaningfulness* of *r*.

Meaningfulness of the Correlation Coefficient

The coefficient of determination r^2 is often used as a measure of the "meaningfulness" of r. This is a measure of the amount of variance that the variables share.

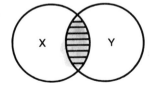

The circle containing X represents all the variability or variance of X, and the other circle represents the total variance for Y. The overlapping area indicates their shared variance. It is that area that can be determined by squaring the correlation coefficient r. To determine the meaningfulness of an r of 0.20, square the coefficient, $r^2 = (0.20)^2 = 0.04$, or 4%. You can then say that the variance shared between these two variables equals 4%. When reporting this, researchers usually say that the independent variable, X, accounts for 4% of the variance of the dependent variable. Obviously, that is not very much, because there is another 96% of variance unaccounted for. To account for about half of the variance, you would need an r of 0.70 (since $0.70^2 = 0.49$, or 49%).

Confidence Intervals

We constructed "confidence" intervals around mean scores and stated with 95 (or 99) % "confidence" that the mean of the population would fall between two points. We may also construct confidence intervals around r, stating that we are 95 (or 99) % "confident" that the population r will fall between two given rs. This is another way of determining just what the r you calculate means. We will demonstrate the construction of these intervals after we demonstrate the calculation of r by the most commonly used formula.

CALCULATIONS

Pearson Product Moment Correlation

The following formula is mathematically equivalent to the z-score formula that we have already demonstrated. As was the case with the formula for the standard deviation, this formula looks more complicated than the z-score formula but is actually easier to calculate because we do not have to subtract all the scores from their respective means.

$$r = \frac{\Sigma XY - \frac{(\Sigma X)(\Sigma Y)}{n}}{\sqrt{\left(\Sigma X^2 - \frac{(\Sigma X)^2}{n}\right)\left(\Sigma Y^2 - \frac{(\Sigma Y)^2}{n}\right)}}$$

The calculation of r is demonstrated in Table 5-5. There are two variables, X and Y. To calculate r, we must have the number in the sample, n, that is the number of pairs of scores. We must also calculate the sum of the X-scores (ΣX) and the sum of the Y-scores (ΣY). Each score is squared and summed, resulting in ΣX^2 and ΣY^2. The cross-products (XY) are calculated by multiplying each pair of scores. For subject one, XY equals $2 \times 1 = 2$. The cross-products are added up, giving us ΣXY. Those components are listed on the lower left side of the table and are inserted in the formula to their right. The result is a correlation of 0.90, which rates a label of "very high."

To determine the statistical significance of the correlation, use the table in Appendix C. The degrees of freedom for r are $n - 2$, that is, the number of subjects

Table 5-5   Calculation of the Pearson Product Moment Correlation Coefficient

Subjects	X	Y	X^2	Y^2	XY
1	2	1	4	1	2
2	5	6	25	36	30
3	7	9	49	81	63
4	3	2	9	4	6
5	10	8	100	64	80
6	1	3	1	9	3
7	9	10	81	100	90
8	4	3	16	9	12
9	8	9	64	81	72
10	6	7	36	49	42
	55	58	385	434	400

$n = 10$
$\Sigma X = 55$
$\Sigma Y = 58$
$\Sigma X^2 = 385$
$\Sigma Y^2 = 434$
$\Sigma XY = 400$

$$r = \frac{\Sigma XY - \frac{(\Sigma X)(\Sigma Y)}{n}}{\sqrt{\left(\Sigma X^2 - \frac{(\Sigma X)^2}{n}\right)\left(\Sigma Y^2 - \frac{(\Sigma Y)^2}{n}\right)}}$$

$$r = \frac{400 - \frac{(55)(58)}{10}}{\sqrt{\left(385 - \frac{(55)^2}{10}\right)\left(434 - \frac{(58)^2}{10}\right)}}$$

$$r = \frac{400 - 319}{\sqrt{(385 - 302.5)(434 - 336.4)}} = \frac{81}{\sqrt{(82.5)(97.6)}}$$

$$= \frac{81}{\sqrt{8052}} = \frac{81}{89.73} = .90$$

minus two. In our example, we had 10 subjects, so the df = 8 (10 − 2 = 8). For a two-tailed test with eight degrees of freedom, we can see that r must equal or exceed 0.632 in order for it to be significant at the 0.05 level, and we see that r must equal or exceed 0.765 to be significant at the 0.01 level. (Note that the levels would change if we had a one-tailed test. With a one-tailed test, the tabeled levels are 0.549 for the 0.05 level, and 0.716 for the 0.01 level.) The correlation of 0.90 exceeds 0.765; therefore, r is "significant" at the 0.01 level, whether this is a one- or two-tailed test.

Confidence Intervals

To set up the confidence interval around a given r, r must first be transformed into what is called a *Fisher's* z_r, through the use of the table in Appendix D. For example, let us assume that we had 103 subjects and an r or 0.90.

The first step is to convert r to z_r. In Appendix D, note that an r of 0.900 equals a z_r of 1.472.

The second step is to determine the standard error. The formula for the standard error is $1/\sqrt{n-3}$. In this example, that is $1/\sqrt{103-3} = 0.1$.

The third step is to determine what confidence interval we will choose. The 95% and 99% levels are commonly used. The formulas are:

a. $95\% = z_r \pm (1.96)$ (standard error)
b. $99\% = z_r \pm (2.58)$ (standard error)

For our example they become:

a. $95\% = 1.472 \pm (1.96)(0.1) = 1.276$ and 1.668
b. $99\% = 1.472 \pm (2.58)(0.1) = 1.214$ and 1.730

The fourth step is to transform the z_rs back to rs using Appendix D. When using the table, you will see that not every possible z_r is listed. Select the one closest to the number you calculated.

a. 95%, z_rs = 1.276 and 1.668; after transformation back to rs, they become 0.855 and 0.930, respectively.
b. 99%, z_rs = 1.214 and 1.730; after transformation back to rs, they become 0.840 and 0.940, respectively.

The fifth step is to set up the confidence intervals.

Level	Bounds for r
a. 95%	0.855–0.930
b. 99%	0.840–0.940

What you are saying is that from your sample data you have calculated an r of 0.90 and you are (1) 95% confident that the population r is between 0.855 and 0.930, and (2) 99% confident that the population r is between 0.840 and 0.940.

EXAMPLES OF COMPUTER PRINTOUTS

Figure 5-6 contains examples of computer printouts generated by the SPSS program. Included in the tables are six measures used by the Admissions Committee at Yale School of Nursing in their decision making, and the final grade point average at

Figure 5-6 Correlation coefficients produced by SPSS program.

Procedure Cards

For one-tailed probabilities:

```
1                      16
PEARSON CORR           GREV GREM BACH AUTO REFTOT TOT OVERGPA
```

For two-tailed probabilities:

```
PEARSON CORR           GREV GREM BACH AUTO REFTOT TOT OVERGPA
OPTIONS                3
```

Output

One-Tailed Probabilties

- - - - - - - - - - - P E A R S O N   C O R R E L A T I O N   C O E F F I C I E N T S

	GREV	GREM	BACH	AUTO	REFTOT	TOT	OVERGPA
GREV	1.0000 (0) P = *****	0.5484 (425) P = 0.000	0.2034 (141) P = 0.008	0.2464 (180) P = 0.000	0.0829 (187) P = 0.130	0.2174 (190) P = 0.001	0.2162 (364) P = 0.000
GREM	0.5484 (425) P = 0.000	1.0000 (0) P = *****	0.3063 (141) P = 0.000	0.1120 (180) P = 0.067	0.0508 (167) P = 0.245	0.0963 (190) P = 0.093	0.1697 (364) P = 0.001
BACH	0.2034 (141) P = 0.008	0.3063 (141) P = 0.000	1.0000 (0) P = *****	0.1627 (139) P = 0.028	0.1904 (142) P = 0.012	0.1647 (143) P = 0.025	0.1922 (133) P = 0.013
AUTO	0.2464 (180) P = 0.000	0.1120 (180) P = 0.067	0.1627 (139) P = 0.028	1.0000 (0) P = *****	0.2724 (181) P = 0.000	0.0978 (182) P = 0.095	0.2775 (171) P = 0.000
REFTOT	0.0829 (187) P = 0.130	0.0508 (187) P = 0.245	0.1904 (142) P = 0.012	0.2724 (181) P = 0.000	1.0000 (0) P = *****	0.1010 (190) P = 0.083	0.0752 (179) P = 0.159
TOT	0.2174 (190) P = 0.001	0.0963 (190) P = 0.093	0.1647 (143) P = 0.025	0.0978 (182) P = 0.095	0.1010 (190) P = 0.083	1.0000 (0) P = *****	0.0199 (181) P = 0.395
OVERGPA	0.2162 (364) P = 0.000	0.1697 (364) P = 0.001	0.1922 (133) P = 0.013	0.2775 (171) P = 0.000	0.0752 (179) P = 0.159	0.0199 (181) P = 0.395	1.0000 (0) P = *****

(COEFFICIENT / (CASES) / SIGNIFICANCE)

(Continued)

Figure 5-6 (*continued*)

Two-Tailed Probabilities

- - - - - - - - - - - P E A R S O N   C O R R E L A T I O N   C O E F F I C I E N T S

	GREV	GREM	BACH	AUTO	REFTOT	TOT	OVERGPA
GREV	1.0000	0.5484	0.2034	0.2464	0.0829	0.2174	0.2162
	(0)	(425)	(141)	(160)	(187)	(190)	(364)
	P = *****	P = 0.000	P = 0.016	P = 0.001	P = 0.260	P = 0.003	P = 0.000
GREM	0.5484	1.0000	0.3063	0.1120	0.0508	0.0963	0.1697
	(425)	(0)	(141)	(180)	(187)	(190)	(364)
	P = 0.000	P = *****	P = 0.000	P = 0.135	P = 0.490	P = 0.186	P = 0.001
BACH	0.2034	0.3063	1.0000	0.1627	0.1904	0.1647	0.1922
	(141)	(141)	(0)	(139)	(142)	(143)	(133)
	P = 0.016	P = 0.000	P = *****	P = 0.056	P = 0.023	P = 0.049	P = 0.027
AUTO	0.2464	0.1120	0.1627	1.0000	0.2724	0.0978	0.2775
	(180)	(180)	(139)	(0)	(181)	(182)	(171)
	P = 0.001	P = 0.135	P = 0.056	P = *****	P = 0.000	P = 0.189	P = 0.000
REFTOT	0.0829	0.0508	0.1904	0.2724	1.0000	0.1010	0.0752
	(187)	(187)	(142)	(181)	(0)	(190)	(179)
	P = 0.260	P = 0.490	P = 0.023	P = 0.000	P = *****	P = 0.166	P = 0.317
TOT	0.2174	0.0963	0.1647	0.0978	0.1010	1.0000	0.0199
	(190)	(190)	(143)	(182)	(190)	(0)	(181)
	P = 0.003	P = 0.186	P = 0.049	P = 0.189	P = 0.166	P = *****	P = 0.790
OVERGPA	0.2162	0.1697	0.1922	0.2775	0.0752	0.0199	1.0000
	(364)	(364)	(133)	(171)	(179)	(181)	(0)
	P = 0.000	P = 0.001	P = 0.027	P = 0.000	P = 0.317	P = 0.790	P = *****

(COEFFICIENT / (CASES) / SIGNIFICANCE)

the end of the Master's program. These data were collected from students in the Yale Master's program in nursing over a 10-year period. The six measures used by the Admissions Committee are the GRE-Verbal and Quantitative scores (GREV and GREM), the undergraduate grade point average (BACH), a score on an essay that each applicant submits (AUTO), a score for the three references (REFTOT), and a score for the inteview (TOT).

The intercorrelations among all the measures are shown in the tables. There are three numbers in each group. The top number is the correlation coefficient, the next is the number of subjects included in the calculation of the coefficient, and the lowest of the three is the probability. In the last column of the first row, you see that the correlation between the GRE-Verbal and final GPA is 0.2162. There were 364 subjects involved in the analysis, and the significance level is 0.000 (which also means that p is less than 0.001, because the computer program only carries the probability to three decimal places). The number of subjects included in each computation varies due to missing data. In this case, most of the missing data are a result of the fact that admissions procedures changed over the 10 years, and new systems of rating were added. There were no ratings of essays, references, and interviews in the older data.

The two tables are the same except for the *p* values. The top table reports a one-tailed test of significance, whereas the bottom table reports a two-tailed test. Note the differences in probabilities.

EXAMPLE FROM PUBLISHED RESEARCH

Noreen E. Mahon (1982) studied the relationship of self-disclosure, interpersonal dependency, and life changes to loneliness in young adults. She stated four hypotheses and used Pearson correlations to test the first three, which will be presented here. For the fourth hypothesis, she used multiple regression, which will be presented in the next chapter.

Hypotheses

Her first three hypotheses were:

    I. The lower the self-disclosure, the higher the level of loneliness.
    II. The higher the interpersonal dependency, the higher the level of loneliness.
    III. The higher the life changes, the higher the level of loneliness. The author is posing a negative relation in hypothesis I and positive relations in hypotheses II and III. *inverse*

Data Gathered

Data were gathered from 209 college students, aged 18 to 25. The four variables under study were measured by the Jourard Self-Disclosure Questionnaire, Interpersonal Dependency Inventory, Recent Life Change Questionanire, and the revised UCLA Loneliness Scale.

Tabular Presentation of Results

Table 5-6 contains the intercorrelations of the predictor (independent) and criterion (dependent) variables. Numbers are used rather than names of variables across the top of the table. Thus, 1 is self-disclosure, 2 is interpersonal dependency, and so on. Although the author used the SPSS program to calculate the *r*s, she does not include the exact probabilities generated by the program. She uses asterisks to indicate which are significant at $p < 0.005$. She does not state whether she used a one- or two-tailed test of significance. Since she hypothesized apriori, the one-tailed test would have been appropriate.

Table 5-6   Intercorrelations of the Predictor and Criterion Variables

	1	2	3	4
Self-disclosure	1.0	.023	−.111	−.336*
Interpersonal dependency		1.0	.117	.239*
Life changes			1.0	.039
Loneliness				1.0

*$p < .005$
From: Mahon, N. E. (1982). The relationship of self-disclosure, interpersonal dependency, and life changes to loneliness in young adults. *Nursing Research 31* (6), 343–347.

Description of Results

The first hypothesis—that there would be an inverse (negative) relationship between self-disclosure and loneliness—was supported ($r = -0.336$, $p < 0.005$). Subjects who had higher rates of self-disclosure generally had lower levels of loneliness, and vice versa.

The second hypothesis—that those with higher interpersonal dependency would be more lonely—was also supported ($r = 0.239$, $p < 0.005$).

The third hypothesis—that more life changes would be related to higher loneliness—was not supported ($r = 0.039$, $p = 0.238$). The number of life changes did not relate to the level of loneliness. However, the author points out that this group of individuals reported relatively few life changes; thus, the variance of that variable was restricted.

Conclusions

The author reports that her study suggests that "explanations for loneliness are complex and include personal characteristics such as self-disclosure and interpersonal dependency and external support systems such as relationships with friends and loved ones" (Mahon, 1982, p. 346).

BRIEF DESCRIPTION OF OTHER MEASURES OF RELATIONSHIP

There are measures other than the Pearson r for measuring relationships. An overview of these will be given here, but computational formulas will not be represented. Three "short-cut" versions of r are *phi, point-biserial,* and *Spearman rho.*

Short-Cut Versions of r

There tends to be some confusion about short-cut versions of r, with many researchers assuming that they are different from Pearson's r and that if you applied r

and one of these formulas to a set of data, you would get different results. Actually, these measures usually give exactly the same result as r. The only advantage for using them is when doing hand calculations. They are really short-cut versions of r that can be used with specific types of data.

Phi. When both variables being correlated are _dichotomous,_ that is, with only two levels, a short-cut version of r can be used. Examples of dichotomous variables include sex (male and female), a yes/no response choice, and pass/fail. If you are using the computer to analyze your data, you can use r and will get exactly the same result as if you had used phi.

Point-Biserial and Spearman Rho. When you want to correlate one dichotomous variable with one continuous variable, you can use the point-biserial formula. When you have two sets of ranks, you can use the Spearman rho formula. You might ask two groups to rank a list of stressors from most stressful to least stressful. You could compare the rankings of the two groups by using the Spearman rho formula. Again, you could also calculate r with these data and get the same result. Spearman rho is often referred to as a "nonparametric" test, as though it were distribution-free, which is not quite true. It is better thought of as a short-cut version of r.

Nonparametric Measures

Kendall's Tau. This measure is a nonparametric measure and is not a short-cut formula for r. It was developed as an alternate procedure for Spearman rho. It is sometimes used when measuring the relation between two ranked (ordinal) variables. But as previously noted, r can usually be applied to such data. Kendall's tau might be an alternative if your data seriously violated the assumptions underlying r. It can be calculated using most of the major computer packages, such as SAS or SPSS.

Contingency Coefficient. One nonparametric technique can be used to measure the relationship between two nominal level variables. The variables need not be dichotomous variables but may have multiple levels. For example, this technique could be used to determine the relationship between race and political affiliation.

Calculating this coefficient requires use of the Chi-Square statistic, which will be discussed in Chapter 7.

Estimating r

There are two formulas that are not short-cut versions of r, but instead "estimate" results that might be obtained using r. Nunnally (1978) recommends that, in general, these techniques _not_ be used. Since they are sometimes reported in the literature and often mentioned in statistics texts, they will be outlined here.

Biserial. This technique can be used when one variable is _dichotomized_ and the other is _continuous._ Dichoto_mized_ means that the variable has been _made_ dichotomous, cut into two levels from a variable that would have been naturally continuous.

For example, scores could be divided into high and low, creating a dichotomized variable. A biserial correlation might be used if you had a scale on which people rated the items with agree or disagree (a dichotomized variable) and another variable that was continuous, such as age, and you wanted to know what the correlation would be if you changed the dichotomized variable into a continuous variable (perhaps by adding response categories). If you calculated the biserial correlation between the dichotomized variable (agree/disagree) and the continuous variable (age), you would have an estimate of what r would be if the dichotomized variable was changed to a continuous one. Nunnally (1978) argues against such a use, stating that the resulting coefficient is usually artificially high.

Tetrachoric. This coefficient estimates r from the relationship between two dichotomized variables. If there are serious problems with estimating r from one dichotomized variable (biserial), there are obviously even more difficulties with estimating r from two dichotomized variables.

"Universal" Measure

Thus far, we have been discussing the relationship between two variables that have a linear relationship. When we graph those relationships, we see that they suggest a straight line across the graph. Although the relationship may be positive or negative, the relationship is the same across all the scores. An example of a nonlinear relationship can be seen in Figure 5-1. In that case, low scores on the X variable are related to low scores on the Y variable, but high scores on X are also related to low scores on Y. Such a relationship is called *curvilinear*. An example might be the possible relationship between anxiety and test scores. In this graph, those with moderate anxiety could tend to perform the best on tests. Those with very low or very high anxiety perform poorly. There is a real advantage to having your data plotted to determine whether a nonlinear relationship exists, because r cannot be used to test such a relationship.

Eta. Eta, sometimes called the *correlation ratio,* can be used to measure a non-linear relationship. The range of values for eta goes from 0 to +1. It can be used with all variables, whether nominal or continuous. Eta is closely related to r and has been called a "universal" relationship because it can be used "regardless of the form of the relationship" (Nunnally, 1978, p. 147). When it is used with two continuous variables that have a linear relationship, it reduces to r.

PARTIAL CORRELATION

When discussing research design, we confront the notion of "control." How do we "control" variance that will distract or mislead us? There are, of course, several ways. If we are concerned about the impact of a variable, such as age, we might use random assignment of subjects to groups as a method of control, we might select only one age group, or we might match subjects by age before assigning them to groups. There are also statistical measures of control: we can record the age of the subjects and use that as a variable in the study. One method of statistical control is *partial correlation.*

This technique also allows us to describe the relation between two variables (or more, if you go to multiple partial correlation) after statistically controlling for the influence of some third variable. In studying research design, you learned that the relationship between two variables may be unclear due to the "confounding" influence of another variable. For example, if you calculate the correlation between mental age and height in children 1 to 10 years of age, you will find a high correlation. Does that mean that height causes intelligence? Of course the key factor is age, not height. Once you control for age, the relationship between height and mental age becomes trivial.

One study was done to determine whether the number of hours studied was related to grades; the reseachers found a negative correlation. Did this mean that if you studied less, you would get higher grades? No, once they controlled for intelligence they found a significant positive relation between grades and hours of study. (Although that study indicates that "smarter" people study fewer hours, more recent evidence suggests that in most cases, brighter students study more.)

Partial correlations may be written as $r_{12.3}$. This indicates that you are measuring the correlation between variables 1 and 2 with the effect of variable 3 removed from *both* the variables being correlated. Let's see the example of college grades (variable 1) with hours of study (variable 2) and intelligence (variable 3). If we used partial correlation to study this relationship, the correlation between intelligence and grades (r_{13}) is removed and the correlation between intelligence and hours of study (r_{23}) is also removed. The confounding influence of intelligence is thus removed statistically, and the relationship between the two variables, grades and hours of study, can be accurately measured. Partial correlation may also be written as $r_{y1.2}$, which would indicate the correlation of an independent variable 1, with a dependent variable, y, with the effect of variable 2 removed from both the independent and the dependent variable.

SEMI-PARTIAL CORRELATION

This is the correlation of two variables with the effect of a third variable removed from only *one* of the two variables being correlated. It is closely tied to multiple correlation, as we shall show in the next section. Semi-partial correlation may be written as $r_{1(2.3)}$ or $r_{y(1.2)}$. The first way would indicate the correlation between variables 1 and 2 with the effect of variable 3 removed from 2 alone; the second way would indicate the correlation between the dependent variable, y, and an independent variable, 1, with the effect of variable 2 removed from 1 alone. We will use the diagram below to explain further.

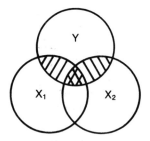

The circles represent the amount of variance of each of the variables. Remember that the variance shared by two variables is measured by r^2. If we take variable X_1 into account first, the variance accounted for in Y equals the variance contributed by X_1 (r_{y1}^2), plus the unique variance accounted for X_2. That unique variance is the variance shared between Y and X_2 after the effect of X_1 on X_2 has been removed (or after the cross-hatched area has been subtracted). The squared semi-partial correlation between X_2 and Y is the unique variance contributed by X_2 ($r_{y(2.1)}^2$). So, in this case, R^2 (the squared multiple correlation, which will be explained more fully in the following section) = the r^2 between X_1 and Y, plus the semi-partial correlation squared between X_2 and Y, or $R^2 = r_{y1}^2 + r_{y(2.1)}^2$.

MULTIPLE CORRELATION

Thus far, we have been discussing correlation as measuring the relationship between two variables. It is possible to extend the concept to one in which the relationship is measured between one variable and a combination of other variables. When discussing r, we were talking about one independent variable (X) and one dependent variable (Y). In multiple correlation (R), we are talking about more than one independent variable (X_1, X_2, X_3, and so on) and one dependent variable (Y). It is also possible to have more than one dependent variable (Y_1, Y_2, Y_3, and so on); this is called *Canonical Correlation* and will be discussed in Chapter 14.

The multiple correlation, R, can go from +0.00 to 1.00. There are no negative Rs, because the method of least squares is used to calculate R, and squaring numbers eliminates negatives. R^2 is the amount of variance accounted for in the dependent variable by the combination of independent variables. In reporting multiple correlations, it is R^2, rather than R, that is often presented.

As we demonstrated in the discussion of semi-partial correlation, the calculation of the squared multiple correlation, R^2, may require more than simply adding up the squared correlation of each independent variable with the dependent variable. Let us see why this is so. If there were no correlation between the independent variables, the correlations might be as follows:

	X_1	X_2	Y
X_1	1.00	0.00	0.40
X_2	0.00	1.00	0.30

and could be depicted as

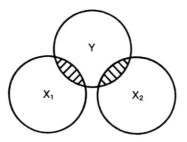

In that case, there is no overlap between variables X_1 and X_2. They are not correlated; thus, each accounts for a different portion of the variance in Y. We could add up their squared correlation (r^2s) with Y ($(0.40)^2 + (0.30)^2$) and determine that $R^2 = 0.25$, or $R^2 = r^2_{x_1y} + r^2_{x_2y}$.

Usually, however, in behavioral research, the independent variables are correlated among themselves as depicted below.

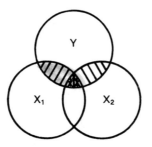

In that case, there is correlation between X_1 and X_2, and if you added up the squared correlation of X_1 with Y ($r^2_{x_1y}$) and the squared correlation of X_2 with Y ($r^2_{x_2y}$), you would add in the cross-hatched area twice. The variance accounted for in Y is actually all that explained by one of the variables plus the *additional* variance explained by the second variable. The additional variance is measured by the squared semi-partial correlation of the second variable with the dependent variable. If X_1 is counted first, it accounts for all of its shared variance with Y, and X_2 adds the variance that it alone contributes (its shared variance with Y minus the cross-hatched area). The first variable gets "credit" for the first piece of variance accounted for, even though it shares some of that with X_2. The order of entry of variables into a multiple correlation may be important when we try to understand the relationships being studied. This will be discussed in more detail in Chapter 6. Multiple correlation, then, is a technique for measuring the relationship between a dependent variable and a weighted combination of independent variables.

The following example comes from the Munro (1985) study of the predictors of success in graduate nursing education.

	Essay Score	GREV	Master's GPA
Essay	1.000	0.246	0.278
GRE-Verbal	0.246	1.000	0.216

The pre-admission essay has a correlation of 0.278 with the final Master's grade point average, that is, it accounts for almost 8% of the variance in GPA ($(0.278)^2 = 0.077$). The essay is also correlated with the GRE-Verbal score ($r = 0.246$). The GRE-Verbal accounts for about 5% of the variance in GPA ($(0.216)^2 = 0.047$), but part of the variance is shared with essay. When the multiple correlation is calculated, it shows that the essay accounts for 7.7% of the variance, and GRE-verbal adds another 2.3% of unique variance. $R^2 = 0.10$ or 10%, which is more than either of the variables could have accounted for alone. Because the essay was counted first, GRE-verbal was only credited with its squared semi-partial correlation with Master's GPA, rather than with its squared correlation with GPA $(0.216)^2$. The contribution of the essay to the explained variance was significant, but the 2.3% added by the GRE-verbal was not a significant addition ($p = 0.069$).

We will not give you computational formulas for multiple correlation, because they require a knowledge of matrix algebra or the ability to solve simultaneous equations. We assume that you would use the computer for the analysis of multiple correlations. Examples of computer printouts containing multiple correlations will be given in Chapter 6.

SUMMARY

Correlation is a procedure for quantifying the relationship between two or more variables. It measures the strength and indicates the direction of the relationship. Multiple correlation measures the relationship between one variable and a weighted composite of the other variables. Partial correlation is a statistical method for describing the relationship between two variables, with the effect of another confounding variable removed. In semi-partial correlation, the influence of a third variable is removed from only one of the variables being correlated.

EXERCISES FOR CHAPTER 5

1. What should the action be regarding the *null hypothesis* (accept/reject) for each of the following:

	$p < 0.05$	$p < 0.01$
a. $r = 0.190$, $n = 102$	_____	_____
b. $r = 0.240$, $n = 47$	_____	_____
c. $r = 0.410$, $n = 30$	_____	_____
d. $r = 0.605$, $n = 20$	_____	_____
e. $r = -0.605$, $n = 20$	_____	_____

2. If you hypothesized that there would be a *positive* relationship between two variables, what would your action be regarding *that* hypothesis? Use the *rs* and *ns* hypothesis? Use the *rs* and *ns* from Exercise 1.

	$p < 0.05$	$p < 0.01$
a.	_____	_____
b.	_____	_____
c.	_____	_____
d.	_____	_____
e.	_____	_____

3. Which indicates a stronger relationship, $r = 0.90$, or $r = -0.90$?

4. You plot two variables to determine their relationship. The variables have a curvilinear relationship. What is the appropriate technique to use to measure their relationship?

5. You want to determine the relationship between postoperative complications and the following factors: age, psychological well-being, and preoperative stress levels. What would be the appropriate technique to use?

6. You want to measure the relationship between the pain reported by the patient and number of visitors, but you think that age might be related to both of these factors. What statistical technique should you use?

7. You want to study the relationship between infant's apgar score and nutritional status of the mother with the effect of mother's age removed from her nutritional score. The appropriate technique to use is _____ .

8. Given the following numbers, calculate *r*. Given a two-tailed test and a significance level of 0.05, is it significant?

X	Y
2	1
3	4
4	3
5	2
6	7
6	7
8	5
8	6
9	8
9	8

9. Calculate 95% and 99% confidence intervals when $r = 0.70$ and $n = 200$.

CHAPTER 6
Regression

Barbara Hazard Munro

OBJECTIVES FOR CHAPTER 6

After reading this chapter and completing the exercises, you should be able to

1. Understand the statistics generated by the regression procedure.
2. Calculate a simple linear regression.
3. Set up and solve a prediction equation.
4. Construct confidence intervals around a predicted score.
5. Explain the difference between testing the significance of R^2 and the significance of a b-weight.
6. Code categorical variables.
7. Apply the Scheffé formula for comparisons among means.
8. Discuss methods for selecting variables for entry into a regression equation.
9. Discuss the strengths and weaknesses of multiple regression.
10. Critically analyze a research report that uses multiple regression.

We are constantly interested in predicting one thing from another. We want to predict the weather to plan our weekend. We want to predict how well a student will do in nursing practice. We want to predict how long a patient may remain ill. Countless predictions are necessary for us simply to move through life.

A brilliant statistical invention is regression, which permits us to make predictions from some known evidence to some unknown future events. Only about a century old, regression is the basis of many statistical methods, and, in this book, there is nothing more important to understand.

Regression is a technique that makes use of the correlation between variables and the notion of a straight line to develop a prediction equation. Once a relationship has been established between two variables, it is possible to develop an equation that will allow you to predict the score of one of the variables, given the score of the other. In the case of a multiple correlation, regression is used to establish a prediction equation (the independent variables are each assigned a weight based on their relationship to the dependent variable). Regression may be used in relation-searching and association-testing studies.

Many studies have used regression to predict how well students would do in school, based on various predictors. Scholastic Aptitude Test scores (SATs) have been found to be predictive of academic success in college and Graduate Record Examinations (GREs) have been found useful in predicting success in graduate school. One such study has shown that GRE-verbal examinations, undergraduate grade point average, and an essay rated by the Admissions Committee are predictive of success in Yale's graduate program in nursing (Munro, 1985).

Mahon (1982), in her study on the relationship of loneliness to self-disclosure, interpersonal dependency, and life changes, used regression to test the hypothesis: "Lower scores on self-disclosure together with higher scores on interpersonal dependency and higher scores on life changes will be a better predictor of a higher level of loneliness than any single variable alone" (p. 344). Her results indicated that self-disclosure was the best predictor of loneliness and that adding interpersonal dependency to the equation significantly increased the variance explained in loneliness. Life changes did not add significantly to the prediction of loneliness. Seventeen percent of the variance in loneliness was explained by those three variables.

Regression is a very useful technique that allows us to *predict* outcomes and to *explain* the interrelationships among variables. The *type of data required* and the underlying *assumptions* are the same for regression as for correlation (see Chapter 5).

SIMPLE LINEAR REGRESSION = 2 variables correlated

We will begin by explaining *simple* regression. A correlation between two variables will be used to develop a prediction equation. The techniques described in this chapter are for predictions based on a *linear* relationship between variables. If the relationship is curvilinear, other techniques, such as trend analysis, must be used. For a discussion of trend analysis, see Pedhazur (1982).

If the correlation between two variables were perfect (+1.00 or −1.00), we would be able to make a perfect prediction about the score on one variable, given the score on the other variable. Of course, we never get perfect correlations, so we are never able to make perfect predictions. The higher the correlation, the more accurate the prediction. If there were no correlation between two variables, knowing the score of one would be of no help in estimating the score on the other. When you have no information to aid you in predicting a score, your best guess for any subject would be the mean, because that is the center of the data.

To be able to make predictions, the relationship between two variables, the independent (X) and the dependent (Y), must be measured. If there is a correlation, a regression equation can be developed that will allow prediction of Y, given X. If we want to be able to predict number of days in the hospital (Y') based on a pre-hospitalization stress score (X), we must first measure in a sample of patients, who are similar to those for whom we will eventually make predictions, pre-hospitalization stress scores and the number of days they spend in the hospital. If these two factors are related, we could develop an equation that would allow us to measure the stress levels of patients on admission and from that information, we could estimate how long they will be in the hospital. The accuracy of that prediction is based on the strength of the correlation between the two variables. In this example, it is obvious that we would need more information than just stress level to make a very accurate prediction. The use of multiple regression would allow us to use other factors, such as diagnosis and age, in addition to stress, to predict hospital stay.

Understanding Regression Through the Use of Standard Scores

In previous chapters, standard scores (z-scores) were used to explain the concepts of standard deviation and correlation. Remember that once scores have been converted to z-scores, they have a mean of 0 and a standard deviation of 1 (Fig. 6-1). Direct comparisons between sets of z-scores can be made, because they are measured on the same scale. Given z-scores, the formula for a prediction (regression) equation is quite simple. It is $Y' = rX$, where Y' is the predicted score and X is the "known" or predictor variable. Given a perfect positive correlation, Y' would equal X. For example, someone with a z-score of $+2$ on X would also score $+2$ on Y.

$$Y' = (1)(2).$$

In Chapter 5, it was shown that with a perfect positive correlation ($r = +1$), everyone received exactly the same z-score on Y as on X. It was shown that with a perfect

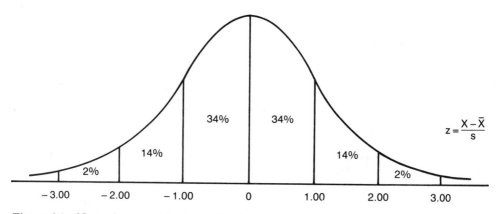

Figure 6-1 Normal curve with standardized scores.

negative correlation ($r = -1$), each subject received exactly the opposite z-score on Y as on X. For example, someone with a -3 on X would get a $+3$ on Y'.

$$Y' = (-1)(-3) = +3.$$

As previously mentioned, if there is *no* correlation between the variables, *no* prediction can be made, and our "best guess" for Y' is the mean. Using the formula for Y', with $r = 0$ and $X = +3$, we calculate Y' as $(0)(3) = 0$. Zero is, of course, the mean of a z-score distribution. These extreme cases, perfect correlations and zero correlations, are, however, most uncommon in the world of research! Therefore, consider what happens with more reasonable correlations. Suppose an individual, Jill, scored $+2$ on X. Given the following rs, what Y score would you predict for Jill? Work these equations, before reading on.

$r = -0.20$ $Y' = rX = (-.20)(2) = -.40$

$r = 0.60$ $= (.60)(2) = 1.20$

$r = 0.20$ $= (.20)(2) = .40$

$r = -0.60$ $= (-.60)(2) = -1.20$

For $r = -0.20$, our equation wold be $Y' = (-.20)(2)$ or $-.40$. The other answers are, respectively, 1.20, .40, and -1.20. If you predicted each Y score correctly, you have mastered this simplest type of prediction, where you have only the standard scores and the correlation coefficient.

"Regression" means literally a falling back toward the mean. With perfect correlations, there is no "falling back"; the predicted score is the same as the predictor. With less than perfect correlations, there is some error in the measurement, and we would "expect" that in the case of an individual who received an extremely high score, "chance" may have been working in her favor, and, therefore, on a second measure, her score would be somewhat less, that is, it would have fallen back toward the mean. In the same way, an individual with an extremely low score perhaps had all the fates against her and, on a second measure, would do better, thus moving her score closer to the mean.

Each prediction "regresses" back toward the mean, depending on the strength of the correlation. As the correlation rises toward 1.00, Y' moves proportionately outward from the mean, toward the position of the X predictor. The correlation coefficient indeed tells us exactly what percentage of this distance Y' moves.

Figure 6-2 shows predictions based on an r of .50. Note on the figure that all the predicted scores (Y's) are halfway between the mean and the X-score. This is because the correlation is .5. (If the correlation had been 0.7, the Y'-scores would have moved .7 the distance between the mean and X.) If the X-score is above the mean, the predicted score will be lower than the X-score and closer to the mean. With an r of .5 and an X-score of $+2$, Y' would equal $(.5)(2) = 1.0$. With a correlation of .5, an individual who was 2 standard deviations above the mean would be predicted to be 1 standard deviation above the mean on Y.

If the X-score is below the mean, the predicted score is higher and closer to the mean. An X-score of -3 would result in a predicted score of $(.5)(-3) = -1.5$.

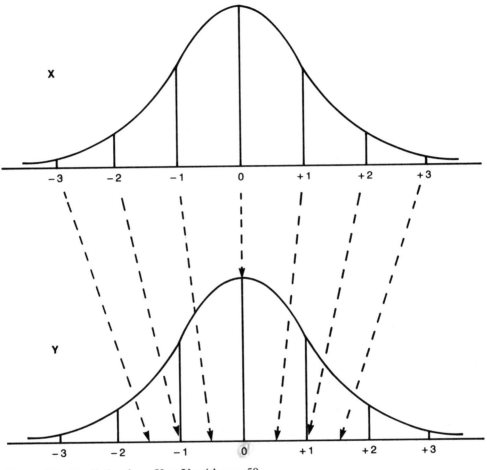

Figure 6-2   Predicting from X to Y, with $r = .50$.

Remember that these are predictions based on a correlation of .5, so you would not be able to predict perfectly an individual's score. The person's actual score will differ from the predicted score. This discrepancy between predicted and actual scores reflects the error in the prediction and will be discussed more fully in the next section of this chapter. Because most measures will not be in z-scores, the more general regression equation will now be presented.

Prediction Equation

The regression equation is the equation for a straight line and is written as

$$Y' = a + bX.$$

Y' is the predicted score.

Given data on X and Y from a sample of subjects called the *regression sample,* a and b can be calculated. With those two measures, Y can be predicted, given X. The letter a is called the *intercept constant* and is the value of Y when $X = 0$. It is the point at which the regression line intercepts the Y axis. The letter b is called the *regression coefficient* and is the rate of change in Y with a unit change in X. It is a measure of the slope of the regression line.

An example is given in Figure 6-3. The intercept constant, a, is equal to 3; you can see that is the value of Y when $X = 0$. It is the point where the regression line connects with the Y axis. The regression coefficient, b, is equal to 0.5. This means that the value of Y goes up 0.5 of a point for every 1 point change in X. When $X = 0$, $Y = 3$, and when X goes up to 1, Y goes up to 3.5. As you will see when we are calculating a and b, a is based on the means of the two variables, and b is based on the correlation between them.

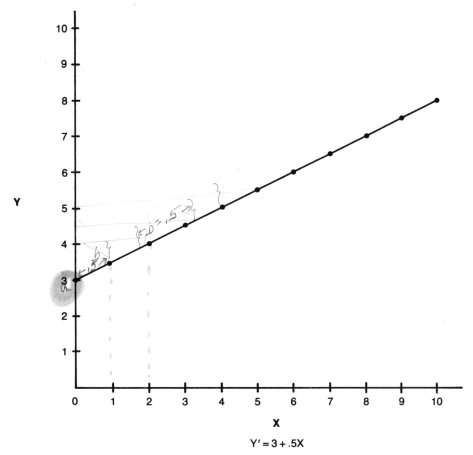

$$Y' = 3 + .5X$$

Figure 6-3 The regression line.

The regression line is the "line of best fit" and is formed by a technique called the *method of least squares.* When the concept of least squares was presented, characteristics of the mean were discussed. Because the mean is (in one sense) the center of the data, the sum of the deviations of the scores around the mean, $\Sigma(X - \overline{X})$, adds up to 0. Also, if you square those deviations and add them, that number will be smaller than the sum of the squared deviations around any other measure of central tendency. In the same way, the regression line pases through the exact center of the data in the scatter diagram. Therefore, it is the "line of best fit." There are deviations around the regression line, just as there are deviations around the mean. The regression line represents the predicted scores (Y's), but since a prediction is not perfect, the actual scores (Ys) would deviate somewhat from the predicted scores. Because the regression line passes through the center of the pairs of scores, if you add up the deviations from the regression line ($Y - Y'$), they will equal 0. Also, if you square those deviations and add them, the sum of the squared deviations around the regression line is smaller than the sum of the squared deviations around any other line drawn through the scatter diagram.

If you predicted days of hospitalization (Y') based on stress scores and then, after the patients left the hospital, recorded their actual days of hospital stay (Y), you would find differences between Y and Y'. $Y - Y'$ would equal the deviations from the predicted scores just as $X - \overline{X}$ equals the deviations around the mean. The regression equation minimizes the squared differences ($(Y - Y')^2$) of the predicted score from the actual score.

Given a regression equation of $Y' = 4 + 0.2X$ and three individuals with scores of 5, 10, and 20, respectively, on X, the predicted scores for the three would be calculated as follows:

	a	$+$	bX	$=$	Y'
1.	4	$+$	(.2) (5)	$=$	5
2.	4	$+$	(.2)(10)	$=$	6
3.	4	$+$	(.2)(20)	$=$	8

Confidence Intervals

Because there is error in predictions, we need to know how "good" a prediction is. The standard error of estimate can be used to construct confidence intervals around predicted scores. The standard error of estimate is the standard deviation of the errors of prediction. We use that in the same way that we use the standard errors of the mean and the correlation coefficient to construct confidence intervals. Given a predicted score, we can then say with some degree of confidence (probably 95% or 99%) that the actual score would fall between two points. The calculation of these intervals will be presented after the calculation of a regression equation is presented.

MULTIPLE REGRESSION

Multiple regression is possible when there is a measurable multiple correlation between a group of predictor variables and one dependent variable. The prediction equation is

$$Y' = a + b_1X_1 + b_2X_2 + b_3X_3 + \ldots b_kX_k.$$

There is still one intercept constant, a, but each independent variable (e.g., X_1, X_2, X_3) has a separate b-weight. Given a prediction of

$$Y' = 2 + .5X_1 + .2X_2 + .4X_3$$

and three individuals with the following scores:

	X_1	X_2	X_3
1.	8	4	7
2.	12	3	5
3.	10	6	9

their predicted scores would be calculated as:

1. $2 + (.5)\ (8) + (.2)(4) + (.4)(7) = \ 9.6$
2. $2 + (.5)(12) + (.2)(3) + (.4)(5) = 10.6$
3. $2 + (.5)(10) + (.2)(6) + (.4)(9) = 11.8$

If adding extra variables increases the amount of variance accounted for in the dependent variable, that will also increase the accuracy of our prediction. Multiple regression simply extends the multiple correlation into the computation of the regression equation.

SIGNIFICANCE TESTING

When doing a simple linear regression, the correlation between the two variables is tested for significance, and r^2 represents "meaningfulness." With multiple correlation, we are interested not only in the significance of the overall R and thus the amount of variance accounted for (R^2) but also in the significance of each of the independent variables. Just because R^2 is significant does not mean that all the independent variables are contributing significantly to the variance accounted for. In multiple regression, the multiple correlation is tested for significance and each of the b-weights is also tested for significance. Testing the b-weight tells us whether or not the independent variable associated with it is contributing significantly to the variance accounted for in the dependent variable.

The F-distribution is used for testing the significance of the R^2s, and either the F- or t-distribution is used to test the significance of the bs. See Appendix E for the

F-distribution. When using the computer packaged programs, the Fs or ts and associated probabilities are printed out for you. The F-distribution will be used for demonstration here.

The calculation of F will be presented later in this chapter. When testing for the significance of R^2s, the degrees of freedom (df) are calculated as $k/(n - k - 1)$, that is, there are two df a numerator, k, and a denominator, $n - k - 1$. The k stands for the number of independent variables, and n stands for the number of subjects. When testing the significance of a b-weight, the df are $1/(n - k - 1)$.

We will start with examples of testing the Fs associated with R^2s for significance. If we had two independent variables and a sample size of 63, the df would be $2/(63 - 2 - 1)$, or 2/60. In Appendix E, the df for the numerator are listed across the top of the page. The numerator is also known as the greater mean square. The df for the denominator are listed down the left side of the page. The denominator is also called the *lesser mean square*. In our example, there are 2 df in the numerator and 60 df in the denominator. The tabled values for 2/60 df, which must be equaled or exceeded, are: 3.15 at the 0.05 level, and 4.98 at the 0.01 level. Note that the 0.05 level is in light print, and the 0.01 level is in dark print. An F of 4.50 would be significant at the 0.05 level but not at the 0.01 level. Two additional examples follow:

F	k	n	df	p
4.05	3	129	3/125	<0.01
2.00	6	207	6/200	ns

To test the b-weights, the procedure is the same except that the numerator of the df is always 1. Some examples for testing b-weights follow:

F	k	n	df	p
5.25	2	68	1/65	<.05
8.00	3	154	1/150	<.01

CALCULATIONS

Simple Linear Regression Equation

The example used here to demonstrate the calculation of the regression equation is the same example we used for the Pearson Product Moment Correlation (Table 5-5). See Table 6-1 for the calculations. To solve the formulas for the regression equation, we need the means of X and Y and the elements that were used to solve the formula for correlation (n, ΣX, ΣY, ΣX^2, ΣY^2, ΣXY). These elements are listed on the lower left side of the table.

Three formulas for deviation sums of squares are listed. The sums of squares for X (Σx^2) and the sums of the cross-products (Σxy) are used in the calculation of the b-weight. The sums of squares for Y (Σy^2) is called the *total sums of squares* and

Table 6-1   Calculation of the Simple Linear Regression Equation

Subjects	X	Y	X^2	Y^2	XY
1	2	1	4	1	2
2	5	6	25	36	30
3	7	9	49	81	63
4	3	2	9	4	6
5	10	8	100	64	80
6	1	3	1	9	3
7	9	10	81	100	90
8	4	3	16	9	12
9	8	9	64	81	72
10	6	7	36	49	42
Σs	55	58	385	434	400

$\overline{X} = 5.5$
$\overline{Y} = 5.8$
$n = 10$
$\Sigma X = 55$
$\Sigma Y = 58$
$\Sigma X^2 = 385$
$\Sigma Y^2 = 434$
$\Sigma XY = 400$

$$\Sigma xy = \Sigma XY - \frac{(\Sigma X)(\Sigma Y)}{n} = 400 - \frac{(55)(58)}{10} = 81$$

$$\Sigma x^2 = \Sigma X^2 - \frac{(\Sigma X)^2}{n} = 385 - \frac{(55)^2}{10} = 82.5$$

$$\Sigma y^2 = \Sigma Y^2 - \frac{(\Sigma Y)^2}{n} = 434 - \frac{(58)^2}{10} = 97.6$$

$$b = \frac{\Sigma xy}{\Sigma x^2} = \frac{81}{82.5} = 0.982$$

$$a = \overline{Y} - b\overline{X} = 5.8 - (0.982)(5.5) = 0.399$$

$$Y' = a + bX$$

$$Y' = 0.399 + 0.982X$$

is a measure of the total variation in the dependent variable. These formulas are all part of the correlation formula. The deviation sums of cross-products is calculated as

$$\Sigma xy = \Sigma XY - \frac{(\Sigma X)(\Sigma Y)}{n}.$$

Note that Σxy is the numerator of the correlation equation. The deviation sums of squares for X and Y are calculated as

$$\Sigma x^2 = \Sigma X^2 - \frac{(\Sigma X)^2}{n}$$

$$\Sigma y^2 = \Sigma Y^2 - \frac{(\Sigma Y)^2}{n}$$

These sums of squares were included in the denominator of the correlation formula.

Given $\Sigma\chi y$, $\Sigma\chi^2$, $\overline{Y}$, and $\overline{X}$, we can calculate a and b. (Note that $\Sigma\chi y$ is *not the same as* ΣXY and that $\Sigma\chi^2$ is *not the same* as ΣX^2.) The formula for b is $\Sigma\chi y / \Sigma\chi^2$, so in our example,

$$b = \frac{81}{82.5} = .982.$$

The formula for a is $\overline{Y} - b\overline{X}$, therefore,

$$a = 5.8 - (.982)(5.5) = .399.$$

The prediction equation is

$$Y' = .399 + ..982X.$$

Because there is only one independent variable in this example, the test for significance is simply the test of the significance of the correlation between X and Y, which we found was .90 (see Table 5-5). The amount of variance accounted for is $(.90)^2$, or 81%.

The calculation of a regression in which there is more than one independent variable will not be worked through, because that would require knowledge of matrix algebra or the ability to solve simultaneous equations. We would expect you to use the computer for such calculations.

We do, however, demonstrate the calculation of R^2 and the F-value that is used to test the significance of R^2 as an aid to your understanding of these statistics when you examine a computer printout. The figures from the example of simple linear regression will be used. Thus, R^2 will be the same as r^2, or 0.81.

We have used the "sum of squares" since we calculated the standard deviation. The symbol χ was used to denote the deviation of a score from the mean $(X - \overline{X})$. It was demonstrated that the sum of those squared deviations, $\Sigma\chi^2$, equaled $\Sigma X^2 - \dfrac{(\Sigma X)^2}{n}$. In regression, the concern is with explaining the variance in the dependent variable, Y. The formula for the sum of the squared deviations for the dependent variable, also called the total sum of squares, is

$$\Sigma y^2 = \Sigma Y^2 - \frac{(\Sigma y)^2}{n}.$$

In any measurement situation, there is variability due to error. In regression, then, the total sums of squares (Σy^2) is made up of the sums of squares (ss) that are due to the regression and the sums of squares that are due to error (also called *residual*). This is symbolized as

$$ss_{total} = ss_{regression} + ss_{residual}$$

The higher the correlation between the independent and dependent variables, the lower the residual, or error portion. The amount of variance accounted for is that percentage of the total variance that is explained by the regression. This is depicted as

$$R^2 = \frac{SS_{regression}}{SS_{total}}$$

To return to the numbers in the example, the total sums of squares (Σy^2) is 97.6. In order to calculate R^2, we also need the sums of squares for the regression. The formula for that is

$$SS_{regression} = \frac{(\Sigma xy)^2}{\Sigma x^2}$$

So,

$$SS_{regression} = \frac{(81)^2}{82.5} = 79.53.$$

Now

$$R^2 = \frac{79.53}{97.6} = .81.$$

To test R^2 for significance, the following formula can be used:

$$F = \frac{R^2/k}{(1 - R^2)/(n - k - 1)},$$

where k stands for the number of independent variables. In our example,

$$F = \frac{.81/1}{(1 - .81)/(10 - 1 - 1)}$$

$$F = \frac{.81}{.19/8} = \frac{.81}{.02} = 40.5$$

An F value with one and eight df is significant at less than 0.01 (see Appendix E).

When more than one independent variable is included, each is tested to determine whether or not it is contributing significantly to the variance accounted for. When the t-test is used, each b-weight is divided by its standard error, and the resulting figure is tested for significance.

Standard Error of Estimate

The formula for the standard error of estimate of the regression is

$$s_{y \cdot x} = \sqrt{\frac{SS_{residual}}{n - k - 1}}$$

The ss residual is the error in the total sums of squares. Since we have the total sums of squares, $\Sigma y^2 = 97.6$, and the sums of squares for the regression, 79.53, we can calculate the residual sums of squares as total ss − regression sums of squares or $97.6 - 79.53 = 18.07$. Substituting into the formula we have

$$\sqrt{\frac{18.07}{8}} = 1.50$$

We could also write the formula for the standard error as

$$s_{y \cdot x} = \sqrt{\frac{\Sigma y^2 - \frac{(\Sigma xy)^2}{\Sigma x^2}}{n - k - 1}}$$

where

$$\Sigma y^2 = \text{total sums of squares}$$

$$\frac{(\Sigma xy)^2}{\Sigma x^2} = \text{regression sums of squares}$$

$$\Sigma y^2 - \frac{(\Sigma xy)^2}{\Sigma x^2} = \text{residual sums of squares}$$

Confidence Intervals

With the standard error of estimate, confidence intervals can be constructed around a predicted score. The prediction equation is $Y' = .399 + .982X$. If an individual scored 100 on X, her predicted score for Y would be $.399 + (.982)(100)$, or 98.599. The formulas for the confidence intervals are:

95% $Y' \pm 1.96 \, (s_{y \cdot x})$
99% $Y' \pm 2.58 \, (s_{y \cdot x})$

In this example, $s_{y \cdot x} = 1.50$; therefore, the confidence intervals are:

95% $98.599 \pm (1.96)(1.50) = 95.659$ to 101.539
99% $98.599 \pm (2.58)(1.50) = 94.729$ to 102.469

We could say that we are 95% confident that this individual's actual Y score would fall between 95.659 and 101.539, and we are 99% confident that it would fall between 94.729 and 102.469.

CODING

Nominal level variables can be included in a regression analysis, but they must be coded to allow for proper interpretation. You might collect information on the marital status of your subjects, and, when entering the information into the computer, let us say, you decide on some arbitrary code numbers, such as, single = 1, married = 2, and divorced = 3. If you entered that variable into a regression equation, it would be treated as though the numbers really meant something, that two was twice as big as 1, and so on. Such coding is *not recommended*. Instead, coding methods have been developed to allow us to enter such variables; three of those techniques, *dummy, effect,* and *orthogonal* coding, will be presented here.

In all the coding methods, variables are coded into "vectors," and the rule is that $n - 1$ vectors are used to describe the categories. If the variable has two categories, as does sex, one vector $(2 - 1 = 1)$ is enough. With dummy coding, which will be described below, all the members of one sex would be given a 1, and all the members of the other group would be given a 0 on the vector. If there were four categories, three vectors would be required, and so on.

Dummy Coding

This system uses 1s and 0s. If sex is a variable, you could code all males as 1 and all females as 0 (or vice versa). Correlational techniques applied to such a variable would tell you whether or not the sex of the individual was related to some measure. The 1, 0, simply says either you belong to the chosen group or you do not. There is no distinction among members of a group, that is, all the 1s are considered equally male, and all the 0s, equally female.

Suppose you had three groups, experimental group 1, experimental group 2, and a control group. You would need $n - 1 \, (3 - 1)$ vectors to describe those categories (Table 6-2). To code those groups, start with the first vector, which we may label $X1$. All the subjects in the first experimental group gets a 1 on that vector, and all others get a 0. On the second vector, $X2$, all subjects in the second experimental group get a 1, and all the other subjects get a 0. The control group has received 0s on both vectors. On these two vectors, each group has a different pattern, that is, the first experimental group has 1,0; the second experimental group has 0,1; and the control group has 0,0.

This form could be extended for any number of categories. When the regression is run, the vectors $X1$ and $X2$ are entered to represent group membership. When such dummy coding is used, the intercept constant, *a,* in the prediction equation equals the mean of the dependent variable for the group that is assigned 0s throughout. In our example, that would be the control group. So, in this form of

Table 6-2   Dummy Coding

	Vectors	
Groups	*X1*	*X2*
Experimental 1	1	0
Experimental 2	0	1
Control	0	0

analysis, we are testing the means of the other groups against the mean of a control group. In addition to "a," the prediction equation would contain a b-weight for each of the vectors, that is, the prediction equation would look like

$$Y' = a + b_1X_1 + b_2X_2$$

The regression weight, b_1, represents the difference between the group assigned 1s on $X1$ and the group assigned 0s throughout. In our example, testing b_1 for significance would be testing to see whether there is a significant difference between the first experimental group and the control group on some dependent variable, Y. Testing b_2 for significance tells us whether or not there is a significant difference between the second experimental group and the control group. Although it is most clear when used with a control group, dummy coding may be used to code categorical variables, whether or not a control group exists. You can use dummy coding for race, marital status, and so on, but it is important that you understand what testing the b-weights mean. In addition to comparing a group with the control group, you may want to compare it with some other group. In our example, you might want to compare experimental group 1 with experimental group 2. In order to do that, you would need to apply a method that allows you to make multiple comparisons between means. Such comparisons will be explained later in this chapter.

Effect Coding

Effect coding looks like dummy coding except that the last group gets -1s throughout, instead of 0s (Table 6-3). Five categories of marital status are coded into four vectors. We proceed in the same way as with dummy coding, but we give the last group -1 on each vector. Vectors $X1$ through $X4$ would then be entered into the regression equation to represent marital status.

When using effect coding, the "a" in the prediction equation represents the mean of the dependent variable. It is not the mean of one particular group on the dependent variable, but the overall mean for all the subjects in the analysis. This is referred to as the *grand mean*. What you are testing with this type of coding is how each group's mean differs from the grand mean.

Table 6-3   Effect Coding

	Vectors			
Marital Status	*X1*	*X2*	*X3*	*X4*
Single	1	0	0	0
Married	0	1	0	0
Divorced	0	0	1	0
Widowed	0	0	0	1
Separated	-1	-1	-1	-1

In our example, the regression equation would be

$$Y' = a + b_1X_1 + b_2X_2 + b_3X_3 + b_4X_4.$$

If you tested b_1 for significance, you would be testing to see whether the mean score on the dependent variable for single people differed from the overall or grand mean. We could compare the means for single, married, divorced, and widowed against the grand mean, but what about the separated group? There is no b-weight to represent the fifth group. That b-weight can be calculated rather easily when you know that all the b-weights add up to zero, that is, in the example, $b_1 + b_2 + b_3 + b_4 + b_5 = 0$. Given the b-weights for the first four categories from the regression, the fifth b-weight can be obtained by subtracting the sum of the first four from zero. For example, if the following b-weights were obtained: $b_1 = 1$, $b_2 = 3$, $b_3 = -2$, $b_4 = 2$, then $1 + 3 + (-2) + 2 = 4$ and $0 - 4 = -4$. So the b-weight for the "separated" category would be -4. To compare specific pairs of means, a test for multiple comparisons between means must be applied.

Orthogonal Coding

As previously mentioned, when you hypothesize ahead of time, you are able to use more powerful statistical tests. Orthogonal coding allows you to code your hypotheses so they can be tested. To use this technique, you must have hypothesized, "a priori," that is, before the data were collected. Here, orthogonal means that the comparisons that you want to test are independent of each other; that is, knowing the answer to one does not give you the answer to the other.

To have comparisons that are independent, only $n - 1$ comparisons can be made; that is, if there were three groups (experimental 1, experimental 2, and control), there could only be two orthogonal contrasts. Let's suppose that you were trying to decrease the number of postoperative complications and you had three groups. Subjects in experimental group 1 (EG1) were given special preoperative instruction by a nurse and a booklet that they could refer to later. EG2 received instruction only, and the control group just received the usual care. You would want to know whether the special instructions reduced postoperative complications and whether providing a booklet and instruction was better than instruction alone. We could compare the mean for groups EG1 and EG2 with the mean of the control group to see whether there was a difference between experimental and control groups. We could also compare the means of EG1 and EG2 to see whether the booklet made a difference. Table 6-4 contains the vectors necessary to code such a contrast. On vector $X1$, subjects in both experimental groups receive a -1, and the control group subjects receive 2. That contrast tests the difference between the mean number of postoperative complications for all the experimental subjects and the mean for the control group subjects. Testing b_1 for significance would tell you whether that difference was statistically significant. The second contrast is given in vector $X2$. There, the first experimental group is compared with the second. Testing

Table 6-4   Orthogonal Coding

	Vectors	
Groups	X1	X2
Experimental 1	−1	1
Experimental 2	−1	−1
Control	2	0

b_2 for significance would tell you whether there was a significant difference in the mean number of postoperative complications between those who received the booklet and those who did not within the experimental group.

To ensure that hypothesized contrasts are orthogonal, there are three tests that must be applied:

First, there must be only $n - 1$ contrasts.

Second, the sum of each vector must equal zero. In the example, the sum of $X1$ is $-1 + (-1) + 2 = 0$, and the sum of $X2$ is $1 + (-1) + 0 = 0$.

Third, the sum of the cross-products must equal zero. In the example, that is, $(-1 \times 1 = -1) + (-1 \times -1 = 1) + (-2 \times 0 = 0) = 0$.

In Table 6-5, there are some other examples of possible contrasts, given three groups. Are they all orthogonal? The vectors $X1$ and $X2$ reflect an orthogonal contrast, as do the vectors $Y1$ and $Y2$. Vectors $Z1$ and $Z2$ do not reflect an orthogonal contrast; group one is compared to group two and to group three. The sum of the cross-products does not equal zero $((-1 \times 1) + (0 \times -1) + (1 \times 0) = -1)$.

In the regression equation with orthogonal coding, a is the grand mean of the dependent variable, and each b represents an hypothesized contrast.

Summary of Coding

Regardless of the method of coding used, the overall R^2 will remain the same, and so will its significance. Predictions based on the resulting prediction equations will be identical. The differences lie in the meaning attached to testing the b-weights for significance. With *dummy coding,* the b-weight represents the difference between the mean of the group represented by that b and the group assigned 0s throughout.

Table 6-5   Contrasts

	Pairs of Vectors					
Groups	X1	X2	Y1	Y2	Z1	Z2
1	2	0	−1	1	−1	1
2	−1	1	2	0	0	−1
3	−1	−1	−1	−1	1	0

In *effect coding,* the *b*s represent the difference between the mean of the group associated with that *b*-weight and the grand mean. With *orthogonal coding,* the *b*-weight measures the difference between two means specified in an hypothesized contrast.

As you will learn in studying analysis of variance, it is possible to study the interaction among variables. Interactions among variables may be coded and entered into the regression equation. Suppose you had two categorical variables to code, group membership and sex. Dummy coding will be used in this example, but any of the coding methods could be used. Figure 6-4 shows the basic design of the study. There are six mutually exclusive groups. We can now look at the effects of group membership, the effects of sex, and whether or not there is any interaction between group and sex. For example, does the booklet reduce postoperative complications for women, but not for men? The idea of interaction will be explained in Chapter 10. Here it is used simply to demonstate coding. In Table 6-6, M and F are used for male and female. The six groups formed by the design are listed. First, we will code group membership. In doing that, ignore the sex variable. We need two

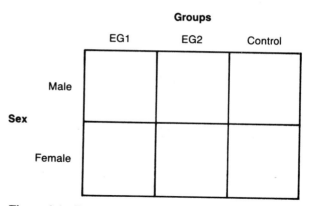

Figure 6-4   Design of study.

Table 6-6   Coding Interactions

Groups	Vectors				
	G1	*G2*	*S1*	*I1*	*I2*
EG1, M	1	0	1	1	0
EG1, F	1	0	0	0	0
EG2, M	0	1	1	0	1
EG2, F	0	1	0	0	0
Control, M	0	0	1	0	0
Control, F	0	0	0	0	0

group vectors and will call them $G1$ and $G2$. All EG1 subjects will be assigned 1 on $G1$; all other subjects will be assigned 0. All EG2 subjects will receive a 1 on $G2$; all other subjects will receive a 0. Only one vector ($S1$) is needed to code sex. Males are assigned 1s; females are assigned 0s.

In this example, there are two vectors for group and one for sex, so there must be two (2×1) vectors to code the interaction between these two variables. These vectors are labeled $I1$ nd $I2$. For $I1$, multiple $G1$ times $S1$, and, for $I2$, multiply $G2$ times $S1$.

As shown in these examples, coding is the way that categorical variables are entered into the regression equation.

MULTIPLE COMPARISONS AMONG MEANS

None of the coding methods allows us to make all the comparisons among mean scores that we might like. If we have three groups A, B, and C, and use dummy coding, we can compare the means of A and B with the mean of the control group C to see whether they are statistically different, but we cannot compare the means of A and B by testing the b-weights. With effect coding, we could compare the means of each of the three groups with the grand mean, but we could not compare A with B, A with C, and so on. With orthogonal coding, we are restricted to $n - 1$ orthogonal hypothesized contrasts.

There are contrasts that can be measured "after the fact," that is, after the overall F is found to be significant. We can then compare each group with every other group, or compare two groups with one group, and so on. Given our two experimental groups (preoperative teaching plus booklet and preoperative teaching alone) and a control group, we could compare each experimental group with the control group, the two experimental groups, the two experimental groups taken together with the control group, and so on.

Tests applied after finding that the overall F is significant, are called *post hoc* tests. Post hoc means "after the fact." There are several such tests, and they will be discussed in Chapter 9. Here we will demonstrate the use of the Scheffé method of post hoc comparison of means. The Scheffé method is quite conservative and is widely used.

First, the difference between the means must be calculated. Let us say that we had the following means on days in the hospital:

Average Hospital Stay

Experimental group 1 (EG1)—		6
Experimental group 2 (EG2)—		7
Control group	—	10

Group membership is significantly related to length of stay in the hospital, and we now want to make the following comparisons:

EG1 with EG2
EG1 with Control
EG2 with Control
EG1 and EG2 with Control

A simple comparison of means tells us that the differences are

EG1 − EG2 = 6 − 7 = −1
EG1 − Control = 6 − 10 = −4
EG2 − Control = 7 − 10 = −3
EG1 and EG2 − Control = (6 + 7)/2 − 10 = −3.5

Group 1 spends one less day in the hospital than group 2 and four fewer days than the control group, and so on. Are these differences significant? They are if the absolute value of the difference *exceeds* a certain value of Scheffé, which is defined below. "Absolute" value means that we ignore which one is larger than the other. For example, there is a difference of four days between group 1 and the control group. In the example, a minus sign occurs because we subtracted the control group mean from the experimental group mean; however, it would be +4 if we had subtracted the experimental mean from the control group mean. The subtraction was arbitrary in direction, so it played no role in the test of significance.

Because we will need to use coefficients in the Scheffé formula, we must complicate, somewhat, the simple measures of difference between groups. The formula for measuring differences that includes coefficients is

$$D = C_1\overline{Y}_1 + C_2\overline{Y}_2 + \ldots C_j\overline{Y}_j.$$

This says that the difference (D) is equal to a coefficient (C) times its associated mean $(\overline{Y})$. $C_j\overline{Y}_j$ represents the last coefficient and mean. If you had six means, $C_j\overline{Y}_j$ would become $C_6\overline{Y}_6$.

To compare two groups, use +1 and −1 for the coefficients. The rule is that the coefficients must equal zero. To compare the two experimental groups, we would have

$D = (1)(\overline{Y}EG_1) + (-1)(\overline{Y}EG_2)$
$D = (1)(6) + (-1)(7)$
$D = -1.$

To compare group 1 with the control group,

$D = (1)(\overline{Y}EG_1) + (-1)(\overline{Y}\text{Control})$
$D = (1)(6) + (-1)(10)$
$D = -4.$

To compare group 2 with the control group,

$D = (1)(\overline{Y}EG_2) + (-1)(\overline{Y}\text{Control})$
$D = (1)(7) + (-1)(10)$
$D = -3.$

To compare both experimental groups with the control group,

$D = (\frac{1}{2})(\overline{Y}EG_1) + (\frac{1}{2})(\overline{Y}EG_2) + (-1)(\overline{Y}\text{Control})$
$D = (\frac{1}{2})(6) + (\frac{1}{2})(7) + (-1)(10)$
$D = 3 + 3.5 - 10$
$D = -3.5.$

These are, of course, the same differences that were calculated in the more straightforward manner of simply subtracting one mean from another. The purpose of this demonstration was to indicate what coefficients mean in the Scheffé formula.

The Scheffé formula is

$$S = \sqrt{(k)(F \text{ table value (df} = k, n - k - 1))} \sqrt{\text{MSR}\left[\Sigma \frac{(C_j)^2}{n_j}\right]}$$

Let's start at the left side of the formula and work through it. The "k" equals the number of vectors required to code the variable. Remember that it takes $n - 1$ vectors to code a categorical variable. In this example, there are three groups, so there would be two vectors. To obtain the tabled value, you must decide on your probability level, probably .05, and then look in the F table (Apppendix E) for the tabled value at the .05 level with the df equal to $k/(n - k - 1)$. In this example, let us suppose that we had 30 subjects (10 in each group). Then, $n - k - 1$ would equal $30 - 2 - 1$, or 27. With 2,27 df and $p = .05$, the tabled value equals 3.35. Then

$$S = \sqrt{(2)(3.35)} \sqrt{\text{MSR}\left[\Sigma \frac{(C_j)^2}{n_j}\right]}$$

MSR stands for the mean square residual. That figure comes from the calculation of the regression and can be found on the computer printout, or may be calculated by hand. To demonstrate the mean square residual, we will digress and repeat an example given previously.

$$F = \frac{R^2/k}{(1 - R^2)/(n - k - 1)}$$
$$F = \frac{.81/1}{(1 - .81)/(10 - 1 - 1)} = \frac{.81}{.19/8} = \frac{.81}{.02} = 40.5$$

When you divide R^2 by k, you get the *mean square regression* (.81 in our example). Dividing the error term, $1 - R^2$ by its df, $n - k - 1$, gives the *mean square residual* (MSR). In this example, the MSR is .02. Dividing the mean square regression (.81) by MSR (.02) gives the overall F (40.5). If you were to use this example in calculating a Scheffé test, you would use the 0.02 as the MSR.

In this example, let us say that MSR turned out to be 2.0. Now let us write up the formula for Scheffé (S) that would stand for the comparison between any two of our groups.

$$S = \sqrt{(2)(3.35)} \sqrt{2.0\left[\frac{(1)^2}{10} + \frac{(-1)^2}{10}\right]}$$

In the portion of the formula in brackets, each coefficient is squared and divided by the number of subjects in that particular group (n_j). Then, all these numbers are totaled. With two groups, we use $+1$ and -1, and, because there are 10 subjects in each group, the S figure remains the same for any comparison between two groups. The Scheffé can also be used with groups of unequal size. In that case, of course, the n_js would not all be the same. To continue with the example,

$$S = \sqrt{6.7} \sqrt{2[.1 + .1]}$$
$$S = 2.59 \sqrt{2[.2]}$$
$$S = (2.59)(.63) = 1.63$$

If D exceeds S, D is significant at (in this example) the .05 level. The D between groups 1 and 2 was -1, so that difference is not significant. The differences between group 1 and the control group and group 2 and the control group were -4 and -3, respectively. Both of these differences were significant. (Remember that the minus does not matter here.)

To test the difference between both experimental groups and the control group, we would calculate Scheffé as

$$S = \sqrt{(2)(3.35)} \sqrt{2.0 \left[\frac{(\frac{1}{2})^2}{10} + \frac{(\frac{1}{2})^2}{10} + \frac{(-1)^2}{10} \right]}$$

We use the coefficients that express that difference. Now

$$S = \sqrt{6.7} \sqrt{2.0[0\ .15]}$$
$$S = (2.59)(.55) = 1.42$$

The D between the experimental groups and the control group was -3.5, so the difference was significant at the .05 level.

Measures for multiple comparisons among means allow us to explore all the interesting differences in our data once we have an overall F that is significant. In Chapter 8, you will learn that t-tests allow you to test the difference between two means and you may wonder why we do not apply that test to these multiple comparisons. The difficulty is that the t-test is set up for independent means. When multiple comparisons are made, the means are related. When using Scheffé, we do not limit ourselves to $n - 1$ orthogonal comparisons. Because of that, the t-test would tend to give false significant results, and the more of them that one calculates, the more likely it would be that error would work in such a way as to give some significant results. Those difficulties are avoided by using post hoc tests specifically designed to make multiple comparisons among means.

To illustrate, suppose that there are three means, A, B, and C. A is found to be larger than B, and B is found to be larger than C. It would not be necessary to test to find out that A is larger than C; that result is evident from the other two comparisons. Why? Because the third test is not *independent* of the other two tests.

There is still another way to look at this problem. Suppose there were seven different means to be compared. We could have six tests for the first variable, five more tests for the second variable, and so on. In fact, there could be $7(7-1)/2$ different tests, or $42/2 = 21$ possible tests. At the 0.05 level, 1 of 20 comparisons may be significant by chance alone; thus, a significant result among 21 tests would have no meaning.

SELECTING VARIABLES FOR REGRESSION

Because there is so much intercorrelation among variables used in behavioral research, we may want to "select" a subset of variables that do the "best" job of predicting a particular outcome. Usually, we want to find the smallest group of variables that will account for the greatest proportion of variance in the dependent variable. In using such information, we may make practical decisions. If two predictors are equally good, we will probably decide to use the one that is easiest to administer, most economical, and so on. Outlined here are some of the more commonly used methods for selecting variables, including *forward, backward,* and *stepwise* solutions; R^2 *improvement technique;* and *forced entry.*

Forward Solution

The independent variable that has the highest correlation with the dependent variable is entered first. The second variable entered is the one that will increase the R^2 the most over and above what the first variable contributed. Let's say that we have four independent variables and that we calculated the correlations between each independent variable and the dependent variable and found the highest correlation to be .50. That independent variable enters the equation and accounts for $(.50)^2$, or 25% of the variance. Now we want to know which of the three remaining variables will add the most to the 25% that is already explained. We cannot simply select the one with the next highest correlation with the dependent variable, because there is intercorrelation among the independent variables. So, we, or more likely the computer, calculate either partial or semi-partial correlations between each of the three remaining independent variables and the dependent variable. Thus, the effect of the first variable is removed from the correlation. Then the variable that has the highest semi-partial (or partial) correlation with the dependent variable enters next. Then the semi-partials between the two remaining independent variables and the dependent variable, taking out the effects of the first two variables in the equation, would be calculated. The one with the highest semi-partial correlation would be entered next. Various criteria may be set for entry into the regression equation. The .05 level of significance is often used. In that case, a variable would have to contribute a significant ($p = .05$) amount of variance in order to be included in the analysis. Once the point is reached where none of the remaining independent variables can contribute significantly to the R^2, the analysis is ended.

Backward Solution

In this method we start with the overall R^2 generated by putting all of our independent variables in the equation. Then each variable is deleted, one at a time, to see whether the R^2 drops significantly. Each variable is tested, therefore, to see what would happen if it were the last one entered into the equation. With four independent variables, the following differences would be tested:

$R^2y.1234 - R^2y.234$ tests for variable 1
$R^2y.1234 - R^2y.134$ tests for variable 2
$R^2y.1234 - R^2y.124$ tests for variable 3
$R^2y.1234 - R^2y.123$ tests for variable 4

If, for any of these variables, there is a significant drop in R^2, that variable is contributing significantly and will not be removed. If all the variables contribute significantly, the analysis would end with all four variables remaining in the equation. If one is not significant, there would be three variables left in the equation. Then, each of those three variables would be tested to see whether it would contribute significantly if entered last. The analysis continues until all variables in the equation contribute significantly if entered last.

Stepwise Solution

The stepwise solution combines the forward solution with the backward solution and, therefore, overcomes difficulties associated with the other two solutions. With the forward solution, once a variable is in the equation, it is not removed. No attempt is made to reassess the contribution of a variable once other variables have been added. The backward solution remedies that problem, but there, the order of entry is not clear, that is, which variable enters first and contributes most to the explained variance.

With the stepwise solution, variables are entered in the method outlined under forward solution and are assessed at each step using the backward method to determine whether or not their contribution is still significant, given the effect of other variables in the equation.

Maximum R^2 Improvement Technique

This technique is available in the SAS package program but not in the SPSS program. It is considered superior to the stepwise method in that in addition to what occurs with the stepwise method, at each step, every variable in the equation is compared with each variable that has not yet been entered into the equation, and, if an exchange of a variable in the equation for one of the remaining variables would increase the R^2, that exchange is made. "With this method, *all* exchanges are evaluated before any change is made. In the stepwise method, the 'worst' variable may be removed without considering what adding the 'best' variable might accomplish" (Helwig and Council, 1979, p. 392).

Forced Entry

The researcher may want to force the order of entry of variables into the equation. Suppose you wanted to know whether a particular intervention would improve pregnancy outcomes. You already have some "givens," such as age, socioeconomic status, and nutritional status, and you would like to know whether your intevention makes a difference over and above factors that you cannot change. You might then enter the "givens" first and add your intervention last. As will be shown in Chapter 14, this technique is used in developing "path" models.

EXAMPLE OF A COMPUTER PRINTOUT

Figure 6-5 contains a stepwise solution generated by the SPSS packaged program. First, ① note the correlations between the independent variables (which are predictors of success in graduate school) and the dependent variable, OVERGPA (which is the final grade point average in a 2-year graduate nursing program). AUTO (an essay written by each graduate program applicant) has the highest correlation with OVERGPA, $r = .278$. That correlation is significant ($p = .000$ means that $p < .001$), and there were 171 subjects involved in the analysis.

On the first step, ② AUTO was entered, and, as you can see, the multiple R was .27752. That is the same as the correlation between the two variables ($r = 0.278$). $R^2 = .07702$; thus, 7.7% of the variance was accounted for. The adjusted R^2 takes into account the number of variables and subjects and makes corrections. The standard error can be used for constructing confidence intervals. The R^2 "change," F "change," and significance of F "change" are useful only when there is more than one variable in the equation.

Moving to the right, ③ we see the Analysis of Variance table. The overall F is 10.93146, significant at the 0.0012 level. The F is the test of the overall R^2, that is, it tells us whether a significant amount of variance is accounted for in the dependent variable.

Go back to the left side of Figure 6-5, ④ and look at the variables in the equation. The B refers to b-weight, since only capital letters are printed. SE B is the standard error of the b-weight. Beta is the standardized regression weight, that is, it is the weight that results when all the variables have been converted to standard scores (z-scores) and the regression is calculated. Beta is easier to interpret than b, because all the variables are measured on the same scale. As you can see, with one independent variable, beta equals the correlation between the two variables (.27752). Squaring beta tells you how much of the variance is accounted for by that particular variable. When there is more than one independent variable in the equation, beta represents semi-partial correlations. Although we can determine the relative importance of the variables by examining the betas, they should be interpreted with caution, because they are not stable, that is, they are very likely to change, depending on what variables are in the equation, and they are very likely to change from sample to sample, even when the same variables are used. T (really t) is the test of the significance of the b-weight (or beta) and measures whether or not the variable associated with that b-weight is contributing significantly to the R^2. Here, $t = 3.306$, and that is significant at the .0012 level (the same probability as that for the overall F). Because there is only one variable in the equation, it is the only one contributing to the R^2, so the significance of R^2 and the individual variable is, of course, the same. We mentioned that either t- or F-tests can be used to test the significance of the b-weights. They give exactly the same results, as the ps demonstrated. $F = t^2$ ($10.93146 = (3.306)^2$). The intercept constant, a, is 0.66940.

The remaining independent variables are listed under the heading VARIABLES NOT IN THE EQUATION ⑤. They are GRE-Verbal, GRE-Math, Bachelor's GPA, a score on references, a score on an interview (TOT), and a general impression score. Partial correlations between each of these variables and OVERGPA are calculated, removing the effect of the essay score (AUTO). The highest partial correlation is between GREV (GRE-Verbal) and OVERGPA (.15871). The significance of that variable's contribution to R^2 is .0691. Because the criteria for entry into this equation had been set at $p = .10$, the GREV enters the equation at the second step. ⑥ R is now 0.31665, and R^2 is .10027. The change in R^2 from step one to step two is .02325 (2.3%). The significance of that change is .0691. The overall R^2 (10%) is significant at the .0010 level.

With two variables in the equation, ⑦ we see that the b-weight for AUTO is significant at the .0062 level, but the b-weight for GREV is not significant ($p = .0691$). This points out that even though the overall R^2 is significant, not all of the independent variables may be contributing significantly to the R^2.

Partials are again calculated between the variables not in the equation and OVERGPA ⑧, that is, the correlations between these variables are measured with the effects of AUTO and GREV removed. None of the partials reach the 0.10 level of significance, so no more variables are added to the equation.

Although GREV did not contribute significantly, we will keep it in the prediction equation to demonstrate how that is applied. The prediction equation with two independent variables is $Y' = a + b_1X_1 + b_2X_2$. From our printout, we take the a- and the b-weights from the final step ⑦. The b-weights change as variables are added, so you use those at the last step when all variables are in the equation. For simplicity, we have rounded the numbers. Our equation would be

$$Y' = 2.4 + .04X_1 + .0006X_2,$$
$$\text{or } Y' = 2.4 + .04(\text{AUTO}) + .0006(\text{GREV}).$$

Note that the b-weight for GREV is written as .62705D—03, which is scientific notation used to allow more non-zero numbers to be printed. The D—03 means that you move the decimal place three places to the left. Then, .62705D—03 is really

(*Text continues on page 114*)

Figure 6-5   Stepwise multiple regression solution generated by SPSS.

Procedure Cards

```
1                      16
NEW REGRESSION         DESCRIPTIVES = DEFAULTS,SIG,N/
                       MISSING = PAIRWISE/
                       VARIABLES = GREV GREM BACH AUTO REFTOT TOT GENIMP
                       OVERGPA/
                       CRITERIA = PIN (.1) POUT (.15)/
                       STATISTICS = DEFAULTS,CHA/
                       DEPENDENT = OVERGPA/
                       STEPWISE/
```

Output

****MULTIPLE REGRESSION****

CORRELATION,SIGNIFICANCE,N OF CASES

	GREV	GREM	BACH	AUTO	REFTOT	TOT	GENIMP	OVERGPA
①								
OVERGPA	0.216	0.170	0.192	0.278	0.075	0.020	0.048	1.000
	0.000	0.001	0.027	0.000	0.317	0.790	0.520	0.999
	364	364	133	171	179	181	181	372

****MULTIPLE REGRESSION****

EQUATION NUMBER 1.
DEPENDENT VARIABLE.. OVERGPA   OVERALL GPA
BEGINNING BLOCK NUMBER 1. METHOD: STEPWISE
VARIABLE(S) ENTERED ON STEP 1.. AUTO

②

MULTIPLE R	0.27752	R SQUARE CHANGE	0.07702
R SQUARE	0.07702	F CHANGE	10.93146
ADJUSTED R SQUARE	0.06997	SIGNIF F CHANGE	0.0012
STANDARD ERROR	0.38881		

④

-----------VARIABLES IN THE EQUATION-----------

VARIABLE	B	SE B	BETA	T	SIG T
AUTO	0.04360	0.01319	0.27752	3.306	0.0012
(CONSTANT)	0.66940	0.20314		13.141	0.0000

③

ANALYSIS OF VARIANCE

	DF	SUM OF SQUARES	MEAN SQUARE
REGRESSION	1	1.65256	1.65256
RESIDUAL	131	19.80391	0.15117

F = 10.93146   SIGNIF F = 0.0012

⑤

----------VARIABLES NOT IN THE EQUATION----------

VARIABLE	BETA IN	PARTIAL	MIN TOLER	T	SIG T
GREV	0.15733	0.15871	0.93928	1.833	0.0691
GREM	0.14040	0.14522	0.98746	1.673	0.0966
BACH	0.15102	0.15510	0.97351	1.790	0.0758
REFTOT	−0.440D-03	−0.00044	0.92578	−0.005	0.9960
TOT	−0.00731	−0.00757	0.99044	−0.086	0.9313
GENIMP	0.03353	0.03485	0.99722	0.398	0.6915

(Continued)

Figure 6-5 (*continued*)

⑥

```
DEPENDENT VARIABLE..    OVERGPA      OVERALL GPA
VARIABLE(S) ENTERED ON STEP NUMBER 2..      GREV          GRE VERBAL

MULTIPLE R                0.31665
R SQUARE                  0.10027    R SQUARE CHANGE       0.02325
ADJUSTED R SQUARE         0.08643    F CHANGE              3.35938
STANDARD ERROR            0.38536    SIGNIF F CHANGE       0.0691
```

⑦

```
- - - - - - - - - - - V A R I A B L E S   I N   T H E   E Q U A T I O N - - - - - - - - - - -

VARIABLE              B            SE B          BETA         T      SIG T

AUTO              0.03751       0.01348       0.23876     2.781    0.0062
GREV           0.62705D-03    0.3421D-03      0.15733     1.833    0.0691
(CONSTANT)        2.40320       0.24825                   9.680    0.0000


FOR BLOCK NUMBER 1 PIN = 0.100 LIMITS REACHED.
```

.00062705. If we had a student who had a score of 16 on her essay (AUTO) and 700 on her GRE-Verbal, her predicted final grade point average would be

$$Y' = 2.4 + (.04)(16) + (.0006)(700)$$
$$Y' = 3.46$$

Once you understand one printout, you can usually, fairly easily, read the printout produced by another program. The format may be different, but the essential ingredients are there.

Figure 6-6 contains an excerpt from a Maximum R^2 Improvement Solution produced by SAS. This was an analysis done in a study on job satisfaction by Munro (1983). This type of solution is very sophisticated and, therefore, quite expensive to run. Only steps 3 and 4 are included here. On Step 3 ①, we see that two variables are already entered and have been reassessed for their contributions against others in the equation, as well as against the independent variables not yet in the equation. A variable called FT14G is entered, the R^2 is .486, which is significant at .0001. The three variables now in the equation are FT14C, FT14D, and FT14G. They are all significant at .0001. Note that an F-test is used to test the significance of the b-weights in SAS.

On the fourth step ②, variable FT14L is entered, and when the reassessment occurs, ③, the variable entered at step 3, FT14G, is replaced by one of the remaining variables, FT14I. So the variable that entered at step 3 gets removed

```
ANALYSIS OF VARIANCE
                         DF                      SUM OF SQUARES    MEAN SQUARES
REGRESSION                2                          2.15143         1.07572
RESIDUAL                130                         19.30504         0.14850

    F = 7.24386                                   SIGNIF F = 0.0010
```

⑧

```
- - - - - - - - - -VARIABLES  NOT  IN  THE  EQUATION- - - - - - - - - -

VARIABLE         BETA IN       PARTIAL     MIN TOLER          T      SIG T

GREM             0.08115       0.07151     0.66461        0.814     0.4170
BACH             0.12837       0.13157     0.91190        1.507     0.1341
REFTOT          -0.00312      -0.00316     0.87533       -0.036     0.9714
TOT             -0.03961      -0.04071     0.90156       -0.463     0.6443
GENIMP           0.01422       0.01484     0.92389        0.169     0.8664
```

during step 4. If that were the last step in this regression, we could say that $R^2 = .52$ and was significant at the .0001 level. Four variables contributed significantly to that R^2. The prediction equation would be

$$Y' = .31 + .29(FT14C) + .20(FT14D) + .16(FT14I) + .24(FT14L).$$

EXAMPLE FROM PUBLISHED RESEARCH

Research Question

A study by Ballard and McNamara (1983) sought to determine what factors are most predictive of services required by cardiac and cancer patients in home care agencies. The researchers investigated factors related to both nursing care and total agency care.

Data Gathered

Data were collected in a retrospective chart review from almost 400 patients' charts in nine randomly selected home care agencies in Connecticut. Data from cancer and cardiac patients were analyzed separately.

Figure 6-6   Maximum R^2 improvement solution produced by SAS.

Procedure Cards

1
```
PROC STEPWISE;
    MODEL FT14K = DUMSEX JOBTIME SES SELF FT14A--FT14J FT14L FT65/MAXR;
    TITLE REGRESSION OF JOB SAT ON PREDICTORS;
```

REGRESSION OF JOB SAT ON PREDICTORS
MAXIMUM R-SQUARE IMPROVEMENT FOR DEPENDENT VARIABLE FT14K

THE ABOVE MODEL IS THE BEST 2 VARIABLE MODEL FOUND.

STEP 3   VARIABLE FT14C ENTERED   R SQUARE = 0.48600152   C(P) = 57.29307642

①

	DF	SUM OF SQUARES	MEAN SQUARE	F	PROB > F
REGRESSION	3	44.35188678	14.78396226	88.88	0.0001
ERROR	282	46.90685448	0.16633636		
TOTAL	285	91.25874126			

	B VALUE	STD ERROR	TYPE II SS	F	PROB > F
INTERCEPT	0.64432108				
FT14C	0.25492050	0.04553957	5.21217425	31.34	0.0001
FT14D	0.25884549	0.04045212	6.81060824	40.94	0.0001
FT14G	0.26532611	0.04842434	4.99366999	30.02	0.0001

THE ABOVE MODEL IS THE BEST 3 VARIABLE MODEL FOUND.

STEP 4   VARAIBLE FT14L ENTERED   R SQUARE = 0.51618629   C(P) = 39.60285390

②

	DF	SUM OF SQUARES	MEAN SQUARE	F	PROB > F
REGRESSION	4	47.10651092	11.77662773	74.95	0.0001
ERROR	281	44.15223034	0.15712537		
TOTAL	285	91.25874126			

	B VALUE	STD ERROR	TYPE II SS	F	PROB > F
INTERCEPT	0.31394482				
FT14C	0.22192128	0.04495693	3.82869681	24.37	0.0001
FT14D	0.24563653	0.03944250	6.09401326	38.78	0.0001
FT14G	0.20669127	0.04910370	2.78395508	17.72	0.0001
FT14L	0.19746531	0.04716098	2.75462414	17.53	0.0001

(Continued)

STEP 4   FT14G REPLACED BY FT14I   R SQUARE = 0.51976622   C(P) = 37.26758113

③

	DF	SUM OF SQUARES	MEAN SQUARE	F	PROB > F
REGRESSION	4	47.43321108	11.85830277	76.03	0.0001
ERROR	281	43.82553018	0.15596274		
TOTAL	285	91.25874126			

	B VALUE	STD ERROR	TYPE II SS	F	PROB > F
INTERCEPT	0.31475555				
FT14C	0.29030040	0.04124853	7.72501260	49.53	0.0001
FT14D	0.20023639	0.04177296	3.58357440	22.98	0.0001
FT14I	0.15669780	0.03508709	3.11065523	19.94	0.0001
FT14L	0.24497004	0.04508106	4.60530686	29.53	0.0001

- -

Tabular Presentation of Results

Table 6-7 shows the results of their study on the regression of nursing visits per day for cancer patients on a set of independent variables, which included the agency, age, sex, payment source, marital status, primary care provider, support system (a rank order of the amount of support required), discharge status, type of surgery, number of diagnoses, use of other services, and score on Health Status Scale (where a higher score indicates more problems). Stepwise regression was used. Dummy coding was used for categorical variables.

Description of Results

The overall R^2 was 19.5% and was significant at <.001. Five of the independent variables were entered into the equation. The first entered was the Health Status Score, which accounted for 8% of the variance. The use of physical therapy and the number of diagnoses were negatively correlated to nursing visits per day (negative b-weights), that is, individuals with more diagnoses and more physical therapy required fewer nursing visits. Those who required the least support (group 1) required the most visits, and there was a difference across agencies in the number of visits.

The Health Status Score was the best predictor of nursing visits and total service by agency for both cardiac and cancer patients. If other agency resources were used, such as physical therapy, the nursing visits were reduced. The negative correlation between number of diagnoses and number of nursing visit seems odd. The researchers point out that since several subdiagnoses were condensed into one main diagnosis, this may be a function of the definitions used. "It may also reflect

Table 6-7 Stepwise Multiple Regression Analysis—Cancer Patients—Selected Independent Variables with Dependent Variables (n = 212)

Dependent Variable—Nursing Visits per Day

Step	Variable Entered	Final Step				Multiple R	R^2	Cumulative		
		b wt	SE	t	Sig t			R^2 Change	SE	F Value
1	Health Status Score	.001	.002	4.699	.000	.282	.080	.080	.245	18.187*
2	Use of physical therapy	−.149	.044	−3.402	.001	.356	.127	.047	.239	15.183*
3	Number of Diagnoses	−.049	.017	−2.810	.005	.392	.154	.027	.236	12.589*
4	Support Group 1, Not Required	.160	.068	2.362	.019	.420	.176	.023	.234	11.092*
5	Agency #4	.146	.067	2.167	.031	.441	.195	.018	.232	9.971*

Constant = 0.095
*$p < 0.001$
From: Ballard, S., & McNamara, R. (1983). Quantifying nursing needs in home health care. *Nursing Research, 32*(4), 236–241.

the tendency for referrals to contain long lists of diagnoses that do not necessarily reflect the degree of illness or disability. Clearly, the number of diagnoses is not a predictor of resource utilization." (Ballard & McNamara, 1983, p. 240)

Another unexpected outcome was that individuals who needed less support had more nursing visits. "These patients, 3.3% of the total sample, may reflect the nurse's questions concerning the patient who appears to be managing independently, but who, in fact, may not be." (Ballard & McNamara, 1983, p. 240)

In summary the researchers report

> The Health Status Scale was useful in predicting utilization of resources. The scale should be refined in any future research in order to minimize redundancy in the ADL measurements. Those agencies that do not have an initial assessment tool might find such an instrument helpful in projecting resource needs. Utilization of resources for cardiac patients depended more upon the agency providing the service than it did for cancer patients. Replication of the study with other diagnostic groups might clarify this issue.

> The study demonstrates that home care is not monolithic. The differences in the agencies reflect the needs of the communities they serve and the financial and emotional commitment these communities are willing to provide, as well as the philosophy and focus of care of the agency itself. (Ballard & McNamara, 1983, p. 241)

SUMMARY

Multiple regression may be used for explanation and prediction. It is a flexible technique that allows the use of categorical, as well as continuous, variables. It is possible to increase the accuracy of the prediction by adding predictor variables to the equation. The best additional variables to add are those that are highly correlated with the dependent variable, but not highly correlated with the other independent variables. Usually four or five predictors are enough. Adding more than that adds little to the R^2 because of intercorrelation among the predictors.

Because the analysis uses error variance as well as true variance, the multiple correlation is usually inflated by such error variance. One way to check on that is to calculate the R^2 with a second sample. That technique is called *cross-validation*. There is also a formula that can predict how much the R^2 is likely to "shrink." The "shrinkage" formula is

$$R^2 = 1 - (1 - R^2)\frac{n - 1}{n - k - 1}$$

That is the formula used to calculate the "adjusted R^2" given on the SPSS printout. This is always smaller than the first R^2. As you can see, the formula is based on the number in the sample (n) and the number of independent variables (k). The more variables compared to subjects, the greater the shrinkage will be. If you put in the same number of subjects as independent variables, you will get a perfect R (1.00) no matter which variables you use. (But the *adjusted R* will be zero!) Thus, you must always consider the number of subjects and independent variables. Very high and seemingly impressive R^2s may be an artifact of too few subjects. Nunnally (1978, p. 180) suggests 30 subjects per independent variable. With only 10 subjects per variable, chance can greatly distort the results.

A weakness of multiple regression is a tendency to throw variables into the equation. There should be some rationale for each variable included. Overall, this is one of the most powerful techniques in our field, and, used wisely, it can be of great assistance in studying many problems related to human behavior and the health professions.

EXERCISES FOR CHAPTER 6

1. You want to develop a technique for predicting who is likely to develop post-operative complications. What statistical technique should you use?

2. Two prediction equations have been developed. In (A), $R = 0.60$, and in (B), $R = 0.75$. In which case can we make the more accurate prediction?

3. Given the following prediction equation, calculate a predicted score for each of the subjects.

$$Y' = 10 + 0.8X1 - 0.4X2$$

SUBJECTS	$X1$	$X2$	Y'
A	40	64	
B	34	57	
C	65	72	
D	58	84	

4. You calculate two standard errors of estimate, $A = 7.2$ and $B = 6.4$. Will you get a more accurate prediction with A or B?

5. To increase the amount of variance accounted for and to decrease the error, which of the following is probably better?
   a. Simple linear regression
   b. Multiple regression

6. Using the following data, calculate the *prediction equation* and the *standard error of estimate*.

SUBJECTS	X	Y
A	7	8
B	5	4
C	10	9
D	2	5
E	1	3
F	6	10
G	3	2
H	4	1
I	9	10
J	8	8

7. Using a standard error of estimate of 2.2 and a predicted score of 8, set up the 95% and 99% confidence intervals.

8. Rate each of the following F values as significant or not, at both the 0.05 and 0.01 levels.

F	df	$p < .05$	$p < .01$
a. 2.00	5/150		
b. 4.10	2/60		
c. 9.43	1/42		
d. 3.00	3/125		

SECTION 3
Analyzing Differences Among Groups

The next four chapters present statistical methods that are designed to analyze differences among groups. As such, these tests still measure a relationship, but it is the relationship that exists between a selected variable and group membership. The question answered by these methods is, How different are subjects in one group from subjects in another group in regard to this characteristic? These methods are important for examining differences between groups (*e.g.*, by illness, diagnosis, ethnic group, social class).

By understanding such tests of difference, we can select our data analysis methods accurately and creatively. Various techniques can be used for the same data sets, so choosing the best test for the specific question becomes an important primary step in research.

In general, such tests are most useful when there are theoretically meaningful groups to be compared on some other variable. For example, diagnostic categories of illness provide a way of placing people into groups. We are then interested in these groups—in their symptoms, response to treatment, prognosis, and so on. Sometimes we need to compare groups on particular variables. Which group of coronary patients misses the most work days? Which has the longest hospitalization? For psychiatric patients, do "manic-depressives" have a lower level of activity than "schizophrenics"?

As discussed in earlier chapters, tests of relationship are preferred when one variable is to be compared with one or more other variables. For example, is age related to level of functioning in cardiac disorders? Is fluctuation in blood glucose levels related to the degree of neuropathy? Is the amount of premenstrual symptomatology related to postpartum depression? In such cases, an important part of the analysis depends on the degree to which both (or all) factors vary. In such variables, there may be no meaningful cutoffs by which to define groups. What is important is the amount of variation in both variables and the way in which the variation is related.

The two classes of statistical techniques are formal ways of representing everyday observations. For example, we may note that one chain of stores is typically more expensive than another (difference); we may also make the observation that the larger the quantity of something we buy, the cheaper the unit price (correlation). Often the two methods in combination give us two different views of the same data. Consider the hypothetical exchange at a cocktail party:

One person says: "We all know that the farther from the East Coast a man lives, the more conservative his politics."

Another person says: "I beg to differ: People on the East Coast are more liberal; however, they think the same as those on the West Coast. Those from the heartland are the conservatives."

The first speaker stated an opinion that there was a correlation (relationship) between variable 1, distance from the East Coast, and variable 2, political conservatism. According to this formulation, the further from the East Coast a person lived, the more conservative his or her view. The second speaker expressed an opinion that viewed persons by *category*—area of country in which they lived—and cited a difference among those categories on political views. This person was describing group differences.

The appropriateness of either set of techniques for data analysis depends on the specific research question asked. Each method provides information that can be used to make predictions about life situations. Consider the following example. Suppose that we knew that there was a positive correlation between the age of a particular brand of wine and the richness of its taste. Based on this information, we would most likely choose the wine based on its age, selecting the oldest bottle available. Now, suppose that in addition to the correlation information that we have, we also know that the richest-tasting wine is that more than 5 years old, that is, the greatest variation occurs between wine 5 years old or under and that over 5 years. Now when we select, we will be more likely to work on that group distinction: We will try to get the oldest wine that has been bottled more than 5 years. The additional information from the group differences now tells us *where the significant difference occurs* in the relationship between age and richness of taste.

In the next four chapters, new tests will be described that can be added to the correlational techniques. Together the tests provide a wide repertory of tools for retrieving information from clinical data and for targeting the analysis to provide answers to our questions. The usefulness of such tests of difference will be shown through examples.

CHAPTER 7

Chi-Square

Madelon A. Visintainer

OBJECTIVES FOR CHAPTER 7

After reading this chapter and completing the exercises, you should be able to

1. Identify the uses of chi-square analysis.
2. Select appropriate data for chi-square analysis.
3. Calculate chi-square analyses for one dimension and 2×2 analysis.
4. Calculate degrees of freedom for use with one dimension and 2×2 and larger chi-square.
5. Interpret the chi-square to draw statistical conclusions.
6. Explain the assumptions that underlie the appropriate use of chi-square.

This chapter deals with a common technique for examining both relationships and differences in nominal level data, that is, categorical data. Nominal level data, as explained in Chapter 1, describe group membership, such as male, female; Catholic, Protestant, Jewish; Black, Caucasian, Oriental; smokers, nonsmokers; and diabetics, hypertensives.

Many research questions concern the way in which membership in one group is related to membership in another. For example, we can ask, How is sex related to occurrence of diabetes? What is the relationship between religious affiliation and marital status?

The research question answered by chi-square analysis deals with the relationship that exists among selected categories. More precisely, the question asks whether membership in one category affects membership in another. If there is no relationship, the categories are considered *independent* of one another. If there is a relationship, the categories are considered *contingent upon* one another.

Consider these examples of independent and contingent relationships. First, if we examine the relationship between gender and melanoma, we would find that the two categories are independent, that is, the disorder is equally distributed among

127

males and females and there is no relationship between gender and the disorder. Therefore, membership in one category (gender) does not affect membership in the other category (melanoma).

Now consider the relationship between breast cancer and gender. Here we find a strong contingency, or relationship. The occurrence of breast cancer is significantly higher in women than in men. It is important to note that the relationship in chi-square is similar to the one defined in Pearson correlation. It does *not* imply causality. In our example, the strong relationship does not show that being female causes breast cancer. Because chi-square tests the nonrelationship between categories, it is sometimes called the *test of independence*.

The question addressed by chi-square is an important one in health science and patient care research because it deals with the connection that exists among variables. Once a connection is established between a disease and some other personality, environmental, genetic, or social variable, we are able to identify risk factors, predictors, and sometimes causal factors. A number of studies have used chi-square analysis to establish a relationship among factors.

One important investigation conducted by Schmale and Iker (1964) showed that women who felt "helpless" at the time of a cervical biopsy were more likely to be diagnosed with cervical cancer than women who did not feel helpless. The study involved two nominal measures that grouped women into two classifications: (1) feelings of helplessness (either they did experience it or they did not), and (2) presence of cancer (either they had cancer or they did not). Chi-square analysis determined the significant difference in the occurrence of cancer between women who felt helpless and those who did not, that is, there was a significant relationship between feeling helpless and having cancer.

We emphasize once again that these findings do not establish that feeling helpless *causes* cancer. Although current investigation is examining whether feelings of helplessness contribute to the development of cancer, the answer must come from strategic methodology.

TYPE OF DATA REQUIRED

In these questions, the relationship between groups is examined, using two (or more) sets of nominal level data. To examine data in this way, a statistical technique called *chi-square* (symbol: X^2) is used. The X^2 is based on the relationship between the *expected* number of subjects that fall into a category and the actual, or *observed*, number of subjects. The use of frequencies (number of subjects) makes the X^2 technique different from the tests of correlation that have been described and the tests that will be discussed in the next few chapters. The other techniques are based on the *distribution of scores*, using the means and variance of the distribution within the group of subjects to describe the relationship. With nominal level data, there is no distribution of scores. There is a frequency count, that is, the number of subjects provide the data to be analyzed. There is no variation within groups to consider.

ASSUMPTIONS

There are four main assumptons. These will be outlined here, and a more detailed explanation will be given later in the chapter after the X^2 statistic has been fully explained.

1. Data must be frequency data.
2. There must be an adequate sample size.
3. Measures must be independent of each other.
4. There must be some theoretical basis for the categorization of the variables.

CALCULATION OF CHI-SQUARE

To introduce the X^2, consider the following research example:

An investigator is interested in the variables affecting smoking in a college population. After collecting a "smoking history" from the entire freshman population on campus, she categorizes the subjects into "smokers" or "nonsmokers" based on their responses on the questionnaire. The first research question she asks is, What is the relationship between the sex of the student and his or her smoking behavior? That is, Are women or men (on this campus) more likely to smoke?

Expected Frequencies

In this example, the investigator is using nominal data to identify a relationship between the students' sex and whether or not they smoke. The statistical question is, Are there more smokers in either sex than would be *expected?*

What do we mean by *expected?* Our expectation is based on the *null hypothesis,* which assumes that the categories are independent of one another, that is, there is no relationship between them. In this example, the null hypothesis assumes no difference in the rate of smoking between men and women. Assuming the null hypothesis, we can calculate the *expected frequencies (fe)* and compare them to what actually occurred in our sample, the *observed frequencies (fo).*

The smoking-on-campus study produced the data in Table 7-1. An eyeball examination of the data shows that more men are smokers than women: 115 men smoke, 100 women smoke. However, there are more men on campus than women; 59% of the students are men (311 men/527 total students), 41% are women (216 women/527 total students). Therefore, the absolute numbers cannot answer the research question.

We can look at the data in another way: 37% of the men are smokers (115/311) compared with 46% of the women (100/216). Viewing the data in this way, we find a higher percentage of smokers in the female group. However, we cannot tell whether the percentage is higher than we are likely to get by chance alone.

In order to determine whether the rate of smoking is different between women

Table 7-1   Contingency Table for Chi-Square
2 × 2

		Sex of Student		
		Males	*Females*	
Smoking Group	Smokers	115	100	215 Total Smokers
	Nonsmokers	196	116	312 Total Nonsmokers

311 Total   216 Total
Males   Females

Total Students = 527

and men, we compare the observed frequencies with the expected frequencies. If we assume the null hypothesis that there is no difference in smoking behavior between the sexes, we would *expect that the proportion of male smokers to female smokers would be the same as the overall proportion of men to women in the sample.* That is, since 59% of the students are men, we would expect that 59% of the smokers would also be men. Similarly, since 41% of the students are women, we would expect that 41% of the smokers would be women. We would have the same expectations for the nonsmokers. These percentages will give us our expected frequencies.

In the sample, the total number of smokers is 215; the total number of nonsmokers is 312. Applying the proportion of men to women on campus to the smoker and nonsmoker group, we can calculate the expected frequencies:

Expected number of male smokers = 59% of 215 total smokers, or .59 × 215 = 126.85

Expected number of male nonsmokers = 59% of 312 total nonsmokers, or .59 × 315 = 184.08

Expected number of female smokers = 41% of 215 total smokers, or .41 × 215 = 88.15

Expected number of female nonsmokers = 41% of 312 total nonsmokers, or .41 × 312 = 127.92

This discussion has presented the logic for determining the expected frequencies. There is a simple formula for calculating expected frequencies (*fe*) for any χ^2 table. For the expected frequency in each cell, multiply the total of the row containing the cell by the total of the column containing the cell, then divide by the total *N*. This formula may be represented as

$$fe = \frac{T \text{ row} \times T \text{ column}}{\text{Total number of subjects}}$$

The following schematic illustrates the calculation:

$$
\begin{array}{ccc}
A & B & T(r1) \\
C & D & T(r2) \\
T(c1) & T(c2) & \\
& & T(N)
\end{array}
$$

where

$T(r1)$ = total of row 1
$T(r2)$ = total of row 2
$T(c1)$ = total of column 1
$T(c2)$ = total of column 2
$T(N)$ = total sample

According to the formula,

$$fe \text{ for cell A} = \frac{T(r1) \times T(c1)}{T(N)}$$

$$fe \text{ for cell B} = \frac{T(r1) \times T(c2)}{T(N)}$$

and so on for each of the cells.

See Table 7-2 for an example of the calculation of expected frequencies (*fes*) using this schema.

The first cell is for male smokers ($n = 115$). To calculate the expected frequency, we multiply the total of the row that includes this cell (T row $= 215$) by the total of the column containing that cell (T column $= 311$) and divide by the total number of subjects in the sample (overall total $= 527$).

For the cell containing female smokers, the expected frequency equals the row total (215) times the column total (216) divided by the total N (527) and equals 88.12. Note that we could also have found this expected frequency by subtracting the expected frequency for male smokers (126.88) from the row total, that is, $215 - 126.88 = 88.12$.

The calculation of the other *fes* is conducted in the same way and is demonstrated in Table 7-2. The slight variations in expected frequencies between the two examples is due to rounding off the percentages in the first example. Although the calculation for each *fe* is given in the table, it is only necessary to calculate one *fe* using that formula; the others can be derived by subtraction, since the expected frequencies add up to their respective row and column totals. This will always be the case in calculating a X^2: *The sum of the expected frequencies and the sum of the observed frequencies must be equal.* The calculation of additional *fes* by subtraction is demonstrated in Table 7-3.

Although our example is a 2×2 table, many X^2 analyses will have more than 4 cells. A general formula to calculate expected frequencies for any number of cells is

$$fe(k) = \frac{T(rk) \times T(ck)}{T(N)}$$

where k equals any one of the cells. The formula can be repeated for each of the cells in the table.

Chi-Square Formula

Once the expected frequencies for all the cells have been calculated, they are compared to the observed frequencies using the X^2 analysis. The formula for the X^2 is

$$X^2 = \Sigma \frac{(fo - fe)^2}{fe}$$

Table 7-2   Demonstration of Calculation of Expected Frequencies (fe)

	Sex of Student		
Smoking Group	Males	Females	Row Totals
Smokers	115 (A)	100 (B)	215 T (r1)
Nonsmokers	196 (C)	116 (D)	312 T (r2)
Column Totals	311 (c1)	216 (c2)	Overall Total 527

$$fe \text{ (male smokers)} = \frac{215 \times 311}{527} = \frac{66865}{527} = 126.88$$

$$fe \text{ (female smokers)} = \frac{215 \times 216}{527} = \frac{46440}{527} = 88.12$$

$$fe \text{ (male nonsmokers)} = \frac{312 \times 311}{527} = \frac{97032}{527} = 184.12$$

$$fe \text{ (female nonsmokers)} = \frac{312 \times 216}{527} = \frac{67392}{527} = 127.88$$

Table 7-3   Demonstration of Calculation of Remaining Expected Frequencies After One is Known

	Sex of Students		
Smoking Group	Males	Females	Row Totals
Smokers	115 (126.88)	100 (88.12)	215
Nonsmokers	196 (184.12)	116 (127.88)	312
Column Totals	311	216	Overall Total 527

Given fe for male smokers = 126.88

Then, fe for female smokers = 215 − 126.88 = 88.12
fe for male nonsmokers = 311 − 126.88 = 184.12
fe for female nonsmokers = 312 − 184.12 = 127.88

where

$$fo = \text{observed frequency}$$
$$fe = \text{expected frequency}$$
$$\Sigma = \text{overall sum, for all cells.}$$

Following this formula, we first *subtract* each expected frequency from its respective observed frequency to obtain the difference. Next, we *square* each difference and then *divide* the result by the appropriate expected frequency (in each case the one used to find the difference). Finally, we *sum the quotients*. The result is the chi-square value. See Table 7-4 for calculations. Note that in squaring the differences, all values become positive. The sign values of the differences are irrelevant to the chi-square calculation. The important factor is the extent of deviation between the expected and observed frequencies.

The X^2 value of 4.58 is interpreted by using the table that shows the significance of chi-square values (Appendix F). The interpretation of X^2 follows the same steps that were used with other statistical tests: The calculated value is compared with the values required to reach various levels of significance (*e.g.,* the .05 level, the .01 level). First we need to determine the degrees of freedom.

Degrees of Freedom in Chi-Square

In Chapter 3, the concept of degrees of freedom (df) was defined as the extent to which values were free to vary given a specific number of subjects and a total score.

Table 7-4   Contingency Table for Chi-Square: 2 × 2 Analysis

Smoking Group	Sex of Students		
	Males	*Females*	
Smokers	115 (126.88)	100 (88.12)	215 Total Smokers
Nonsmokers	196 (184.12)	116 (127.88)	312 Total Nonsmokers
	311 Total Males	*216 Total Females*	*527 Total Students*

Calculations:

$$\Sigma \frac{(fo - fe)^2}{fe}$$

$$\frac{(115 - 126.88)^2}{126.88} + \frac{(100 - 88.12)^2}{88.12} + \frac{(196 - 184.12)^2}{184.12} + \frac{(116 - 127.88)^2}{127.88}$$

$$= \frac{(-11.88)^2}{126.88} + \frac{(11.88)^2}{88.12} + \frac{(11.88)^2}{184.12} + \frac{(-11.88)^2}{127.88}$$

$$= \frac{141.13}{126.88} + \frac{141.13}{88.12} + \frac{141.13}{184.12} + \frac{141.13}{127.88}$$

$$= 1.11 + 1.60 + 0.77 + 1.10$$

$$= 4.58$$

$$X^2 = 4.58$$

In the tests that use scores to calculate means, the *df* depend on the number of scores involved in the analysis. Because each subject usually contributes a score, the *df* are based on the sample size.

In X^2 analysis, however, frequencies rather than scores are used. No means are calculated. The values that are free to vary in X^2 are the *cell frequencies* in a X^2 table. The number of cells that are free to vary depends on the number of cells found in the table. In our example, we have a 2×2 table and, therefore, 4 cells with frequencies. We can use the schematic representation shown in Table 7-5. The fixed values are the total *N* and the totals for each row and each column. In other words, the "marginal values." In reference to our example, this means that the number of men $(A + C)$, women $(B + D)$, smokers $(A + B)$, and nonsmokers $(C + D)$ is determined. We are interested in the way in which these totals are related to each other; that is, we are interested in the *cell frequencies* and the way in which they vary. How many cell frequencies would we need to know in order to derive the others? The answer to that question will be equal to the *df*. We have already demonstrated that given one expected frequency, we can determine the other frequencies by simple subtraction. Similarly, we can see from our example that given the row and column totals, if we knew *one* of the cell frequencies, we could calculate the others. For example, if we knew that there were 116 female non-smokers, the number of female smokers would equal all the females (216) minus the nonsmokers, or $216 - 116 = 100$. The male smokers would equal the total number of smokers (215) minus the female smokers (100), or $215 - 100 = 115$. In this way, we could determine the rest of the cell frequencies. By knowing one cell value (regardless of the cell) in a 2×2 table, we know all the other cell values. Therefore, only *one* cell is free to vary; the others are dependent on that value. The *df* for a 2×2 chi-square analysis is always 1, *regardless of the sample size*.

There is an easy formula for calculating the *df* for X^2 analysis. It is

$$df = (r - 1)(c - 1)$$

where *r* = number of rows, and *c* = number of columns. In the example, there are 2 rows and 2 columns, a 2×2 table. Using the formula, the degrees of freedom are calculated as

$$df = (2 - 1)(2 - 1)$$
$$df = 1$$

Now look up the significance of $X^2 = 4.58$ in Appendix F using the appropriate *df*.

INTERPRETING THE CHI-SQUARE

As shown in Appendix F, with one *df*, a X^2 value of 3.841 is significant at the .05 level; a value of 6.635 is significant at the .01 level. The value of 4.56 is greater than the 3.841 needed to reach significance at the .05 level but less than the 6.635 needed to reach significance at the .01 level. Using the convention of rejecting the null

**Table 7-5   Schematic for Degrees of Freedom
in 2 × 2 Contingency Tables**

| Smoking Group | Sex of Student | | Row Totals |
	Males	Females	
Smokers	A (115)	B (100)	A + B (215)
Nonsmokers	C (190)	D (116)	C + D (312)
Column Totals	A + C (311)	B + D (216)	Total N = A + B + C + D (527)

hypothesis if the .05 level of significance is reached, we do reject the null hypothesis that there is no relationship between gender and smoking.

The results showed that there was a significant relationship between the gender of the college students and their smoking ($X^2 = 4.56$, $df = 1$, $p < .05$). We can describe the relationship in several ways: The smoking rate is higher in women than in men in this sample. The proportion of women who smoke is significantly greater than the proportion of men who smoke. We can also describe the results in terms of a difference. Women and men differed in their rate of smoking: A greater proportion of women are smokers. The various expressions are all based on the significant difference obtained in the X^2 analysis.

A FURTHER LOOK AT THE ASSUMPTIONS
FOR THE USE OF CHI-SQUARE

All X^2 analyses essentially follow the calculations and interpretation described above. There are some additional concepts and techniques that make the test more versatile and ensure its appropriate use. Most of the assumptions upon which the X^2 is based have already been implied. To the extent that the assumptions are met, the test can provide valid analysis of the data. Four main conditions are important for appropriate X^2 analysis.

The *first* condition requires that the data analyzed must be frequency data. The test cannot validly measure the difference between scores or their means. If the data are not at the nominal level, they must first be categorized in order to be used with X^2. For example, suppose from a study of what factors influenced subjects' selection of a nurse practitioner versus a physician as primary caregiver, we have the subjects' ages in years. This is ratio level data and cannot be used in X^2. However, if we choose to use X^2 to determine whether persons of different age groups made different choices of caregivers, we would first be required to convert the measure of age in years to categories of age; that is, we would place the subjects into age groups based on their age in years, such as, 21 to 40, 41 to 60, and 61 to 80. The age is now a category measure, and we have the frequency of subjects per category. We can now use the X^2 analysis. The advantages and disadvantages of converting the data will depend on the particular purpose of the analysis and the research question we are addressing. This point is considered in more detail later in this chapter.

Second, there must be an adequate sample size for analysis. This assumption is much less definite than the first. The size of the sample determines how closely the result will approximate the distribution of X^2; that is, the sample size influences the validity of the results. As is true in all statistical tests, the larger the sample, the more valid the results of the test. In X^2, the desired sample size depends on the *df* (based on the number of cells in the table). A generally agreed upon rule of thumb for sample size is that when the *df* are *greater* than 1, all expected frequencies in any cell should be at least 5; when there is only 1 *df,* the expected frequencies should be at least *10.* Note that the requirement is for *expected frequencies* and not the observed frequencies.

This rule of thumb is a relatively conservative restriction on the use of the X^2. It is useful to know that the greatest discrepancy in the distribution of X^2 occurs in cases with small *df.* Therefore, in tables with large number of cells (more than 4) the X^2 can validly be used, even if some expected frequencies are less than 5. This is true as long as no more than 20% of the expected frequencies are that small (Hays, 1973; Spence, Cotton, Underwood & Duncan, 1976). In general, in X^2, the fewer the cells, the relatively larger the sample size required.

The *third* condition requires that the measures be independent of one another. This means two things: (1) no subject can be *counted* more than once, and (2) no subject can *influence* any other subject. Let's consider the first problem, which is the easier of the two to solve. Of course, each subject is measured on each of the variables, but no subject can appear in more than one cell. This assumption is critical to the validity of the analysis, and any violation renders the test useless.

Consider the following example. Suppose a clinical specialist in psychiatric nursing was studying treatment programs for substance-abuse patients. She conducted a survey in a Drug and Alcohol Treatment Center to determine whether drug-dependent patients differed from alcohol-dependent patients in their interest in attending a group. Her sample included all the patients registered in the outpatient department: 40 drug patients and 32 alcohol patients. Each day patients coming into the center filled out a brief questionnaire in which they stated that they would or would not be interested in attending a group. They also stated whether they were drug or alcohol dependent. The planned analysis was a 2 × 2 chi-square to determine whether there was a difference in the preference for a therapeutic group between the two types of patients.

Preference for Group	Type of Patient	
	Drug	*Alcohol*
Yes	55	23
No	32	35
Column Totals	87	58

Although the table might appear appropriate for X^2 analysis, there is a violation of the assumption of independence of the measures. In the drug group, there are 87 responses, but only 40 drug patients attend the clinic! Clearly, some patients had completed the questionnaire several different times; in addition, they had different opinions on the matter from day to day. The same is true for the alcohol group, in which there were only 32 patients. In this example, there is a clear breach of the assumption that each subject is represented only once. An interpretation of the results of the X^2 analysis on this data would be meaningless.

The second problem is trickier: "Independence" means, in principle, that the response of *one* subject must not influence the response of any other subject. Technically, if two friends discuss an opinion and then mark their papers in the same way, independence is violated. This results in experimenters preferring to test subjects *individually*.

In the smoking example on a college campus, it is obvious that data should not be collected more than once from the same student. But, in addition, limiting the sample to one sorority and one fraternity house might create problems, because friends may influence smoking habits. *Random selection* of subjects should be used to avoid this problem.

The *final* assumption for the X^2 is that there is some theoretical reason for categories of data. The basis for the categories can be obtained from previous research or from some logical consideration. This assumption helps to ensure that the analysis will be meaningful. It also prevents so-called fishing expeditions wherein data are analyzed in random groupings until some combination reaches statistical significance. For example, in the earlier case in which we grouped subjects into age categories and compared their selection of a caregiver by considering all possible age groups, we are likely to stumble upon one combination that will show a significant difference in choice. We might even try enough different groupings to find the particular difference that we most desire (*i.e.,* selection favoring nurse practitioners or one favoring physicians). However, such a random grouping is merely a statistical exercise and offers little meaningful information. What random "fishing" is most likely to yield is a healthy catch of Type I errors, that is, falsely rejecting the null hypothesis!

The concept of the X^2 requires that the age groups used have some logical basis (*i.e.,* the age of young adults, one of the child-bearing years, *etc.*). A further requirement is that the categories have a uniform basis. For example, we might use age groupings that match the different stages of the family: new couples, couples in the child-bearing years, families with teenage children, elderly couples. We might also use categories that reflect adult development: late adolescent, young adults, and so on. Although these categorizing systems overlap, it is important to use only one at a time in the analysis.

These assumptions provide the guidelines for appropriate use of the X^2. When met, they result in valid results and allow meaningful interpretation of data. In situations in which they cannot be met, other techniques should be used. In particular, when the sample size is too small to meet the assumptions, tests that calculate exact probabilities can provide the same information as the chi-square. For 2×2 tables, Fisher's Exact Test is often used. Further information on these techniques is available in books in which nonparametric analyses are described, for example, in Hays' (1973) *Statistics for the Social Sciences,* and in Siegel's (1956) *Nonparametric Statistics for the Behavioral Sciences.*

YATES' CORRECTION FOR CONTINUITY

In this section, we will present a technique that enhances the validity of the chi-square analysis in cases in which the *df* is one. The 2×2 contingency table deserves special attention in chi-square. Not only is it a popular way to analyze either/or data, but it also has special statistical significance in the chi-square distribution. As we discussed earlier, the 4-cell table requires *relatively* higher cell frequencies than do tables with more cells. Whereas larger tables can be analyzed appropriately with expected frequencies of 5 (and under), a 4-cell table requires expected frequencies of at least 10 for the most reliable analyses. The 2×2 X^2 has a different requirement, because the distribution of X^2 for 1 *df* is different from the distributions of X^2 with *df* greater than 1 (Hays, 1973; Hinkle, Wiersma & Jurs, 1979). The distributions for the X^2 are represented in the table of values of X^2 (Appendix F). As we can see from the table, the widest deviations between values at different levels of significance occur at 1 *df*. The result of the 2×2 analysis, therefore, is the most sensitive when the expected frequencies fall below those upon which the X^2 distribution is based.

Moreover, the X^2 distribution is based upon continuous data, even though the data that we use are discrete. The continuous data provide a smooth, continuous curve for the distribution. In contrast, the X^2 calculation is not continuous, because it is based on frequencies that must be whole numbers. When we compare our results to the X^2 table, we are comparing a discrete value to a continuous curve. In most X^2 distributions, this creates little difficulty in interpretation. However, in the X^2 with 1 *df,* the curve is especially steep when the expected frequencies are below 10. This would create problems in interpretation.

To lessen the problem, a correction factor is added in the calculation of X^2 for 2×2 tables when the expected frequency is less than 10 in one or more cells. The correction factor is usually called the *Yates Correction factor* or the *Correction for Continuity factor* or some similar phrase. The correction involves subtracting .5 from the *absolute value* of the difference between each *fo* and *fe* pair. Absolute value means that you do not consider whether the number is positive or negative, that is, you use the number and ignore the sign. In other words, we reduce the magnitude of the difference between the observed and expected frequencies by .5. The correction is made *before squaring the differences.*

The formula for the X^2 with Yates correction is

$$\sum \frac{(|fo - fe| - .5)^2}{fe}$$

where *fo* and *fe* again equal the observed and expected frequencies, respectively, and the vertical lines | | indicate the absolute value of the difference.

Consider the following example: Suppose that 40 cardiac patients were randomly assigned to either a relaxation treatment group or to a control group while they were hospitalized for myocardial infarction. Following discharge, they were followed for 1 year, and the rate of reoccurrence in each group was measured. Table 7-6 presents the results. The expected frequencies are in parenthesis. As we can see from the table, 2 of the 4 cells have expected frequencies of less than 10, so we apply the Yates Correction Factor. Table 7-7 shows the calculations for the resulting X^2. With 1 *df,* the X^2 value of 1.69 has a probability level of $> .10$ and $< .20$. Therefore, we accept the null hypothesis and conclude that there was no difference in the recurrence of MIs between the treatment and control groups. The treatment had no demonstrated effect on the rate of recurrence.

Note in the table for this example that all the differences resulted in the same absolute value of 2.05. This will not always be the case in tables with more than 4 cells. However, in 2×2 tables, there is always this pattern across the differences.

Table 7-6 Contingency Table Showing MI Relapse Across Relaxation and Control Groups

| Second MI | Treatment Group | | Row Totals |
	Relaxation	Control	
Yes	6 (8.55)	12 (9.45)	18
No	13 (10.45)	9 (11.55)	22
			Overall N
Column Totals	19	21	40

Table 7-7 Calculation of Chi Square Using Yates Correction for Continuity

$$\Sigma \frac{(|fo - fe| - .5)^2}{fe}$$

$$\frac{(|6 - 8.55| - .5)^2}{8.55} + \frac{(|12 - 9.45| - .5)^2}{9.45} + \frac{(|13 - 10.45| - .5)^2}{10.45} + \frac{(|9 - 11.55| - .5)^2}{11.55}$$

$$= \frac{(2.05)^2}{8.55} + \frac{(2.05)^2}{9.45} + \frac{(2.05)^2}{10.45} + \frac{(2.05)^2}{11.55}$$

$$= .49 + .44 + .40 + .36$$

$$= 1.69$$

The net effect of using the Yates Correction Factor is to reduce the X^2 value. It thereby provides a more conservative estimate of the significance and reduces the likelihood of a Type I error, the incorrect rejection of the null hypothesis.

The recommendations for using the Yates Correction factor vary to some extent across references. The most conservative position holds that the correction factor be used in all 2×2 analyses. However, because there is a negligible discrepancy between the calculated chi-square value and the chi-square distribution in cases in which the expected frequencies are large (10 or more), the most discerning use of the factor is its application in those cases in which any expected frequency falls below 10 (Spence *et al*, 1976, pp. 226–227).

THE PHI (Φ) COEFFICIENT

This section deals with a technique that enables us to interpret the strength of the relationship shown in a significant X^2 analysis. The technique is a statistical test of association derived directly from the value of the X^2. It is called the *phi (Φ) coefficient,* or *phi (Φ) statistic.*

Phi is most useful for 2×2 tables and is interpreted only in cases in which the value of the X^2 reaches a significant probability level. (It can be used for larger tables, but its meaning is somewhat different.) In these cases, phi measures the strength of the relationship that has been identified by the X^2. In this way, phi is very similar to the r^2 measure calculated to show the strength of the relationship in Pearson correlation (Chapter 5).

The formula for the phi coefficient is

$$\Phi = \sqrt{\frac{X^2}{n}}$$

According to this formula, phi is calculated by dividing the X^2 value by the total n and taking the square root. Phi has the value of 0 when there is no correlation and + 1.00 when there is a perfect relationship. Again this is similar to the ranges of the r and is interpreted in the same way: The value of phi equals the strength of association between the variables.

Let us calculate the phi coefficient for the smoking-on-campus example previously discussed. The X^2 value is 4.58. The total n was 527. According to the phi formula our calculations will be

$$\Phi = \sqrt{\frac{4.58}{527}}$$

$$\Phi = \sqrt{.0087}$$

$$\Phi = .09$$

Phi is equal to .09; that is, the strength of the association between gender and smoking behavior is .09. Although we obtained a significant X^2, we can see that the strength of the relationship, or the amount of association between the two variables, is relatively low. We might suggest that the investigator seeking to understand what influenced smoking behavior look for other variables that have a stronger association.

Although we could mathematically calculate phi for the MI/Relaxation example in Table 7-6, its meaning might be clouded. In that example, the X^2 value did not reach an acceptable level of significance (.05 or less). We accepted the null hypothesis. Calculating phi for a nonsignificant X^2 value, some would say, might be the same as measuring the strength of a relationship that may not exist.

The phi coefficient is complementary to the X^2 because it is less sensitive to the total sample size. For this reason, it is another kind of correction factor for X^2. In chi-square analysis, the sample size has a direct effect on the calculated value. By increasing the n without changing the proportionate distribution of the frequencies, the significance of the X^2 will increase. In describing this characteristic of the X^2, we may say that the test is *inflated by large numbers*. The phi coefficient gives an indication of the strength of the association that exists quite independent of the sample size.

Phi has another use in the interpretation of X^2. Often, replications of studies yield a number of similar chi-squares on the same variables. In cases in which the sample sizes differ, the phi coefficient can be used to compare the strength of the relationship found across studies.

In conjunction with X^2, phi allows a sophisticated interpretation of relationships between nominal level variables. Its ready calculation and few restrictions make it a useful tool in evaluating research results.

CHI-SQUARE ANALYSIS
AMONG SEVERAL GROUPS

The foregoing examples have all been based on 2×2 table analyses. The method of analysis for a larger number of groups is identical to that used in the 2×2 tables. The same assumptions hold, and the calculations for the expected frequencies and the *df* follow the same formulas. For an example of a table with more than 4 cells, consider the following study:

In the family planning and sex counseling section of an adolescent clinic in a large city, data on adolescent pregnancies were collected over a number of years to help in planning the delivery of services and evaluating ongoing programs. The data included the number of pregnancies and the outcomes of the pregnancies over time for 1970, 1975, and 1980. These data are shown in Table 7-8.

A X^2 analysis was done to determine whether there was a difference in the outcomes of the pregnancies over the three different periods. Table 7-9 shows the results of the calculations. The large number of cells resulted in many more calculations. However, each step followed exactly the same arithmetic procedure as in

Table 7-8 Outcomes of Adolescent Pregnancies for 1970, 1975, and 1980 (Percentages)

	Years			
Outcomes of Pregnancies	*1970*	*1975*	*1980*	*Row Totals*
Abortion	195 (27)	67 (17)	46 (15)	308
Keeping Baby	88 (12)	53 (14)	51 (17)	192
Family Adoption	154 (22)	100 (26)	85 (28)	339
Agency Adoption	280 (39)	163 (43)	118 (40)	561
Column Totals	*717*	*383*	*300*	*1400*

Table 7-9 Calculation of Chi-Square for 12-Cell Table

$$\frac{(195-157.74)^2}{157.74} + \frac{(67-84.26)^2}{84.26} + \frac{(46-66.00)^2}{66.00} + \frac{(88-98.33)^2}{98.33}$$

$$+ \frac{(53-52.53)^2}{52.53} + \frac{(51-41.14)^2}{41.14} + \frac{(154-173.62)^2}{173.62} + \frac{(100-92.74)^2}{92.74}$$

$$+ \frac{(85-72.64)^2}{72.64} + \frac{(280-287.31)^2}{287.31} + \frac{(163-153.47)^2}{153.47} + \frac{(118-120.21)^2}{120.21}$$

$$= 8.80 + 3.54 + 6.06 + 1.09 + .00 + 2.36 + 2.22 + .57 + 2.10 + .19 + .59 + .04$$

$$X^2 = 27.56$$

the 2×2 analyses. The expected frequencies were each calculated according to the formula discussed earlier.

$$fe(k) = \frac{T(rk) \times T(ck)}{T(N)}$$

For example, to get the expected frequency for the observed frequency of 53 (in the second column, second row of Table 7-8), we multiplied the total of the second row (192) by the total of the second column (383) and divided by 1400 to get $fe = 52.53$.

Similarly, to get the expected frequency for 154 (in the third row, first column of Table 7-8), we multiplied the total of the third row (339) by the total of the first column (717) and divided by 1400 to get $fe = 173.62$.

The df for the example are determined by the formula described previously.

$$df = (r-1)(c-1).$$

In the example, there are 4 rows and 3 columns; so, $df = (3)(2) = 6$.

For 6 df, the X^2 value of 27.56 is significant beyond the .001 level (the tabled value for .001 is 22.457). Therefore, we reject the null hypothesis that there is no difference in the pregnancy outcomes over the three different time periods.

We can conclude that there is a difference and, by inspection, see that the rate of abortion and the number of agency adoptions have tended to decrease the most, whereas the number of adolescent mothers who keep their babies and the number of those who have family members adopt the baby have stayed more stable over time and have even increased in proportion. In fact, the largest increase is in mothers who keep their babies, rising from 12% in 1970 to 17% in 1980.

Note that in a X^2 with more than 4 cells, the X^2 value determines whether there is an overall difference, but not precisely where the difference lies. If we wanted to determine which of the cells were significantly different from others, we would need to calculate a series of 2×2 X^2s, selecting specific cells at a time. The hazard of such a series of analyses is in the risk of making Type I errors. However, the risk is somewhat reduced by first calculating an overall X^2. If significant, it justifies further analyses. We can further reduce the risk by making very selected comparisons instead of running every possible variation of 2×2 combinations.

Even with many-celled tables, the X^2 analysis is arithmetically simple enough to complete with a simple hand calculator.

SPECIAL CASES IN CHI-SQUARE ANALYSIS

The X^2 test is a versatile analysis for categorical data. Although most of the time it is used to determine a difference among category groups, there are other situations in which X^2 is appropriate. This section deals with the way in which the X^2 calculation and interpretation are adjusted to meet the situational requirements. The two situations detailed here are the *one-sample case* and the *additive* X^2. Although the calculations may vary from the 2×2 example described above, the basic assumptions in these situations are very similar to those previously described.

The One-Sample Case

The simplest form of X^2 is one dimensional and involves the distribution of a sample across one category level. For example, we may look at how a sample of persons is divided into diagnostic categories: The number of juvenile onset diabetics compared with the number of adult onset diabetics in a particular clinic. Or, we may use the one-sample case to examine the way in which a group of subjects decides among a set of options: Do women prefer male or female caregivers?

In the one-sample case, the basic X^2 question is still the same as the one in the 2×2 analysis, or in any X^2: How do the observed frequencies compare with the expected? Let us use an example to discuss the particulars of one-dimensional X^2, the one-sample case.

In preparation for establishing a birthing center as an alternative to the routine hospital stay during the birth of a baby, nurse-midwives conducted a marketing survey in the community. The sample included 140 women of child-bearing age who belonged to the three large health plans in the city. One question on the survey asked women to indicate which option they would select as a care site for having their babies: the birthing center (carefully described on the survey) or their favorite hospital. The research question that the midwives addressed with the data was, Would more women prefer a birthing center or a hospital?

The results of the survey showed that 80 women selected the birthing center and 60 chose the hospital (Table 7-10). What can we conclude from the data? Although the absolute count shows that more women preferred the birthing center, the research question asks whether the *difference* in the choices was greater than what could be expected by *chance alone*. In other words, was the difference a "real difference," or a sampling error?

To answer the research question, the appropriate statistical analysis is conducted. The data are frequency level data and appropriate for X^2 analysis. The measures are independent: Each subject answered only one questionnaire and chose only one option. The categories are meaningful: The birthing center and the hospital represent distinct options. With the assumptions met, the X^2 can be calculated.

We begin by determining the "expected" frequencies. Assuming the null hypothesis, we would expect no difference in the selection of the two birthing sites. Therefore, we would expect that the number of women choosing either site would be equal. The expected frequency for each of the choices is 70; that is, half the women would choose the birthing center, and the other half would choose the hospital (Table 7-11). Note that the expected frequencies and the observed frequencies add up to the same total: 140. As we stated before, this is a necessary condition for the analysis.

Table 7-10   Frequency of Selection for Birthing Site

	Choice of Option	
	Birthing Center	*Hospital*
Number of Women	80	60
	Total N = 140	

Table 7-11   Calculation of One-Sample Chi-Square Analysis

	Choice of Option	
	Birthing Center	*Hospital*
	80 (70)	60 (70)
	Total N = 140	
Calculations:		

$$\frac{(80-70)^2}{70} + \frac{(60-70)^2}{70} = 1.43 + 1.43 = 2.86$$

$$X^2 = 2.86$$

With the expected frequencies, the X^2 can be calculated according to the regular formula

$$X^2 = \Sigma \frac{(fo - fe)^2}{fe}$$

The analysis is shown in Table 7-11.

To interpret the X^2 value, we must first determine the *df*. Our table has 2 cells; once we determine one of the cell's values, the other one is no longer free to vary, because the total number of 140 is fixed. Therefore, there is 1 *df*. In one-sample chi-squares, the *df* are equal to the number of cells minus 1:

$$df = n(\text{cells}) - 1.$$

We interpret the X^2 value 2.86 by using Appendix F. With 1 *df*, X^2 of 2.86 falls between the .10 level of significance (at value 2.706) and the .05 level of significance (at value 3.841). The X^2 is less than that required to reject the null hypothesis. We would therefore conclude that there is no demonstrated difference in the selection of a birthing site. In other words, it seems possible that an equal number of women choose either option.

However, we might note that we could use the X^2 table another way. If we had a good reason for predicting the choice of a birthing center over a hospital, we could use a "one-tailed test" (see Chapter 4). In that case, the probability of the X^2 would be halved. In the table, the .10 level is used, and the null hypothesis is rejected at the .05 level. Then there *would* be a demonstrated preference for the birthing center.

The one-sample case for the X^2 is actually easier in its calculation than the larger bi-dimensional analysis, particularly for the calculation of the expected frequencies and *df*. In other ways, the one-sample case is very similar to the 2×2 or larger analyses. One additional similarity is that in a 2-celled one-sample case, as we had in our example, the Yates correction factor can be used if the expected frequencies fall below 10. The phi coefficient, however, is not appropriate for the one-sample case.

Optional Expected Frequencies for One-Sample Chi-Square

There is one additional option available for the one-sample analysis. This option involves the use of theoretical expected frequencies instead of those based on the null hypothesis for the sample. The theoretical frequencies come from norms that have been established for particular variables from previous research. These provide a standard against which to compare the observed frequencies in any given sample.

For many variables, the expected frequencies can be derived from established rates. For example, there are rates for particular illnesses, for deaths across age ranges, for accidents, for church attendance, for unemployment. These rates provide the basis for calculating the expected frequencies for comparison with a given sample. The validity of that comparison, of course, depends on the selection of an appropriate norm.

In addition to theoretical frequencies from standard rates, expected frequencies from previous research can provide a comparison for change over time or differences across samples. This is a convenient technique that increases the versatility of the analysis. Consider the following example:

Suppose that in the marketing study by nurse midwives, there were similar data about preference for birthing site from 3 years before. At that time, nurse-midwifery had just been introduced into the city and the idea of a birthing center was brand new, and, at that time, the women made the choices displayed in Table 7-12. In this earlier survey, women preferred the hospital 2 to 1 over the birthing center. The chi-square for this survey ($X^2 = 6.66$, $df = 1$) was significant, showing that more women selected the hospital. The more recent survey showed no significant difference in preference between the two. This change from a significant difference to no significant difference implies that there is an increasing preference for the birthing center.

That implication can be examined directly by comparing the observed frequencies in the present survey to the frequencies we would expect if the change over time had not occurred; that is, if there had not been a change in preference between the hospital and birthing center over the past 3 years, we would expect that twice as many women would still choose the hospital over the birthing center. These proportions will give us our expected frequencies. The expected frequency for the hospital will be twice as large as that for the birthing center. With a total n of 140, a ratio of 2 to 1 is 93.3 for the hospital and 46.7 for the birthing center ($93.3 + 46.7 = 140$) (Table 7-13).

We can now calculate the chi-square based on these theoretical expected frequencies. Essentially we are asking the question: Are the observed frequencies different from what we would expect from an earlier time. The test is now measuring a change over time. The calculations are shown in Table 7-13.

With 1 df, the chi-square value of 35.6 is significant at less than the .001 level. The analysis shows that there has been a significant change in the pattern of selection over time. These results are more meaningful than those that show no difference in choice at the present time.

Chi-square used in this way can show trends and changes in patterns of nominal level variables. The validity of the analysis depends on the selection of appropriate

Table 7-12   Preference for Birthing Site

	Choice of Option	
	Birthing Center	*Hospital*
Number of Women	20 (30)	40 (30)
	Total N = 60	

theoretical frequencies. One further note on this example: The rate of selection of the hospital and birthing center from the earlier study provided a valid theoretical expectation, because the original study showed a significant difference ($X^2 = 6.66$, $p < .01$) with more women selecting the hospital. However, if the first X^2 had not been significant, the original survey would not have provided a valid comparison. Nonsignificant results indicate that no difference was found.

The Addition of Chi-Square Results

Some research studies are conducted in which a number of different groups of subjects are measured in the same way on the same variables but at different times or in different places or even by different investigators. Although the groups of subjects may be similar, they are still separate samples, and it would violate rigorous methodology to combine the subjects into one sample to complete the analysis. However, with X^2, there is a way to combine the sub-samples by adding up the individual X^2 values calculated for each of the subgroups.

The following conditions must be met in order to make this technique valid:

1. The measurement across subgroups must be equivalent.
2. All assumptions for X^2 must be met in each sample.
3. The studies themselves must be similar in sampling criteria, setting, conduct, and so on.
4. The chi-squares to be added must have the same number of cells.
5. All samples must be independent of each other; that is, no subject can be a member of more than one sample.

If these conditions are met, the X^2 values can be added to give a total X^2. This value is then interpreted in the usual way using the X^2 table. The df for an additive X^2 is equal to the sum of all the df from the individual X^2 analysis. Before using such an

Table 7-13   Theoretical Expected Frequencies for Birthing Study

Choice of Option	
Birthing Center	Hospital
80 (46.7)	60 (93.3)

Total N = 140

Calculations for One-Way Chi-Square Using
Theoretical Expected Frequencies

$$\frac{(80 - 46.7)^2}{46.7} + \frac{(60 - 93.3)^2}{93.3} = 23.7 + 11.9 = 35.6$$

$$X^2 = 35.6$$

approach, the technique should be read about in more detail in a book such as Hays (1973), *Statistics for the Social Sciences*.

CHI-SQUARE AS THE TEST OF CHOICE

An important consideration in data analysis is the choice of the statistical technique. Because many data will lend themselves appropriately to a variety of analyses, choosing the *best* test for the analysis is more complicated than selecting a *correct* test. Certainly, any test we choose must meet the assumptions of the test in order to give valid, interpretable results. In addition, we want to select tests that preserve the most information that the data have to offer. So, for example, if we have ratio-level data we usually prefer to select an analysis that requires ratio-level data, rather than categorizing the data into ordinal or nominal measurement for use with other techniques. Because the tests that use interval and ratio-level data, such as the correlational and regression techniques described in Chapters 5 and 6, are both powerful and versatile, they are often the best tests to use.

There is another consideration when selecting methods of data analysis: the *clinical relevance* of the data. Sometimes mean differences are not as important clinically as are categorical differences. For example, we are less likely to be concerned about fine distinctions in blood sugar than we are about diabetic vs. non-diabetic. The group classification "diabetic" overrides the within-group variation of blood sugar. That is not to say that fine distinctions are not useful in other circumstances (*e.g.,* when determining doses of insulin). However, the category "diabetic" is a useful concept for diagnosis, treatment, and prognosis. It thereby is a meaningful concept for clinical research.

There are categorical classifications other than diagnostic groups that are useful. Many of these classifications describe characteristics of people that cannot be further refined into more precise levels of measurement without losing the meaning and the value of the characteristic; for example, religion, ethnicity, profession, psychological style, avocation, and family structure are categories by which we classify people into groups. At the same time, they are categories that give a great deal of information, and they are the basis for making many assumptions (valid or not).

These nominal categories, both disease- and person-related, often have clinical relevance in the area of patient care research. For example, we study the relationship between ethnicity and pain, between psychological style and disease, and so on. It is here that the chi-square analysis is often the test of choice—in those cases in which between-group differences or relationships are the focus of the research and in which within-group distinctions are not clinically meaningful. In such cases, variance techniques may blur the category boundaries and give misleading results.

An example is a study of children's tonsillectomies (Visintainer & Wolfer, 1975; Wolfer & Visintainer, 1975). In that study, children who received systematic psychological preparation before surgery were compared to children who received no such preparation on a variety of outcome measures. One measure was temperature, recorded for each child 4 hours after return from the recovery room. Because the Fahrenheit scale is an interval measurement, the first analysis studied mean temperatures for each group of children. (The technique used was the t-test, which is described in Chapter 8.) That analysis showed that children who had the preparation showed a significantly lower temperature than children who did not have the preparation.

Consider the group means. The children who received the preparation had a group mean temperature of 98.9 degrees Fahrenheit; the children who did not receive the preparation had a group mean temperature of 99.5 degrees Fahrenheit. The means differed by just 0.6 of a degree, large enough, given the sample size, to show statistical significance.

Was such a statistical difference *clinically* relevant as well? How relevant is variation in a degree of temperature? In caring for children, the importance of a change in tenths of a degree is determined first by the *category of temperature;* that is, the first and most relevant clinical question is: Does the child have a fever? If so, tenths of a degree may be relevant in showing that the temperature is rising or falling. However, if the child is in the normal category for temperature, tenths of a degree are not especially relevant.

In this research, therefore, a more clinically useful analysis was the 2×2 chi-square classifying children into "Preparation-No preparation" by "Fever-No fever" groups. By the chi-square analysis, there was no significant difference between the groups on the presence of fever; that is, preoperative preparation had no demonstrated effect on fevers, even though it made a mean difference in the temperature.

When categories have clinical relevance, statistical analyses that preserve these categories are more likely to give us useful interpretations. They are less likely to give us "differences that do not make a difference."

EXAMPLE OF A COMPUTER PRINTOUT

Although the X^2 is relatively easy to calculate by hand, computer programs provide easy and complete X^2 analysis. Most computer programs also present the data in readable tables, displaying the observed and expected frequencies as well as percentages for each cell. Depending on the package in the computer, the programming for X^2 may require some additional preparation of the raw data to ensure accurate computer analysis.

In all cases, the data used for such tests must be at the frequency level. If it was entered into the computer as nominal level data, no further preparation is required for most packages. However, if the data was entered as higher level data (ordinal, interval, ratio), it must first be transformed into frequencies. In the packaged program SPSS (Statistical Package for the Social Sciences), the transformation is accomplished through the *RECODE* statement. For example, if the subjects' ages had been entered as number of years that are ratio-level data, the data would be recoded into age groups before executing the χ^2.

Figure 7-1 contains an example of a χ^2 analysis produced by SPSS. These data came from a study that compared nurses and aides on their attitudes toward death. There are two nominal-level variables. The first (seen at the top of the cross-

Procedure Cards

```
1              16

CROSSTABS    TABLES = E2 BY TITLE

STATISTICS   1
```

Output

```
ALICES'S DEATH AND DYING STUDY

FILE    NONAME    (CREATION DATE = 06/25/83)

******************C R O S S T A B U L A T I O N   O F****
   E2                                          BY   TITLE
**********************************************************
                       TITLE
               COUNT  I
               ROW PCT I                          ROW
               COL PCT I                          TOTAL
               TOT PCT I      1.I        2.I
E2             -----------------I---------I
          0.  I      23 I        90 I      113
             I    20.4 I      79.6 I     87.6
             I    74.2 I      91.8 I
             I    17.8 I      69.8 I
             -I--------I---------I
          1.  I       8 I         8 I       16
             I    50.8 I      50.0 I     12.4
             I    25.8 I       8.2 I
             I     6.2 I       6.2 I
             -I--------I---------I
           COLUMN     31        98      129
           TOTAL    24.0      76.0    100.0
```

1 OUT OF   4 (25.0%) OF THE VALID CELLS HAVE EXPECTED CELL FREQUENCY
                 LESS THAN 5.0.
MINIMUM EXPECTED CELL FREQUENCY = 3.845
CORRECTED CHI SQUARE = 5.22116 WITH 1 DEGREE OF FREEDOM. SIGNIFICANCE = 0.0223
     RAW CHI SQUARE = 6.74734 WITH 1 DEGREE OF FREEDOM. SIGNIFICANCE = 0.0094

Figure 7-1   Chi-square analysis produced by SPSS.

frequency table) is TITLE. That variable was coded so that registered nurses (RNs) were 1 and aides were 2. The other variable (seen on the side of the table) is E2. That was one of 5 questions at the end of this attitude scale about death and dying that asked what effects the questionnaire itself had on the respondent. E2 was, "It has made me think of my own death." If subjects checked E2, they were coded 1. If they did not check the item, they were coded 0. In the upper left hand corner, note that

COUNT = number of subjects
ROW PCT = row percentage
COL PCT = column percentage
TOT PCT = total percentage

To demonstrate what all that means, look at the upper left cell. It contains subjects who were RNs and did not check E2. The top number, 23, is the count, that is, there were 23 RNs who did not agree that the questionnaire made them think more about their own death. There were 8 (lower left hand cell) RNs who checked E2; thus, the total number of RNs was 31 (column total). If we look across the top row, we can see that 23 RNs and 90 aides did not check E2; thus, the row total was 113.

The row percentages in the bottom cells are both 50%. Thus, of the 16 people who checked E2, half were RNs and half were aides. Looking at the column percentages, we see that 25.8% of the RNs and 8.2% of the aides agreed with E2. A much larger *percentage* of RNs than aides agreed that the questionnaire caused them to think about their own death.

The lowest figures in each cell (TOT PCT) reflect the individual cell percentage; that is, the 17.8% in the top left cell means that of the 129 people in this analysis, 17.8% (23/129) were RNs who did not check E2. The four TOT PCTs add up to 100%. The totals of these cell percentages are given outside the cells. The column total (17.8 + 6.2 = 24.0) is given below the total number of subjects for the column. The row totals are given below the respective total row *n*.

In the analysis, a warning is given that one of the cells has an expected cell frequency less than 5.0. With SPSS, for 2×2 tables, Fisher's exact test is applied if there are fewer than 21 cases, and Yates' corrected X^2 is used for all other 2×2 tables. Here, the "corrected" X^2 is the Yates' corrected X^2 (5.22116), which is significant ($p = .0223$). This analysis shows that significantly more RNs than aides agreed with E2.

EXAMPLE FROM PUBLISHED RESEARCH

A study was conducted by Ziemer (1983) to test the effects of information on post-surgical coping. Only the portion of this study in which X^2 was used will be reported here. Patients were randomly assigned to three groups. Group I received procedure information; Group II received procedure and sensation information;

and Group III received procedure and sensation information, plus information on selected coping strategies.

Research Question

"Did the three groups differ in their perceptions of the amount of information they had received?"

Data Gathered

One hundred and eleven subjects were randomly assigned to the three groups. For each of six behaviors identified in a Physical Coping Behavior Scale, subjects were asked "Were you provided with any information about how to do this prior to surgery?" (Ziemer, 1983, p. 286)

Tabular Presentation of Results

Table 7-14 contains the results of the study. The X^2s are significant for all the behaviors except requesting analgesics. In this table, we see asterisks used to indicate significant results. Although this is acceptable, it is more common to see the actual probabilities given, because the computer programs produce them for us. Moving across row one, we see that 54% of Group I, 56% of Group II, and 97% of Group III stated that they had received information about breathing prior to surgery.

Table 7-14   Physical Coping Behaviors and Patient Responses

			Information Before Surgery				
			Group				
	I		II		III		
Behaviors	N	(%)	N	(%)	N	(%)	X^2
Breathing	21	(54)	18	(56)	34	(97)	19.53*
Coughing	21	(57)	19	(57)	34	(97)	17.95*
Turning	16	(41)	17	(53)	32	(89)	19.10*
Leg exercises	6	(17)	9	(30)	31	(91)	43.50*
Abdominal splinting	22	(58)	19	(59)	34	(97)	17.03*
Requesting analgesics	25	(66)	22	(65)	24	(72)	.58

* Not all subjects responded to these questions. If a subject reported never engaging in a particular behavior, having prior information was seldom reported. Percentages are based on the number of subjects who reponded to this question.
* $p < .000$
From Ziemer, M. M. (1983). Effects of information on postsurgical coping. *Nursing Research*, 32(5), 282–287.

Description of Results

Group III differed significantly from the other two groups on five of the six behaviors. Subjects in Group III were significantly more likely to report having received information about those behaviors prior to surgery than were members of the other two groups. Although they reported having the information, they did not differ from the other two groups when it came to actually carrying out the behaviors.

Conclusions

"Results showed no evidence that the type of information provided for patients prior to surgery increased the reported frequency of coping behaviors or that the reported frequency of coping behaviors was related to improved outcomes as evaluated by pain intensity, distress, or selected physical complications." (Ziemer, 1983, p. 282)

EXERCISES FOR CHAPTER 7

1. The staff of a long-term psychiatric facility for adolescents wishes to evaluate its new intermediate treatment program (ITP) in which a randomly selected group of patients are given more privileges and responsibilities. One way to evaluate the program is to compare the number of elopements (runnings away) that occurred in the ITP with those in the conventional treatment program (CTP). The following table shows the comparison for a 1-year period:

	ITP	CTP	Total
Elopes	6	15	21
Non-Elopes	34	65	99
Total	40	80	120

State the implied research question. Compute the χ^2 analysis and interpret the results. Calculate the strength of the relationship, if applicable.

2. At an ACCN convention, 90 nurses were invited to participate in a survey. They were asked to select which of three different floor plans seemed most functional for an adult intensive care unit. The results of the survey showed the following selections:

Plan A	Plan B	Plan C
33	34	23

What do you conclude from the survey?

3. The infection control unit of a large hospital evaluated the rate of nosocomial infections in their institution by comparing their rate with the JAH estimate of 16%. Of the 16,400 admissions at the institution during the past year, there were 900 suspected hospital-originated infections.

Infection Free	Infections
15,500	900

How does this hospital compare with others nationally?

4. In problem 3, there is the possibility of a violation of one assumption for the χ^2. Which one? How might it be violated? What are the implications for the interpretation of the results?

5. Nursing educators wanted to evaluate the relationship between basic education and selections of specialty areas after graduation. They surveyed 1209 nurses.

	BSN	AD	DIP	Totals
Pediatrics	115	100	130	345
Medical-Surgical	94	185	210	489
Psychiatric	206	76	93	375
Totals	415	361	433	1209

Calculate the χ^2 and interpret the results.

6. In a 2×2 study, $\chi^2 = 5.4$, and $n = 100$. Calculate phi. What information does it provide?

CHAPTER 8

t-Tests: Measuring the Differences Between Group Means

Madelon A. Visintainer and Barbara Hazard Munro

OBJECTIVES FOR CHAPTER 8

After reading this chapter and completing the exercises, you should be able to

1. Determine when the *t*-test is the appropriate technique to use.
2. Discuss how mean difference, group variability, and sample size are related to the statistical significance of the *t*-statistic.
3. Discuss how the results of the homogeneity of variance test are related to choice of *t*-test formula.
4. Select the appropriate *t*-test formula (separate, pooled, or correlated) for a given situation.
5. Carry out the calculations involved for each of the three formulas.
6. Use the appropriate degrees of freedom (*df*) to determine the significance of the results.

Many research projects are designed to test the differences between two groups. When the differences involve interval or ratio data, the analysis requires an evaluation of means and distributions of each group. For example, to compare the heart rates of men and women, we would examine how much the mean and distribution for men differed from those for women. Or in another example, to measure the effect of an intervention to reduce anxiety levels, we might compare the anxiety (measured on a self-report scale) of patients who received the intervention with those patients who did not.

In this chapter, a statistical method for testing the difference between two groups will be presented. This method is the *t*-test, or Student's *t*-test. It is named after its inventor, William Gosset, who published under the pseudonym of Student. Gosset invented the *t*-test as a more precise method of comparing groups. He described a set of distributions of *means* of randomly drawn samples from a normally distributed population. These distributions are the *t* distributions.

The shape of the distributions vary depending on the size of the samples drawn from the populations. However, all the t distributions have a normal distribution with a mean equal to the mean of the population. Unlike the z distributions, which are based on the normal curve, and so estimate the theoretical population parameters μ and σ, the t distributions are based on the sample size and therefore vary according to the df. The use of the t distributions is based on the concepts presented in Chapter 3. Theoretically, when an infinite number of samples of equal size are drawn from a normally distributed population, the mean of the sampling distribution will equal the mean of the population. If the sample sizes were large enough, the shape of the sampling distribution would approximate the normal curve.

In this chapter, we are going to use a set of t distributions to compare the differences between two means. These distributions are described by the sample of *differences between means* obtained from drawing pairs of random samples from a population. If we could draw an infinite number of pairs of samples and plot the differences between the means of all possible pairs of samples, we would find a particular distribution with a mean of zero and a shape similar to the normal curve. The range of the distribution will again depend on the size of the sample pairs; in this case, the larger the sample sizes, the narrower the distributions.

THE RESEARCH QUESTION

When we compare two groups on a particular characteristic, we are asking whether or not the groups are different. The statistical question asks *how different* the groups are; that is, is the difference we find greater than that which could occur by chance alone? Symbolically, the null hypothesis would be written H_0: $\mu_1 = \mu_2$. The null hypothesis for the t-test states that any difference that occurs between the means of two groups is a difference in the sampling distribution. The means are different not because the groups are drawn from two different theoretical populations, but rather because of different random distributions of the samples from such a population. The null hypothesis is represented by the t distributions constructed by the random sampling of one population. When we use the t-test to interpret the significance of the difference between groups, we are asking the statistical question, What is the probability of getting a difference of this magnitude in groups this size if we were comparing random samples drawn from the same population? That is, *What is the probability of getting a difference this large by chance alone?*

An example of the use of the t-test to compare two groups is the study of Williams and Nikolaisen (1982) on parents' perceptions and responses to the loss of a child from sudden infant death syndrome (SIDS). The authors used the t-test to compare two groups (mothers and fathers) on their responses to the SIDS event. Fathers had significantly higher scores on a measure of how they viewed the crisis event. This indicated that they held a more realistic view than the mothers. There was also a significant difference between mothers and fathers on the amount of support they thought they had received, with fathers reporting higher levels of support. Mothers reported significantly more feelings about the event than did the fathers.

To answer research questions through use of the *t*-test, we compare the difference we obtained between our means with the sampling distribution of such differences. In general, of course, the larger the *difference* between our two means, the more likely that the *t*-test will be significant. When we look at the formula for *t*, we see that this difference appears in the numerator. However, two other factors are taken into account: the variability and the sample size. In the *t*-formula, the denominator is the standard error of the *t* statistic. In Chapter 3, when we discussed the standard error of the mean, it was pointed out that the standard deviation (variability) and *n* (sample size) are used in calculating that error term. An increase in variability was shown to lead to an increase in error, and an increase in sample size was shown to lead to a decrease in error. These same principles apply to the *t*-test.

Given the same mean difference, groups with less variability will be more likely to be significantly different than groups with wide variability. Why? Because in groups with more variability, the error term will be larger, reflecting the fact that if the groups have scores that vary widely, there is likely to be considerable overlap between the two groups; thus, it will be difficult to ascertain whether or not a difference exists. Groups with less variability and a real mean difference will have distributions more clearly distinct from each other, that is, there will be less overlap between their respective distributions. With *more* variability (thus larger error), we need a *larger difference* to be reasonably "sure" that a real difference exists.

With a larger sample size, there is a smaller error term. In discussing the correlation coefficient, we pointed out that with a larger *n*, a smaller *r* will be considered significant. This is also the case with *t*, where with a larger sample, a smaller *t* value will be statistically significant.

TYPE OF DATA REQUIRED

For the *t*-test, we need one nominal-level variable, with two levels as the independent variable. A simpler way to say this is that we must have two groups. The dependent variable should be interval or ratio level, although, as previously indicated, ordinal-level data can often be treated as interval-level data and used in *t*-test analysis.

The *t*-test has been the technique commonly used to compare two groups. The mathematics involved is simpler than that required for analysis of variance, which will be discussed in Chapter 9. It should be made clear, however, that when comparing two groups on some continuous variable, it does not matter whether one uses a *t*-test or a one-way analysis of variance. The results will be mathematically identical. The *t*-statistic (derived from the *t*-test formula) is equal to the square root of the *F*-statistic (derived from the one-way analysis of variances). Symbolically then, $t = \sqrt{F}$ and $F = t^2$.

With the use of the computer, ease of calculation is not an issue, so some people will use analysis of variance to compare two groups. Either way is correct; it is a matter of individual preference. The typical *t*-test table has the advantage of clearly presenting the means being compared in the analysis.

ASSUMPTIONS

The assumptions underlying the *t*-test concern both the kind of data used in the test and the characteristics of the distribution of the variables.

First, the *t*-test requires at least *interval-level* data for the dependent measure. *Second,* the test assumes that each subject will contribute one score to the distribution of one specific group; that is, each subject can belong to one and only one of the two groups and contributes one and only one score. This is the assumption of independence.

A *third* assumption of the *t*-test is that the distribution of the dependent measure is normal. If the distribution is seriously skewed, the *t*-test may be invalid. For example, suppose we were investigating nurses' salaries and included in our sample all nurses working in an inpatient setting. If we also include the nursing director in our sample, who by virtue of the administrative position had a much greater salary than the other nurses, we would have a positively skewed sample. The mean of the sample will reflect the single high salary and thereby be less representative of the bulk of the salaries. Now, if we use the sample to calculate the distribution of difference between means, we would have an inflated estimate of the difference.

The *final* requirement for a valid *t*-test interpretation is that the groups that we are comparing be similar in their *variances*. This is related to the assumption implied by the null hypotheses that the groups are from a single population. This assumption is referred to as the requirement of homogeneity of variance. We can test this assumption by comparing the variances of the two groups with the *F* test, prior to calculating the *t* ratio. We use the following formula:

$$F = \frac{\text{larger variance}}{\text{smaller variance}}$$

We will use an example to demonstrate this test of the homogeneity of variance. Suppose we had two groups, an experimental and a control group. In the experimental group, $n = 25$ and the variance, $s^2 = 6.0$. In the control group, $n = 30$, and $s^2 = 4.5$.

We put the larger variance in the numerator and the smaller variance in the denominator, so the formula becomes

$$F = \frac{6.0}{4.5}$$

The *df* for this *F* ratio are based on the *n*s for the groups and equal $n - 1$. For the experimental group, the *df* will be $25 - 1 = 24$, and, for the control group, they will be $30 - 1 = 29$. The *df* for the group with the larger variance are given first, so, here, the *df* for the experimental groups are given first, and we may complete the formula as

$$F_{24, 29} = \frac{6.0}{4.5}$$

$$F_{24, 29} = 1.33$$

Now turn to the *F* table (Appendix E) to determine whether or not an *F* of 1.33 with 24 and 29 *df* is significant: With 24 *df* associated with the greater mean square (across top of table) and 29 *df* associated with the lesser mean square (n_2 in table), we find the tabled values to be 1.90 for the .05 level and 2.49 for the .01 level. There is a complication here in that the *F*-table is set up to test one-tailed tests of significance. With the homogeneity of variance *F*-test, one does not know which group will have the larger variance and thus be in the numerator; therefore, the two-tailed test of significance is appropriate. The simplest way to convert the figures in the *F*-table to those necessary to test a two-tailed test is to double the *probability values*. For a .05 level with a two-tailed test, we would use the tabled values for the .025 level. The *F*-table in Appendix E only contains the .01 and .05 levels (for simplicity of use). A more complete table or a computer printout would give exact values. In this example, the *F*-value of 1.33 is not significant at the .05 level with a two-tailed test. Thus, the variance for the experimental group does not differ significantly from the variance for the control group. The *t*-test would be the appropriate test to use.

Meeting this last assumption protects against type II errors—incorrectly accepting the null hypothesis. When the variances are unequal, that is, when the variation in one sample is significantly greater than the variation in the other, we are less likely to find a significant *t* value. We might, therefore, incorrectly conclude that the groups were drawn from the same population when they were not.

What if the variances are significantly different? What then? There are occasions when groups that we wish to compare do not have equal variances. For example, suppose our imaging intervention in the above study had a diverse effect on the group such that some who received it showed exceptional benefit while others showed an unexpected negative effect. The wide diversity in the group would give a large variance. If it were significantly larger than the variance for the control group, we would be restricted in our use of the *t*-ratio. Fortunately, there is a statistical method that approximates the *t*-test and can be interpreted in the same way using a different calculation for the standard error.

Actually, there are three different formulas based on the *t*-distribution that can be used to compare two groups.

First, there is the basic formula sometimes called the *pooled formula,* which is used to compare two groups when the assumptions for the *t*-test (including the test for homogeneity of variance) are met.

Second, when the variances are *unequal,* a formula called the *separate formula* is used. This takes into account the fact that the variances are not alike. It is a more conservative measure.

Third, if there is correlation between the data taken from the two groups, adjustment must be made for that relationship. That formula is often called the *correlated t-test* or the *t*-test for *paired comparisons.* Comparing a group of subjects on their pre- and post scores is an example of when this technique would be used. Because these are not two independent groups, but rather one group measured twice, the scores will most likely be correlated; thus, the correlated *t*-test should be used. Another example is when the two groups consist of matched pairs. If the pairs are carefully matched, there will be correlation between their scores, and the standard *t*-test would not be appropriate. All three of these formulas will be presented in this chapter.

CALCULATING THE BASIC (POOLED) *t*-TEST

Suppose we were interested in finding ways of increasing the rehabilitation of patients after major injury. One technique we wished to try was a technique of mental imaging in which a patient would imagine moving the particular muscle group or limb that was nonfunctional.

We hypothesize that patients who receive the imaging intervention will show greater recovery as indicated on a recovery measure. To test the hypothesis, we randomly assign patients with similar injuries to either an experimental group or a control group. Those in the experimental group are taught imaging techniques; those in the control group are not. After the prescribed length of time, we measure the amount of flexibility and strength that the subjects in each group have in the injured limbs. Based on these measures, the subjects receive a "recovery score" (Table 8-1).

Now we ask the statistical question: "Is the group of subjects who received the experimental intervention different from the group who did not in terms of the recovery scores?" This question is asked about our specific groups, but the theoretical assumption is that we are using this sample to *infer* something about other patients who are similar to our sample subjects. Therefore, we are using our two samples as representative of two theoretical populations—one that receives imaging techniques and one that does not. By examining the group differences, we are aiming to make projections about the populations.

One further note about the populations. Prior to the intervention, all subjects were assumed to be members of the same population. However, the application of an intervention under experimental conditions essentially attempts to define a new population—the population of subjects who receive the intervention. If the intervention is such that it creates a difference between the groups in terms of the dependent variable, we have a change in the sample. The change is such that the sample now belongs to a different population in terms of the dependent measure.

Table 8-1   Recovery Scores for the Experimental and Control Group

Group 1 Experimental	Group 2 Control
X_1	X_2
21	12
18	14
14	10
20	8
11	16
19	5
8	3
12	9
13	11
15	
$n = 10$ $\overline{X}_1 = 15.10$	$n = 9$ $\overline{X}_2 = 9.78$

For example, in our study, if the group that received the intervention shows a significantly greater recovery than the control group, we would infer that giving patients an imagery intervention places them into a new category (population) of patients who show greater recovery.

How do we determine whether the groups are different? We begin by checking our assumptions. In particular, we must test for homogeneity of variance before deciding whether to use the pooled or separate formula. Remember that the formula for variance is

$$s^2 = \frac{\Sigma x^2}{n-1} \quad \text{or} \quad \frac{\Sigma X^2 - \frac{(\Sigma X)^2}{n}}{n-1}$$

See Table 8-2 for the calculation of the two variances. For group I, the variance is 18.32, and for group 2, it is 16.94. We compare these variances with the *F* test

$$F_{9,8} \quad \frac{18.32}{16.94}$$

$$F = 1.08$$

Using the *F* table in Appendix E, we find the tabled values for 9, 8 *df* to be 3.39 (.05 level) and 5.91 (.01 level). We should double the probability levels for the two-tailed test to .10 and .02. Because an *F* of 1.08 is not significant at the .10 level (3.39), it will not be significant at the .05 level. Thus, the pooled *t*-formula is the appropriate formula to use.

Table 8-2 Data for Pooled t-Test Example

Group 1 Experimental			Group 2 Control	
X_1	$X_1{}^2$		X_2	$X_2{}^2$
21	441		12	144
18	324		14	196
14	196		10	100
20	400		8	64
11	121		16	256
19	361		5	25
8	64		3	9
12	144		9	81
13	169		11	121
15	225		88	996
151	2445			

$$s^2 = \frac{\Sigma X^2 - \frac{(\Sigma X)^2}{n}}{n - 1}$$

$n = 10$ $n = 9$

$\overline{X}_1 = 15.10$ $\overline{X}_2 = 9.78$

$$s^2 = \frac{2445 - \frac{(151)^2}{10}}{10 - 1}$$ $$s^2 = \frac{996 - \frac{(88)^2}{9}}{9 - 1}$$

$s^2 = 18.32$ $s^2 = 16.94$

Next, we compare the group means as an estimate of the means of the two different populations. The mean of the experimental group is 15.10, and the mean of the control group is 9.78. The group means are different, with the treatment group having a higher recovery score mean than the control group. However, the question is whether this difference is a sampling error (*i.e.*, a chance difference) or a true difference (*i.e.*, one that occurred because the groups are different). We answer this question by finding the probability of such a difference assuming that *there is no difference*, that is, when the null hypothesis is true. The *t*-ratio (*t*-test) can compare the difference to the distribution of differences between pairs of means in the theoretical population. The comparison is made through the *t*-formula:

$$t = \frac{(\overline{X}_1 - \overline{X}_2) - (\mu_1 - \mu_2)}{s(\overline{X}_1 - \overline{X}_2)}$$

Before we work out the formula for our example, we can examine the relationship of the *t*-ratio to *z* scores and the normal distribution. We can see that the *t*-formula is very similar to the formula for calculating *z*-scores. Recall the *z* formula where we subtract the mean from the raw score and divide by the standard deviation. In Chapter 3, we gave the formula as

$$z = \frac{X - \bar{X}}{s}$$

We might also write the z-formula in terms of the population parameters as

$$z = \frac{X - \mu}{\sigma}$$

Because we are comparing the *differences between group means* to the distribution of *the population of differences between pairs of means*, our "score" in the case of the *t*-ratio is a difference; specifically, the difference between two means: $\bar{X}_1 - \bar{X}_2$. Our population mean is the theoretical difference between two population means: $\mu_1 - \mu_2$. Therefore, the numerator of the z formula and the *t*-ratio are equivalent.

However, when we use the z-statistic, we typically know the population parameters. In the case of the *t*-ratio, because the population parameters are unknown, we estimate them based on the sample statistics. The parameter that we must estimate is the standard deviation of the population, the term in the denominator of the z-statistic: σ. When we estimate σ, we use the standard error of the *t*-statistic. Simply stated, the *t*-ratio differs from the z in that an estimate of the standard error of the population is used in place of σ. In Chapter 3, we used $s_{\bar{X}}$ as the symbol for the standard error of the mean. Now we use $s(\bar{X}_1 - \bar{X}_2)$ or $s_{\bar{X}_1} - s_{\bar{X}_2}$, as the symbol for the standard error for the *t*-statistic.

Returning to our example, we use the following formula for the *t*-test to analyze the group differences

$$t = \frac{(\bar{X}_1 - \bar{X}_2) - (\mu_1 - \mu_2)}{s(\bar{X}_1 - \bar{X}_2)}$$

In the numerator, $(\bar{X}_1 - \bar{X}_2)$ represents the difference between the means of two groups. In our example, it would be $(15.10 - 9.78)$. The term $(\mu_1 - \mu_2)$ is based upon the null hypothesis, which assumes that the two populations are not different and therefore the difference is equal to zero. So $(\mu_1 - \mu_2) = 0$.

In this formula, the denominator represents the "pooled" variance of both groups and is appropriate, because their variances were not different. The denominator is, then, the appropriate standard errror for this *t*-statistic. The basic formula for this standard error is

$$s(\bar{X}_1 - \bar{X}_2) = \sqrt{\left(\frac{\Sigma x_1^2 + \Sigma x_2^2}{n_1 + n_2 - 2}\right)\left(\frac{1}{n_1} + \frac{1}{n_2}\right)}$$

where

$\Sigma x_1^2 =$ sum of squares of group 1
$\Sigma x_2^2 =$ sum of squares of group 2
$n_1 =$ the number of scores in group 1
$n_2 =$ the number of scores in group 2

When the two groups have equal ns, the formula is simplified to

$$s(\overline{X}_1 - \overline{X}_2) = \sqrt{\frac{\Sigma\chi_1^2 + \Sigma\chi_2^2}{n(n-1)}}$$

To find the sum of squares for each group, we use the familiar formula. For Group 1, we use

$$\Sigma\chi_1^2 = \Sigma X_1^2 - \frac{(\Sigma X_1)^2}{n_1}$$

for Group 2, we use

$$\Sigma\chi_2^2 = \Sigma X_2^2 - \frac{(\Sigma X_2)^2}{n_2}$$

The calculation of these sums of squares and their application in the t-test formula are demonstrated in Table 8-3. The sum of squares for group 1 is 164.90, and the sum of squares for group 2 is 135.56. Entering these figures into the denominator and the means of the groups into the numerator of the t-test formula, we calculate a t of 2.76.

INTERPRETING THE t-STATISTIC

We now compare this value to the distribution of t values for our df. Because we have two groups, each group having a mean, we calculate the df according to the following formula:

$$df = (n_1 + n_2) - 2, \quad \text{or} \quad df = \text{total } n - 2$$

For our example, we have

$$df = (10 + 9) - 2$$
$$df = 19 - 2$$
$$df = 17$$

Using the table in Appendix G, we find that a t-value of 2.76 with 17 df falls between the probability levels of .01 and .005 for a one-tailed test; that is, the difference that occurred between our two group means would occur by chance alone, not even 1 time in 100.

We have used the one-tailed distribution because we hypothesized a difference in a particular direction. We hypothesized that the intervention group would have higher scores than the control group. If we had not made a directional hypothesis, we would have based our interpretation on the two-tailed distribution.

We set our desired alpha level at .05; therefore, we would reject the null hypothesis and conclude that our groups are significantly different. We conclude that the experimental group has significantly higher recovery scores than the control group.

Table 8-3   Calculation of Pooled *t*-test

Group 1 Experimental	Group 2 Control
$\bar{X}_1 = 15.10$	$\bar{X}_1 = 9.78$
$n_1 = 10$	$n_1 = 9$
$\Sigma X_1 = 151$	$\Sigma X_2 = 88$
$\Sigma X_1^2 = 2445$	$\Sigma X_2^2 = 996$
$\Sigma_{X_1^2} = 2445 - \dfrac{(151)^2}{10}$	$\Sigma_{X_2^2} = 996 - \dfrac{(88)^2}{9}$
$= 164.90$	$= 135.56$

$$t = \frac{(\bar{X}_1 - \bar{X}_2) - (\mu_1 - \mu_2)}{\sqrt{\left(\dfrac{\Sigma_{X_1^2} + \Sigma_{X_2^2}}{n_1 + n_2 - 2}\right)\left(\dfrac{1}{n_1} + \dfrac{1}{n_2}\right)}}$$

$$t = \frac{(15.10 - 9.78) - (0)}{\sqrt{\left(\dfrac{164.90 + 135.56}{10 + 9 - 2}\right)\left(\dfrac{1}{10} + \dfrac{1}{9}\right)}}$$

$$= \frac{5.32}{\sqrt{\left(\dfrac{300.46}{17}\right)(0.21)}} = \frac{5.32}{\sqrt{(17.67)(0.21)}}$$

$$= \frac{5.32}{\sqrt{3.71}} = \frac{5.32}{1.93} = 2.76$$

CALCULATING THE "SEPARATE" *t*-TEST

If the variances for the two groups were not the same, we would use a more conservative formula, because it would be an error to "pool" different variances. The formula for this *t*-test is

$$t = \frac{(\bar{X}_1 - \bar{X}_2) - (\mu_1 - \mu_2)}{\sqrt{\dfrac{s_1^2}{n_1} + \dfrac{s_2^2}{n_2}}}$$

where

$$s_1^2 = \text{variance for Group 1}$$
$$s_2^2 = \text{variance for Group 2}$$

To demonstrate the use of this formula we will use the same example that we used for the "pooled" formula.

$$t = \frac{(15.10 - 9.78) - (0)}{\sqrt{\dfrac{18.32}{10} + \dfrac{16.94}{9}}}$$

$$t = \frac{5.32}{\sqrt{1.832 + 1.88}}$$

$$t = \frac{5.32}{1.93}$$

$$t = 2.76$$

Here, because there was no significant difference between the group variances, the t-statistic is the same as that calculated using the pooled formula.

The distribution of this test is not the same as the t-distribution. However, by modifying the df, we can interpret the results as we would the t-statistic. To obtain the appropriate tabled value with which to compare the t-statistic, you take the *average* of the t-values obtained by using the separate df. For example, for Group 1, the df are $9(10 - 1)$, and, for Group 2, they are $8(9 - 1)$.

If we select the .05 level for a one-tailed test, we find (in Appendix G) the tabled value for 9 df is 1.833, and the tabled value for 8 df is 1.860. The tabled value that we should use for the separate formula (if our variances had been unequal) is the average of these two values, or $(1.833 + 1.860)/2 = 1.8465$.

CORRELATED OR PAIRED t-TEST

If the two groups being compared are matched or paired on some basis, we expect that the scores are likely to be similar. Then the chance differences between the two groups will not be as large as when they are drawn independently. In the correlated t-test, a correction is made that has the effect of increasing t, thus making it more likely to find a significant difference if one exists. The formula is as follows:

$$t = \frac{(\overline{X}_1 - \overline{X}_2) - (\mu_1 - \mu_2)}{\sqrt{\dfrac{s_1^2}{n_1} + \dfrac{s_2^2}{n_2} - 2r \left(\dfrac{s_1}{\sqrt{n_1}}\right)\left(\dfrac{s_2}{\sqrt{n_2}}\right)}}$$

Where s_1^2 and s_2^2 are the group variances and s_1 and s_2 are the standard deviations, which of course are the square roots of the variances. The correlated t-test uses the pooled estimate of variance, so we do not have to decide whether to use a separate or pooled formula.

Let us use the data in Table 8-4 to demonstrate the calculation of the correlated t-test. We have 100 subjects who took a pre-test and a post-test. The correlation

Table 8-4   Data for Correlated t-test ($n = 100$, $r = 0.50$)

Pre-test Scores (1)	Post-test Scores (2)
$\overline{X}_1 = 20$	$\overline{X}_2 = 15$
$s_1^2 = 81$	$s_2^2 = 64$
$s_1 = 9$	$s_2 = 8$

$$t = \frac{20 - 15}{\sqrt{\dfrac{81}{100} + \dfrac{64}{100} - (2)(.5)\left(\dfrac{9}{\sqrt{100}}\right)\left(\dfrac{8}{\sqrt{100}}\right)}} = \frac{5}{\sqrt{.81 + .64 - 1(.9)(.8)}}$$

$$= \frac{5}{\sqrt{0.0064 - 0.72}} = \frac{5}{\sqrt{0.7136}} = \frac{5}{0.845} = 5.917$$

between these two measures is .50. Applying those numbers to our formula, we have a t of 5.917. The df associated with this formula are the number of pairs minus 1. Here we have 100 pairs of scores, so our $df = 99$. Although 99 df are not given in the table, a t-value of 5.917 exceeds the tabled values for 60 df and therefore is significant.

EXAMPLE OF A COMPUTER PRINTOUT

The example in Figure 8-1 was produced by SPSS. Here we have two groups. Group 1 is composed of RNs, and Group 2 is composed of aides. The two groups are compared on three variables: UNCOM, FRIEND, and UNCER, which are parts of a scale that measures attitudes toward death and dying. UNCOM contains items relating to feeling uncomfortable when with a dying person, FRIEND contains questions relating to the death of a friend, and UNCER's questions relate to one's attitude about death in general. We see that when the two groups are compared on UNCOM, 27 RNs and 66 aides are included in the analysis. The RNs reported a higher mean score (78.3333) on this variable than did the aides (61.9545). The F-value with its associated two-tailed probability tells us whether or not the variances of these two groups are the same on this variable. For UNCOM, $F = 1.42$ and $p = .323$. Since $p > .05$, the variances are *not* significantly different, and the appropriate formula to use is the pooled variance estimate. There we find a t-value of 4.69 with 91 df and a two-tailed probability of .000 ($< .001$). Therefore, RNs reported significantly higher levels of discomfort with dying patients than did the aides.

On the variable FRIEND, the aides scored higher (24.0270) than the RNs (20.7857). The probability level associated with the F-test (test for homogeneity of variance) was significant ($p = .028$). Therefore, the variances of the two groups were *not* equal, and the separate variance estimate should be used. Thus, for this comparison, $t = -2.13$, $df = 71.37$, and two-tailed probability = .036. Aides re-

Figure 8-1 *t*-Tests calculated by SPSS program.

Procedure Cards

```
1         16
T-TEST    GROUPS = TITLE(1,2)/VARIABLES = UNCOM FRIEND UNCER
```

Output

```
ALICE'S DEATH AND DYING STUDY

FILE    NONAME    (CREATION DATE = 01/29/84)
```

GROUP 1 - TITLE EQ   1.
GROUP 2 - TITLE EQ   2.

- - - - - - - - - - - - - - - - - T-TEST - - - - - - - - - - - - - - - - -

VARIABLE	NUMBER OF CASES	MEAN	STANDARD DEVIATION	STANDARD ERROR	F VALUE	2-TAIL PROB.	POOLED VARIANCE ESTIMATE			SEPARATE VARIANCE ESTIMATE		
							T VALUE	DEGREES OF FREEDOM	2-TAIL PROB.	T VALUE	DEGREES OF FREEDOM	2-TAIL PROB.
UNCOM												
GROUP 1	27	78.3333	13.416	2.582								
					1.42	0.323	4.69	91	0.000	5.04	57.27	0.000
GROUP 2	66	61.9545	15.993	1.969								
FRIEND												
GROUP 1	28	20.7857	5.965	1.127								
					2.15	0.028	-1.80	100	0.074	-2.13	71.37	0.036
GROUP 2	74	24.0270	8.751	1.017								
UNCER												
GROUP 1	30	8.2000	4.180	0.763								
					1.16	0.667	-0.31	112	0.760	-0.32	54.73	0.752
GROUP 2	84	8.4881	4.503	0.491								

ported being more uncomfortable with a dying friend than did RNs. The table gives two-tailed probabilities. If you want one-tailed probabilities, you simply divide the tabled value by 2. For example, if we had hypothesized ahead of time that aides would have higher scores on this variable, we would take the two-tailed probability .036 and divide it by 2 to get the one-tailed level (.036/2 = .018). We could now say that the difference (one-tailed) was significant at the .018 level.

On the UNCER variable, the variances were equal and the groups did not differ significantly. The correlated or paired *t*-test is reported similarly except that the correlation between the two variables is given and only the pooled variance estimate of the *t*-test is given.

EXAMPLE FROM PUBLISHED RESEARCH

A study by Barsevick and Llewellyn (1982) compared the anxiety-reducing potential of two techniques of bathing. The two techniques were the conventional bed bath and the "towel bath." In the latter, a 7-foot towel is soaked in a preheated antiseptic solution that contains both cleansing and softening agents. Rinsing is not required. The sample was further subdivided into two groups: those having invasive procedures, and those with unrelieved pain.

Hypotheses

There were five hypotheses, but only three are presented here.

1. After treatment, the group receiving a towel bath will have lower anxiety scores than patients receiving a conventional bed bath.
2. Within the invasive procedure group, the towel bath group will have lower anxiety scores than the conventional bath group.
3. Within the unrelieved pain group, the towel bath group will have lower anxiety scores than the conventional bath group.

Data Gathered

Patients who fell into one of two categories (having invasive procedures or having unrelieved pain) were identified. Subjects who met the initial criteria were then randomly assigned to either the conventional bath or the towel bath group. One hundred and five hospitalized patients participated in the study. The State-Trait Anxiety Inventory was used.

Tabular Presentation of Results

Table 8-5 contains the results related to the three hypotheses. In the overall results, we see that the groups had similar anxiety scores before bathing ($t = -.74$,

Table 8-5   Two-Sample t-Tests on State Anxiety Scores

Overall Results

	Mean Raw Score Towel Bath Group	Mean Raw Score Conventional Bath Group	t	p
Pre-bath	41.89	44.00	−0.74	0.461
Immediate Post-bath	32.63	37.89	−2.04	0.045*
One Hour Post-bath	35.35	39.35	−1.37	0.175

Invasive Procedure Group

	Mean Raw Score Towel Bath Group	Mean Raw Score Conventional Bath Group	t	p
Pre-bath	38.50	44.08	−1.45	0.15
Immediate Post-bath	31.10	40.46	−2.68	0.01*
One Hour Post-bath	32.79	42.00	−2.40	0.02*

Unrelieved Pain Group

	Mean Raw Score Towel Bath Group	Mean Raw Score Conventional Bath Group	t	p
Pre-bath	45.81	42.62	0.85	0.40
Immediate Post-bath	34.39	36.19	−0.59	0.56
One Hour Post-bath	38.58	38.00	0.15	0.88

* $p = 0.05$
From Barsevick, A., Llewellyn, J. (1982). A comparison of the anxiety-reducing potential of two techniques of bathing. *Nursing Reserach, 31*(1), 22–27.

$p = .461$). Immediately after the bath, the towel group had lower state anxiety scores ($t = −2.04$, $p = .045$). One hour later, there was no significant difference between these two groups.

In the invasive procedure group, the towel group had lower scores immediately after the bath and 1 hour later. In the unrelieved pain group, there were no differences between the two bath groups at any time.

Description of Results

Hypothesis 1 was supported in relation to the immediate post-bath period, but not in terms of 1-hour post-bath. Hypothesis 2 for the invasive group was supported at both time periods. Hypothesis 3 was not supported. Because none of the groups were significantly different in terms of anxiety scores prior to the bath, one can say that the random assignment worked; that is, the groups really were equivalent in terms of their levels of anxiety before the experimental intervention.

Conclusions

"The towel bath cannot be recommended over the conventional bed bath for the relief of anxiety, especially for patients with unrelieved pain. For patients antici-pating invasive procedures, there is evidence that the towel bath may be more effective, but further testing is suggested. The towel bath was evaluated for its effect on anxiety level. From this study, it is not possible to make any judgments concern-ing the value of the towel bath for cleansing or comfort." (Barsevick & Llewellyn, 1982, p. 27)

SUMMARY

The *t*-test is a statistical method for comparing differences between two groups. The *t*-statistic is very similar to the *z*-statistic. It uses an estimate of the population parameters and thereby is substituted for the *z*-statistic when these parameters are unknown. The test requires interval or ratio measurement of the variable on which the groups are being compared. The test assumes that the variable is normally distributed in the populations from which the samples are drawn and that the samples have equivalent variances. The *t*-test is particularly useful in experimental and quasi-experimental designs in which an experimental and control group are compared.

EXERCISES FOR CHAPTER 8

1. A study was designed to evaluate the effects of relaxation therapy on blood pressure in hypertensive patients. In the study, 50 subjects were randomly assigned to either the relaxation group ($n = 25$) or to a control group ($n = 25$). The following results of the measurement of diastolic pressure were obtained:

Experimental Group	Control
$\overline{X} = 77$	$\overline{X} = 82$
$\Sigma \chi^2 = 1536.64$	$\Sigma \chi^2 = 384.16$

Accept the .05 level of significance for alpha and test the following hypothesis: Relaxation therapy significantly reduces diastolic blood pressure.

2. What are the t-values required to reach significance in each of the following cases (assume use of the pooled t-test):

	p	n	Tail	t-Value
Case 1	.05	15	one-tailed	_____
Case 2	.05	15	two-tailed	_____
Case 3	.01	28	one-tailed	_____
Case 4	.01	28	two-tailed	_____
Case 5	.01	122	two-tailed	_____

3. In an experiment on the effects of a particular anti-anxiety drug, the following data were collected on days-at-work for two groups of phobic patients. It was hypothesized that the drug group would work more days than the placebo group.

Drug Group

$\Sigma X_1 = 324$
$\Sigma X_1^2 = 6516$
$n_1 = 17$

Placebo Group

$\Sigma X_2 = 256$
$\Sigma X_2^2 = 4352$
$n_2 = 16$

Using $p = .05$, draw the appropriate conclusions concerning the effect of the drug on days at work.

4. On a developmental scale, children raised in an orphanage were compared with those cared for in foster-care settings. Children were measured in terms of age in months when interaction with others was evident. The following data were collected.

Orphanage Group	Foster-Care Group
9	6
6	7
8	7
8	9
9	8

Write a research question for this study and draw the appropriate conclusions.

5. Suppose you planned an experiment to measure the effectiveness of patient teaching in reducing length of hospital stay in adult diabetics. To conduct the

study, you randomly assigned 29 diabetic patients to either the experimental or control group.

At the conclusion of your study, you presented the data. First you wished to show that random assignment had indeed produced groups equivalent on age, number of years with disease, and general capacity to learn.

For each of these variables, what *t*-value would you hope to get when you did your analysis? Why?

6. You believe that you have developed a cure for baldness. Your subjects are 20 sets of bald, male, identical twins. The twins in each set are randomly assigned to either the experimental or control group. After treatment, an independent observer rates the subjects on a 20-point scale, where 0 equals completely bald, and 20 equals a full head of hair. Using the following data, test the hypothesis that your treatment will significantly increase hair growth.

$$r = .95$$

Experimental Group   **Control Group**

$\overline{X} = 15$ $\overline{X} = 5$

$s^2 = 11$ $s^2 = 9$

CHAPTER 9

Differences Among Group Means: One-Way Analysis of Variance

Madelon A. Visintainer and Barbara Hazard Munro

OBJECTIVES FOR CHAPTER 9

After reading this chapter and completing the exercises, you should be able to

1. Determine when analysis of variance is the appropriate statistical method to use.
2. Calculate a one-way analysis of variance.
3. Explain the use of post-hoc tests.
4. Report the results of one-way analysis of variance in a summary table.
5. Interpret the output produced by the SPSS ONEWAY program.

Many times, a clinical research question involves a comparison of several groups on a particular measure. When the measure is represented by interval- or ratio-level data, we want to determine whether or not the groups vary from one another in their distribution of scores. In Chapter 8, we discussed the *t*-test as a method for examining the difference between *two* groups. The basic *t*-test compared two means in relation to the distribution of the differences between pairs of means drawn from a random sample. When we have more than two groups and are interested in the differences among the set of groups, we are dealing with different combinations of pairs of means. If we chose to analyze the differences by *t*-test analysis, we would need to do a number of *t*-tests. Suppose, for example, that we had four different groups—A, B, C, and D—that we wished to compare on a particular variable. If we were interested in the differences among the four groups we would need to do a *t*-test for each of the possible pairs that exist in the four groups. We would have A vs. B, A vs. C, A vs. D, B vs. C, B vs. D, and C vs. D. In all, we would have six separate comparisons, each requiring a separate analysis.

The problem with conducting such multiple group comparison is related to the underlying concept of statistical analysis. Each test is based on the probability that the *null hypothesis is true*. Therefore, each time that we run a test, we are running the risk of a Type I error. The probability level we set as the point at which we reject the null hypothesis is also the level of risk that we decide we are comfortable with. If that level is .05, we are accepting the risk that 5 of 100 times our rejection of the null hypothesis will be in error.

However, when we calculate multiple t-tests on independent samples that are being measured on the same variable, the rate of error increases exponentially by the number of tests conducted. For example, with our four-group problem, the error rate increases to 18 of 100 times, a substantial increase in risk of incorrectly rejecting the null hypothesis.*

Instead of using a series of individual comparisons, we examine the differences among the groups through an analysis that considers the variation across all groups at once. This test is the Analysis of Variance (ANOVA).

The question answered by the ANOVA test is whether group means differ from each other. For example, Munro and Krauss (1985) studied the success of non-traditional students in a graduate nursing program. The three groups of students admitted to a 2-year Master's program in nursing included RNs with a bachelor's degree in nursing, RNs with a non-nursing bachelor's degree, and college graduates (non-nurses) who had spent 1 year in pre-specialty nursing education. The question was whether or not these three groups of students would do equally well in the Master's program. To answer that question, ANOVA was used to compare the three groups on their clinical and theoretical grade point averages at the end of the first and second year of the Master's program. Essentially, what was done was to determine whether or not the mean scores of these groups differed significantly from each other. In fact, there were no differences; these three groups did equally well in clinical and theoretical courses.

TYPE OF DATA REQUIRED

In ANOVA, the independent variable(s) are at the nominal level. A "one-way" ANOVA means that there is only *one* independent variable (often called *factor*). That independent variable has two or more levels. Sex would be a variable with two levels, whereas race, religion, and so on may have varying numbers of levels depending on how the variable is defined. "Two-way" ANOVA indicates two independent variables, and n-way ANOVA indicates that the number of independent variables is defined by "n."

---

* The calculation of the rate of Type I errors is determined by the following formula:

$$1 - (1 - \alpha)^t$$

where

α = the level of significance for the tests
t = the number of test comparisons used

In our example, the calculation would give us $1 - (1 - .05)^4 = .18$.

The dependent variable should be continuous, that is, should be interval or ratio level. It is possible to extend the concept of ANOVA to multiple analyses of variance (MANOVA) where there is more than one dependent variable. (However, a full description of MANOVA is beyond the scope of this book.)

ASSUMPTIONS

Analysis of variance has been shown to be fairly "robust." This means that even if the assumptions are not rigidly adhered to, the results may still be close to the truth.

The assumptions for ANOVA are the same as those for the t-test; that is, continuous data should be used for the dependent variable, the groups should be mutually exclusive (independent of each other), the dependent variable should be normally distributed, and the groups should have equal variances (homogeneity of variance requirement).

ONE-WAY ANALYSIS OF VARIANCE

Here we have one independent categorical variable with "n" levels and one continuous dependent variable. Let's consider an example. Suppose clinicians in a nursing home were interested in helping patients with Alzheimer's disease to increase orientation and self care. To that end, two experimental conditions were evaluated against the usual conditions in the care facility. The *first* condition involved increased stimulation within the patients' rooms through music and colors, along with clocks and calendars. The *second* experimental condition involved periodic "orienting sessions" with the patients in which they were told the time, day of week, and season and were reminded of where they were, who had visited, and so on. The *control* condition involved the usual care on the unit. One outcome measure was an evaluation of the patient's orientation on a test of memory and problem solving. It was hypothesized that the groups would differ significantly on the outcome measure, but specific group differences were not specified. The investigators randomly assigned 30 patients in the same stage of Alzheimer's disease to one of the three conditions. Table 9-1 contains the results of the evaluation on the test measure.

The question now is whether the groups score differently on the orientation measure. If the groups differ in their scores, the question is "Which groups are different from which other groups?" That is, where is the difference?

THE STATISTICAL QUESTION
IN ANALYSIS OF VARIANCE

To answer the research question, we will use ANOVA. The statistical question in ANOVA is based on the null hypothesis: the assumption that all groups are equal, drawn from the same population. Any difference found comes from a sampling difference that is random in nature.

Table 9-1   Scores on the Orientation Measure Across Groups

Control Condition	Increased Stimulation	Orienting Sessions
68	78	94
63	69	82
58	58	73
51	57	67
41	53	66
40	52	62
34	48	60
27	46	54
20	42	50
18	27	32
$\overline{X} = 42.0$	$X = 53.0$	$\overline{X} = 64.0$
$s = 17.66$	$s = 14.12$	$s = 17.19$

To test the null hypothesis, we will consider the variation in the scores and compare the amount of variation that we find in our groups with that which occurs when random numbers from the same population are used, that is, when the null hypothesis is true. To do this, we must consider the variability of the scores.

SOURCE OF VARIANCE

Under the null hypothesis, all groups are from the same population, and each of their scores also comes from the same population of measures. Any variability of scores can be looked at in two ways: First, the scores vary from each other in their own group, and, second, the groups vary from each other. The first variation is called *within-group variation*; the second variation is called *between-group variation*. Together the two types of variation add up to the *total variation*.

It is often confusing to students when we say that ANOVA tells us whether or not the means of groups differ significantly and then proceed to talk about analyzing variance. The *t*-test was clearly a test of mean difference, because the difference between the two means was contained in the numerator of the *t*-test formula. It is important to understand how analyzing the variability of groups on some measure can tell us whether or not their measures of central tendency (means) differ.

In analysis of variance, the variance of each group is measured separately; then all the subjects are "lumped" together and the variance of the total group is computed. If the variance of the total group (total variation) is about the same as the average of the variances of the separate groups (within group variation), the *means* of the separate groups are not different. That is so because if total variation is the sum of within group variation and between group variation and if within group variation and total variation are equal, there is no between group variation. Hopefully, this will become more clear in the diagrams that follow. If, on the other hand, the variance of the total group is much larger than the average variation within the separate groups, a significant mean difference exists between at least two of the subgroups. In that case, the within group variation does not equal total variation. The difference between them must equal the between group variation.

To visualize the difference in the types of variation, consider the three groups in the experiment described above. Suppose that the three conditions yielded widely different scores, so different that there was no overlap between the three groups in terms of the outcome measure (Fig. 9-1). We could then represent our three groups in terms of their relationship to each other and also in terms of a *total group*. Then each group would have its own mean as well as its own distribution around its mean. At the same time, there would be a *grand mean,* which would be a mean for all the groups combined. Now, as we can see from Figure 9-1, we can look at the variation *within* the groups as well as the variation *between* the groups. The combination of the within group and between group variation equals the *total* variation.

The ANOVA test examines the variation and tests whether the between group variation is greater than the within group variation. When the *between* group variance is greater (statistically greater) than the *within* group variance, the means of the groups must be different. On the other hand, when the within group variance is about the same as the between group variance, the groups means are not importantly different. This relationship between the difference among group and the different types of variance is shown in Figure 9-2.

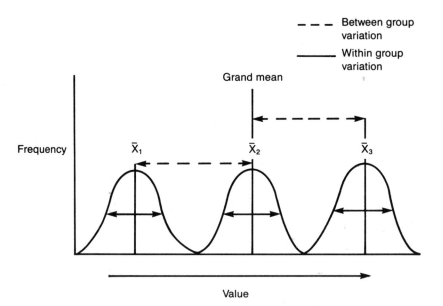

Figure 9-1   Between group and within group variation: the case of no overlap.

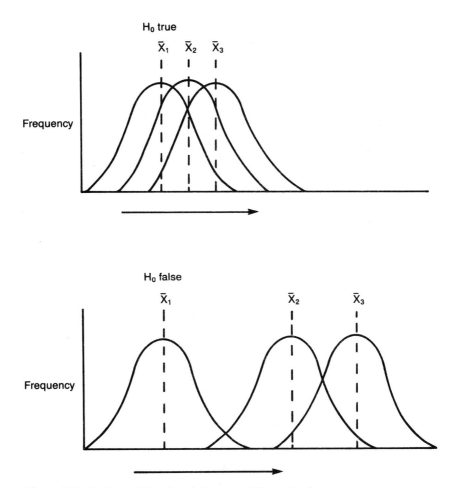

Figure 9-2   Relationship of variation to null hypothesis.

When the null hypothesis is true, the groups overlap to a large extent and the within group variation is greater than the between group variation. When the null hypothesis is false, the groups show little overlapping and the distance between groups is greater.

As we can infer from Figure 9-2, both the group variation and the deviation between group means determine the likelihood that the null hypothesis is true. More explicitly, when the variation within a group or groups is great, the difference between the groups must be greater than when the distribution within groups is narrow in order to reject the null hypothesis (Fig. 9-3). In the same way, when the group distributions are narrow (low within group variance), relatively small between group differences will be significant.

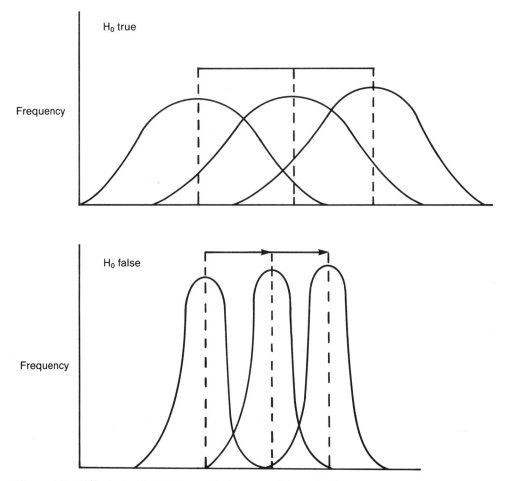

Figure 9-3   Effect of within-group variation on null hypothesis.

THE MEASURE OF VARIANCE:
SUMS OF SQUARES

The concept of the kinds of variation we find when examining scores within groups has an intuitive as well as a statistical meaning. We have discussed the intuitive meaning as the extent to which the scores within a group vary from each other and the extent to which the groups vary from each other. The statistical concept of this variation involves a quantification of the amount of variation of scores around the mean. We have already defined and used this concept with the term *sum of squares*.

The sum of squares is the sum of the squared deviations of each of the scores around a respective mean. In examining the variation that occurs among several groups, we will be considering several different categories of sum of squares, one for each type of variation. In this section, we will define each of the types of sums of squares and consider the formulas.

The Sum of Squares for Total Variation: SS_{tot}

The total sum of squares is equal to the sum of the squared deviations of each score in all groups from the grand mean. The total sum of squares is expressed by the following equation:

$$SS_{tot} = \Sigma(X - \overline{X}_{tot})^2 = \Sigma\chi^2_{tot}$$

To calculate the total sum of squares, we must subtract the mean of the total sample from each individual score, square the deviations, and then sum them. As we can see from the formula, we will have one calculation for each subject in the study. The total sum of squares represents the basis of the null hypothesis that all the subjects belong to one population, which is described by the grand mean.

The Sum of Squares for Within Group Variation: SS_w

The within group variation is the total of the variation that occurs in each subgroup. It is calculated by finding the sum of squares for each group separately and then summing the results. We represent the formula for the within group variation by the following equation:

$$SS_w = SS_{w1} + SS_{w2} + SS_{w3} + SS_{wk}$$

where SS_{wk} equals the last group in the set included in the analysis. The calculation of each individual group sum of squares follows the familiar formula discussed in Chapters 2, 5, and 6. For example, the sum of squares for Group 1 is

$$SS_{w1} = \Sigma(X_1 - \overline{X}_1)^2 = \Sigma\chi^2_1,$$

for Group 2

$$SS_{w2} = \Sigma(X_2 - \overline{X}_2)^2 = \Sigma\chi^2_2$$

and so on.

Applying this formula to our three-group example, we see that the within group variation follows this equation:

$$SS_w = SS_{w1} + SS_{w2} + SS_{w3},$$

or

$$SS_w = \Sigma(X_1 - \overline{X}_1)^2 + \Sigma(X_2 - \overline{X}_2)^2 + \Sigma(X_3 - \overline{X}_3)^2$$
$$= \Sigma\chi^2_1 + \Sigma\chi^2_2 + \Sigma\chi^2_3$$

In calculating the within group variation, we add together the sum of squares of each of the groups.

The Sum of Squares for Between Group Variation: SS_b

The between group variation examines how each of the groups varies from the grand mean. For this calculation, we use group means as representative of the individual groups. The between group variation examines the variation of the group means from the grand mean. First, we find the squared deviation of each group mean from the grand mean: $(\overline{X}_g - \overline{X}_{tot})^2$. We will have one such calculation for each group.

Then, because the weight of the difference of any mean from the grand mean is influenced by the number of the scores in the group, we *weight the difference* by the size of each group $n_g(\overline{X}_g - \overline{X}_{tot})^2$. Finally, we sum the weighted deviations

$$SS_b = \Sigma\, n_g(\overline{X}_g - \overline{X}_{tot})^2$$

where

$$n_g = \text{the } n \text{ size of each group}$$
$$\overline{X}_g = \text{the mean of each group}$$

Considering our three-group example again, we have the following equation:

$$SS_b = n_1(\overline{X}_1 - \overline{X}_{tot})^2 + n_2(\overline{X}_2 - \overline{X}_{tot})^2 + n_3(\overline{X}_3 - \overline{X}_{tot})^2$$

In summary, these three sums of squares define the three different kinds of variation that exist when subjects are members of different groups and measured on a single variable. They include the *total variation* of each of the scores around the grand mean, the variation of scores *within* their respective groups, and the deviation *between* groups measured by the deviation of group means from the grand mean. In the next section, we will examine the computational formulas for calculating the sums of squares.

CALCULATION OF SUMS OF SQUARES
USING COMPUTATIONAL FORMULAS

One obvious fact about the formulas that we have discussed is that they entail a long, tedious calculation. An easier formulation is provided for the calculation of sums of squares that is similar to the one presented for the calculation of variance (see Chapter 2). These formulas are derived from the definitional formulas explained above.

We will describe and apply the computational formulas to our example in which patients with Alzheimer's disease were assigned to different intervention groups and then evaluated on a measure of orientation. See Table 9-2 for the data.

From the information provided in Table 9-2, we can calculate the three sums of squares. First, however, we should check the assumption of homogeneity of variance.

Table 9-2   Data for Calculation of One-Way ANOVA

Control Condition		Increased Stimulation		Orienting Sessions	
X_1	X_1^2	X_2	X_2^2	X_3	X_3^2
68	4624	78	6084	94	8836
63	3969	69	4761	82	6724
58	3364	58	3364	73	5329
51	2601	57	3249	67	4489
41	1681	53	2809	66	4356
40	1600	52	2704	62	3844
34	1156	48	2304	60	3600
27	729	46	2116	54	2916
20	400	42	1764	50	2500
18	324	27	729	32	1024
Σs 420	20448	530	29884	640	43618

$$\overline{X}_1 = 42 \qquad\qquad \overline{X}_2 = 53 \qquad\qquad \overline{X}_3 = 64$$

$$\Sigma X_{tot} = \Sigma X_1 + \Sigma X_2 + \Sigma X_3 = 420 + 530 + 640 = 1590$$

$$\Sigma X_{tot}^2 = \Sigma X_1^2 + \Sigma X_2^2 + \Sigma X_3^2 = 20448 + 29884 + 43618 = 93950$$

$$n_{tot} = n_1 + n_2 + n_3 = 10 + 10 + 10 = 30$$

Homogeneity of Variance

Since one of the assumptions underlying the use of ANOVA is that the variances of the groups do not differ significantly from each other, that assumption should be checked. When using computer programs, tests such as Bartlett's and Cochran's tests of homogeneity of variance can be requested. With hand calculation, a simpler measure is to divide the smallest group variance into the largest group variance.

$$F = \frac{\text{largest group variance}}{\text{smallest group variance}}$$

The degrees of freedom (df) are calculated as $ng - 1$ (number in group minus 1), and the F table is used (Appendix E) to determine the significance of this statistic. Using the information in Table 9-2, we calculate the variance for each group. The formula for variance is

$$s^2 = \frac{\Sigma X^2 - \dfrac{(\Sigma X)^2}{n}}{n - 1}$$

For the control group, we have

$$s^2 = \frac{20448 - \dfrac{(420)^2}{10}}{9} = 312$$

For the Increased Stimulation Group, we have

$$s^2 = \frac{29884 - \frac{(530)^2}{10}}{9} = 199.33$$

and, for the Orienting Sessions Group, we have

$$s^2 = \frac{43618 - \frac{(640)^2}{10}}{9} = 295.33$$

Since each of these groups has 10 subjects, the df for each group is $10 - 1 = 9$. Placing the largest variance over the smallest, we have

$$F_{9,9} = \frac{312}{199.33} = 1.565$$

The tabled value in the F-table (Appendix E) for the .05 level (.10 for a two-tailed test) is 3.18; therefore, the variances of the groups do *not* differ and the assumption of homogeneity of variance has been met. We now calculate the sums of squares using the computational formulas.

First we calculate SS_{tot} using the following formula:

$$SS_{tot} = \Sigma X_{tot}^2 - \frac{(\Sigma X_{tot})^2}{n_{tot}}$$

Note that when we calculate the total sum of squares, we treat the scores as though they belong to one large group. We ignore their individual group membership. Every individual score (X) is squared, and the sum of all the squared scores equals ΣX_{total}^2. In our example, that means adding up all the squared scores in all three groups, or, as shown in Table 9-2,

$$\Sigma X_{tot}^2 = \Sigma X_1^2 + \Sigma X_2^2 + \Sigma X_3^2 = 93950$$

The total of all the X scores is ΣX_{total}. In our example, that is $\Sigma X_1 + \Sigma X_2 + \Sigma X_3 = 1590$. There are 30 individuals, 10 in each group, so $n_{total} = 30$. Inserting these figures into the formula for total sums of squares, we have

$$SS_{tot} = 93950 - \frac{(1590)^2}{30}$$
$$SS_{tot} = 93950 - 84270$$
$$SS_{tot} = 9680$$

The total sum of squares is equal to 9680. Next we calculate the SS_b, the between group variation. The formula is

$$SS_b = \Sigma_g \left[\frac{(\Sigma X_g)^2}{n_g} \right] - \frac{(\Sigma X_{tot})^2}{n_{tot}}$$

According to this formula, we work with each group individually. For each group, we find the sum of its scores ΣX; we square the sum and then divide by the respective n. The resulting values for all the groups are added together

$$\Sigma_g \left[\frac{(\Sigma X_g)^2}{n_g} \right]$$

Finally, we subtract the quantity $\dfrac{(\Sigma X_{tot})^2}{n_{tot}}$ from this sum. The term $\dfrac{(\Sigma X_{tot})^2}{n_{tot}}$ is the same as that previously calculated for the SS_{tot}. The formula for SS_b could also be written as follows:

$$SS_b = \left[\frac{(\Sigma X_1)^2}{n_1} + \frac{(\Sigma X_2)^2}{n_2} + \frac{(\Sigma X_3)^2}{n_3} + \cdots \frac{(\Sigma X_k)^2}{n_k} \right] - \frac{(\Sigma X_{tot})^2}{n_{tot}}$$

Following the formula, in our example, we have

$$SS_b = \frac{(420)^2}{10} + \frac{(530)^2}{10} + \frac{(640)^2}{10} - \frac{(1590)^2}{30}$$

$$SS_b = \frac{176400}{10} + \frac{280900}{10} + \frac{409600}{10} - 84270$$

$$SS_b = \frac{866900}{10} - 84270$$

$$SS_b = 2420$$

The between group sum of squares is equal to 2420. Next we find the within sum of squares by subtracting the between value from the total.

$$SS_w = SS_{tot} - SS_b$$
$$SS_w = 9680 - 2420$$
$$SS_w = 7260$$

SS_w can also be calculated independently of SS_b and SS_{total} by using a formula in which the sum of squares is calculated separately for each group and the individual sum of squares are added up to give the within sum of squares. See Table 9-3 for those calculations. The within sum of squares is equal to 7260. We now have the three sums of squares values and are ready to determine whether or not the groups are different. Remember, we will do this by comparing the size of variation between the groups with the size of variation within the groups. Although we will use the sums of squares to make this comparison, we will not use them directly.

We can see that the size of the sum of squares is related to the number of scores used in the calculation. Because the within sum of squares will always include the total sample, it will always be larger than the between group sum of squares, which is based on the number of groups. To correct for the number of scores involved, we divide the sums of squares by the df. The analysis of the variance from the different sources will give us the test of the null hypothesis.

Table 9-3   Calculation of Within Sum of Squares

$$SS_w = \Sigma_g \left[\Sigma X_g^2 - \frac{(\Sigma X_g)^2}{n_g} \right]$$

$$\Sigma\chi_1^2 = \Sigma X_1^2 - \frac{(\Sigma X_1)^2}{n_1}$$

$$= 20448 - \frac{(420)^2}{10}$$

$$= 20448 - \frac{176400}{10}$$

$$= 2808$$

$$\Sigma\chi_2^2 = \Sigma X_2^2 - \frac{(\Sigma X_2)^2}{n_2}$$

$$= 29884 - \frac{(530)^2}{10}$$

$$= 1794$$

$$\Sigma\chi_3^2 = \Sigma X_3^2 - \frac{(\Sigma X_3)^2}{n_3}$$

$$= 43618 - \frac{(640)^2}{10}$$

$$= 2658$$

Thus, $SS_w = \Sigma\chi_1^2 + \Sigma\chi_2^2 + \Sigma\chi_3^2$

$$= 2808 + 1794 + 2658$$

$$= 7260$$

CALCULATING THE VARIANCE: THE MEAN SQUARE

The first step in using the sums of squares is to convert them to a variance term. As we recall from the calculation of variance for a *sample*, variance is equal to the sum of squares divided by *n*, the size of the sample. Because we are using these samples as estimates of *populations*, we divide by the *df*, rather than by *n*. In this way, we correct for the bias that occurs from the estimate. This corrected estimate of the variance is called the *mean square*. The mean square is simply the term used for variance.

Each of the different sums of squares has its own mean square, or variance, and each has its own *df*. These are based on the way in which the respective sum of squares was calculated. The two variance terms that we are interested in are the *between variance* and the *within variance*. We calculate these by dividing the SS_b and SS_w terms by their respective *df*.

In other words, the between group mean square (variance) is equal to the between group sum of squares divided by the between group *df*. We represent this symbolically by the following:

$$MS_b = SS_b/df_b$$

Likewise, the within group mean square (variance) is equal to the within group sum of squares divided by the within group *df*. We represent this term as

$$MS_w = SS_w/df_w$$

Degrees of Freedom

The *df* for the between group variance is equal to the number of groups minus one. This is represented in the following way:

$$df_b = k - 1,$$

where *k* equals the number of groups. In this example, we have

$$df_b = 3 - 1,$$

or 2 *df* for our between group variance.

The *df* for the within variance is equal to the *df* for each group added together. Each individual group has *df* equal to the *n* size of the group minus one. We can represent that with the shorthand formula:

$$df_w = n_{tot} - k,$$

where n_{tot} equals the total *n* across all groups, and *k* again equals the number of groups. For our example, we have

$$df_w = 30 - 3,$$

or 27 *df* for our within group variance.

Now we can calculate the mean square terms for the between and within variation using the appropriate *df*. The mean square term for the between group variation is calculated following the formula:

$$MS_b = SS_b/df_b$$
$$MS_b = 2420/2$$
$$MS_b = 1210$$

Now we calculate the mean square for the within variation:

$$MS_w = SS_w/df_w$$
$$MS_w = 7260/27$$
$$MS_w = 268.9$$

Note that although the within group sum of squares was much larger than the between group sum of squares, the mean square for the between group is now larger than that for the within group. Indeed, in order for there to be significant group differences, that is in order for the null hypothesis to be false, the between mean square must be substantially larger than the within mean square.

We determine the statistical significance of the difference between the between group and within group variance by using a ratio. We compare the between mean square to the within mean square. The ratio we use is the F ratio, or the F test.

Testing the Difference Among Groups:
The F Ratio

To determine whether the between group difference is great enough to reject the null hypothesis, we compare it statistically to the within group variance. The F ratio, which has been described before and used in Chapter 8 to test for the homogeneity of variance, is the test of choice.

Simply, we create a ratio with the between mean square as the numerator and the within mean square as the denominator. The result is called an F *value*. It is represented in the following way:

$$F = MS_b/MS_w .$$

For our example, we obtain the following F result:

$$F = MS_b/MS_w$$
$$F = 1210/268.9$$
$$F = 4.50$$

We interpret the F value by comparing it to the values obtained when the null hypothesis is true and the scores randomly selected from one single population. To make the interpretation, we use the table that presents the F distributions (Appendix E). We locate the critical values for comparison by using the df for the between and within mean squares.

In the example, the between df were 2 and the within df were 27. We locate the between *df on the row across the top of the table*, and we locate the within *df on the column on the left side of the table*. With these points as coordinates, we locate two critical values for F.

The top value (in light print) is 3.35. This is the value required to reject the null hypothesis at a probability level of .05 (given a one-tailed test). The value below (in bold print) is 5.49, the value required to reject the null hypothesis at the .01 level.

The value of 4.50 is greater than the value required to reach an alpha of .05.

Therefore, we can reject the null hypothesis at the .05 level. We say we have reached a probability level of "less than .05." However, our value is lower than that needed to reject the null hypothesis at the .01 level. Therefore, our probability level is "less than .05 but greater than .01."

In summary, we obtained an F value of 4.50. We therefore rejected the null hypothesis that there were no differences between the groups, and we concluded that the groups were different; that is, the interventions made a difference in the patients' orientation as measured on our assessment.

Before we discuss how we find out which groups are different, let us examine how we display the findings from the ANOVA.

DISPLAYING THE RESULTS: THE SUMMARY OF ANALYSIS OF VARIANCE

The results of the calculations leading to the F ratio are summarized in a table form that is standard for presenting ANOVA results. This presentation of the results is called the *Summary of ANOVA* table. The results for the calculations of our problem are shown in Table 9-4 as a model of the usual table form.

As can be seen from Table 9-4, the three categories of sums of squares are presented, along with the *df* for the between and within variance. The *MS*, or mean square, terms are also presented. This format is a complete presentation of the ANOVA results. As can also be seen, with the sums of squares presented and the respective *df*, we can calculate the *MS* terms and the F directly; that is, we calculate the *MS* by dividing the *SS* term by its respective *df* (e.g., $MS_b = 2420/2$). We calculate the F ratio by dividing the between *MS* value by the within *MS* value ($F = 1220.0/268.9$).

In other standard presentations of ANOVA summary tables, the within variance is sometimes called the *error variance,* or *error term.* This terminology reflects the assumption of the analysis of variance: The within difference is sampling error or random difference. In addition to the summary table, it is often helpful to include a table in your results section that shows the means and standard deviations for the scores of each group. One can then see which group scored higher and by how much. To test for significant differences between the groups, we must use other measures, however.

Table 9-4   Summary of ANOVA for Alzheimer Study

Source of Variance	SS	df	MS	F	p
Between Group	2420	2	1220.0		
				4.50	.05
Within Group	7260	27	268.9		
Total	*9680*				

MULTIPLE GROUP COMPARISONS
AFTER ANALYSIS OF VARIANCE

When a significant F test is obtained, we are able to reject the null hypothesis that all the groups are from the same population or that all the populations are equal; that is, we are able to state that there is a difference among the groups. However, when more than two groups are being compared, we cannot determine from the F test alone which of the groups differ from each other. In other words, a significant F test does not mean that every group in the analysis is different from every other group. A number of patterns of difference are possible. Some of the groups may be similar, forming a cluster that is different from one other select group. Or, depending on the number of groups being compared, there may be wide deviation between each pair of the groups.

To determine where the significant differences lie, further analysis is required. Here we are confronted with the task of comparing group means. However, if we decide to use the standard t-test, we are again confronted with the possibility of an increased rate of Type I errors. To prevent this from happening, a number of secondary analyses following the computation of the F ratio are available to pinpoint the source of the difference. Two methods will be presented here: one for comparisons between groups of equal size, and one for comparisons between groups with unequal ns.

The Tukey Honestly Significant Difference Test

The first method that will be presented here was devised by Tukey. It is called the *Honestly Significant Difference* test (*HSD* test), or the Tukey test for multiple comparisons. It can be used for comparisons of groups with equal size n.

The *HSD* test is calculated only when there is a significant F test overall. The significant F justifies the multiple comparisons to identify the difference. For the test, we calculate a quantity called the *HSD*. We then compare this quantity to the difference we obtain for any pair of means for groups in our analysis. We conclude that the pairs are significantly different at a given alpha level when the deviation between the means is *equal to* or *greater than* the *HSD* value.

The formula for calculating the *HSD* follows:

$$HSD = q_{\text{alpha}} \sqrt{\frac{MS_w}{n_g}}$$

where

$$MS_w = \text{the within variance}$$
$$n_g = \text{the } n \text{ of } each \text{ group}$$
$$q_{\text{alpha}} = \text{the Studentized range statistic for a}$$
$$\text{particular alpha level}$$

The new term in this formula is the *Studentized range statistic*. It is a value based on the t distributions. These values are found in Appendix H. We use the table by locating the q_{alpha} value specific for the df and k in a particular analysis. As in the ANOVA calculations, k equals the number of groups, and the df equal the total n minus k.

We will use the HSD test for our example to identify which of the different patient groups showed greater orientation. We need the following values:

$$\overline{X}_1 = 42, \qquad \overline{X}_2 = 53, \qquad \overline{X}_3 = 64$$
$$MS_w = 268.9, \qquad df_w = 27, \qquad k = 3$$

The first step is to calculate the absolute differences between each pair of means. These differences are shown in Table 9-5.

Now we compute the HSD value. We will set alpha at .05. In Appendix H, we locate the q value for $df_w = 27$, $k = 3$. We find no value for $df = 27$, so we use the next lower value of 24. This provides a more conservative estimate of HSD. Our q value is equal to 3.53. The test equation can be calculated following the HSD formula:

$$HSD = q_{alpha} \sqrt{\frac{MS_w}{n_g}}$$

$$HSD = 3.53 \sqrt{\frac{268.9}{10}}$$

$$= (3.53)(5.19)$$

$$HSD = 18.32$$

We compare the HSD to the differences between the means (Table 9-5).

We find that only one comparison is equal to or greater than the HSD value of 18.32. That comparison is between the mean of Group 1 and the mean of Group 3 (equal to 22). Therefore, we conclude that Group 1 was significantly different from Group 3 at the .05 level.

Our conclusion for the example is that there was a significant difference in levels of orientation among the groups of patients receiving different treatments (the interpretation of the significant F value). The difference was specifically that the patients who received the Structured Orienting Sessions (Group 3) were signifi-

Table 9-5   Absolute Differences Between Means

	X_1	X_2
X_2	11	—
X_3	22	11

cantly more oriented than patients in the Control Group (Group 1). Patients who received the Increased Stimulation (Group 2) were not significantly different from either the Control or the Structured Intervention Group; their results fell some- where between the other two groups.

We were able to use the *HSD* test in our example because we had obtained a significant *F* test indicating that there was a difference among groups. Furthermore, the groups were of equal size (*ns* = 10). In cases in which the groups are of *unequal* size, we calculate the ANOVA and *F* ratio in the same way. However, we need to use another test to look for multiple comparisons.

The Scheffé Method

We use the Scheffé method when we obtain a significant *F* ratio and the groups are not equal in size. (It can also be used with groups of equal size.) The Scheffé test is a type of *F* test that uses the differences between means to calculate an *F* ratio.

In the Scheffé test, we do not use the *F* table, but instead calculate a "critical value" (*cv* of *F* to use as a standard against which to compare the differences between pairs of means. We calculate the critical value of *F* according to the following formula:

$$F_{cv} = (k - 1)(F_{alpha})$$

where

$$k = \text{the number of groups}$$
$$F_{alpha} = \text{the value of } F \text{ needed to gain significance in the}$$
$$\text{ANOVA (With 2, 27 } df \text{ and a .05 level, it equals 3.35.)}$$

In other words, the F_{alpha} is the value that we used in interpreting the *F* ratio in the ANOVA. In our example, $F_{cv} = (3 - 1)(3.35)$, or $F_{cv} = 6.70$.

After calculating the F_{cv}, we find the differences between the means for the selected pairs according to the following formula:

$$\text{Scheffé value} = \frac{(\overline{X}_1 - \overline{X}_2)^2}{MS_w \left(\dfrac{1}{n_1} + \dfrac{1}{n_2}\right)}$$

where

$$\overline{X}_1 = \text{the mean of a selected group}$$
$$\overline{X}_2 = \text{the mean of another group}$$
$$MS_w = \text{the within variance}$$
$$n_1 = \text{the } n \text{ of the group corresponding to the first mean in the}$$
$$\text{comparison}$$
$$n_2 = \text{the } n \text{ of the group corresponding to the second mean in}$$
$$\text{the comparison}$$

In our example, the Scheffé values would be calculated as follows:
To compare Groups 1 and 2,

$$\text{Scheffé value} = \frac{(42-53)^2}{268.9\left(\frac{1}{10}+\frac{1}{10}\right)} = \frac{121}{53.78} = 2.25$$

To compare Groups 1 and 3,

$$\text{Scheffé value} = \frac{(42-64)^2}{268.9\left(\frac{1}{10}+\frac{1}{10}\right)} = \frac{484}{53.78} = 9.00$$

To compare Groups 2 and 3,

$$\text{Scheffé value} = \frac{(53-64)^2}{268.9\left(\frac{1}{10}+\frac{1}{10}\right)} = \frac{121}{53.78} = 2.25$$

We compare the Scheffé value to the F_{cv}. If the Scheffé value is equal to or larger than the F_{cv}, we conclude that the two groups in the comparison are significantly different from each other.

The Scheffé value for the comparison of Groups 1 and 3 equals 9 and that is larger than the F_{cv}, which, in our example, equaled 6.7. The other two Scheffé values are lower than F_{cv}. Thus, our conclusions here are the same: Group 3 was significantly more oriented than Group 1.

The *HSD* and the Scheffé tests are similar in that a standard is calculated and then comparisons between groups are calculated. The between group differences are then compared to that standard. These tests provide the basis for pinpointing the difference that was suggested by the significant ANOVA.

EXAMPLE OF A COMPUTER PRINTOUT
OF A ONE-WAY ANALYSIS OF VARIANCE

Figure 9-4 contains an example of a one-way analysis of variance created by the SPSS program ONEWAY. The advantage of using that program instead of SPSS's ANOVA is that with ONEWAY, you can request post hoc statistics such as *HSD* and Scheffé test. In this example, we compared the graduating classes of 1979, 1980, and 1981 on their scores on an autobiography written for the Admissions Committee. We have one independent variable, graduating class (GRAD), with three levels: 79, 80, and 81. The dependent variable is the score on the autobiography (TOTAL) that had a potential range of one to four.

The summary table is presented first (①). Since we had three groups, the *df* for the between groups sum of squares is $3-1=2$. The within group *df* is the total n minus the number of groups or $191-3=188$. Dividing the sum of squares by their

(*Text continues on page 196*)

Figure 9-4 Analysis of variance produced by SPSS ONEWAY program.

Procedure Cards

```
1

ONEWAY        TOTAL BY GRAD(79,81)/
              RANGES = SCHEFFE/

STATISTICS    1,3
```

Output

```
YSN ADMISSIONS STUDY                                  06/26/82                PAGE 37

FILE    NONAME    (CREATION DATE = 06/26/82)

---------------------------------------O N E   W A Y---------------------------------------
    VARIABLE      TOTAL      AUTOBIOGRAPHY TOTAL
 BY VARIABLE      GRAD       GRADUATING CLASS
```

ANALYSIS OF VARIANCE

	SOURCE	D.F.	SUM OF SQUARES	MEAN SQUARES	F RATIO	F PROB.
①	BETWEEN GROUPS	2	9.9446	4.9723	9.324	0.0001
	WITHIN GROUPS	188	100.2541	0.5333		
	TOTAL	190	110.1987			

②

GROUP	COUNT	MEAN	STANDARD DEVIATION	STANDARD ERROR	MINIMUM	MAXIMUM	95 PCT CONF INT FOR MEAN		
GRP79	43	2.8140	0.7639	0.1165	2.0000	4.0000	2.5788	TO	3.0491
GRP80	70	3.2429	0.7696	0.0920	2.0000	4.0000	3.0593	TO	3.4264
GRP81	78	3.4103	0.6730	0.0762	2.0000	4.0000	3.2585	TO	3.5620
TOTAL	191	3.2147	0.7616	0.0551	2.0000	4.0000	3.1060	TO	3.3234

TESTS FOR HOMOGENEITY OF VARIANCES

③ COCHRANS C = MAX. VARIANCE/SUM(VARIANCES) = 0.3637, P = 0.784 (APPROX.)
  BARLETT-BOX F =   0.767, P = 0.465
  MAXIMUM VARIANCE / MINIMUM VARIANCE =   1.308

           VARIANCE   TOTAL   AUTOBIOGRAPHY TOTAL
  BY VARIANCE   GRAD   GRADUATING CLASS

MULTIPLE RANGE TEST

SCHEFFE PROCEDURE
RANGES FOR THE 0.050 LEVEL -

④   3.49   3.49

THE RANGES ABOVE ARE TABLE RANGES. THE VALUE ACTUALLY CHANGED COMPARED WITH MEAN(J) - MEAN(I) IS..
  0.5164 * RANGE * SQRT(I/N(I) + 1/N(J))

  (*) DENOTES PAIRS OF GROUPS SIGNIFICANTLY DIFFERENT AT THE 0.050 LEVEL

                      G G G
                      R R R
                      P P P
                      7 8 8
                      9 0 1

MEAN   GROUP

2.8140   GRP79
3.2429   GRP80   *
3.4103   GRP81   *

respective *df* gives the mean squares, and the between groups mean square divided by the within groups mean square equals the *F* ratio. Here the *F* ratio is significant at the .0001 level.

Printed below the summary table are the statistics for the three groups (②). We see that there were 43 members in GRP79, and their mean score on the dependent variable was the lowest (2.8140) of the three groups. Moving toward the right, we see confidence intervals for the respective means.

Next we see tests for homogeneity of variance (③). Cochran's and Bartlett's are both nonsignificant; hence, the assumption of homogeneity of variance is met. If you look up the *F* ratio obtained from dividing the maximum variance by the minimum (1.308), you will find that to be nonsignificant also.

We requested a Scheffé test to determine which of these groups differed from which (④). The class of 1979 with a mean score of 2.8140 on the autobiography scored significantly lower than the classes of 1980 and 1981, which scored 3.2429 and 3.4103, respectively. The scores of the classes of 1980 and 1981 were not significantly different, but it appears that each class is improving in their ability to write an admissions autobiography. Perhaps the word was getting around that the autobiography was an important part of the Admissions Committee's decision-making process.

EXAMPLE OF ONE-WAY ANALYSIS OF VARIANCE FROM PUBLISHED RESEARCH

Question Posed

A study by Lamontagne (1984) examined the relationship between children's locus of control and their preoperative coping behavior. The hypothesis tested was that active coping will be related to degree of internality.

Data Gathered

Data were gathered from 51 children between the ages of 8 and 12 years who were admitted for minor elective surgery. Locus of control was measured as a continuous variable, with higher scores indicating more external orientation. Coping was measured on a scale, with a range of scores from 1 to 10. Those children receiving high scores (8–10) were considered to be *active* copers; those with low scores (1–3) were considered to be *avoidant*; and those in the middle (4–7) showed evidence of both types of coping.

The relationship between the locus of the control score and the coping score was examined using Pearson *r*. There was a significant relationship ($r = -.39$, $p < .01$). Therefore, active coping (high score) is associated with internal locus of control (low score). To clarify the relationship, an ANOVA was performed where the independent variable was coping, and the children were classified into one of three groups: avoidant, middle, or active. The dependent variable was locus of control. Table 9-6 contains the results of this analysis.

Tabular Presentation of Results

In looking at the means and standard deviations, we see that avoiders had the highest mean score on locus of control (were more external), middle type copers had lower scores, and active copers scored lowest of all (were the most internal). With 2 and 48 *df,* an *F* of 3.60 is significant at the .05 level (but not at .01).

Description of Results

The author used the Newman Keuls post hoc procedure. (This post hoc test is somewhat less stringent than the Scheffé test.) The results showed that the active copers had significantly lower locus of control scores than either of the other two groups. The scores of the avoidant and middle groups did not differ significantly. Internal locus of control was related to higher socioeconomic status but not to other demographic variables or to gender.

Conclusions

The results of this study show that children's locus of control orientation may be an important dispositional variable related to how children cope with the stresses of surgery. Patients with internal beliefs are more likely to adopt active coping behaviors, whereas patients with an external orientation are more likely to adopt avoidant strategies. This has important implications for nursing intervention. The type of

Table 9-6 Summary of Analysis of Variance Between Coping Groups on Locus of Control

	$\overline{X}$		SD	
Avoidant	15.33		3.75	
Middle	14.61		4.52	
Active	11.00		4.05	

Source	df	SS	MS	F
Between groups	2	130.66	65.33	3.60
Within groups	48	871.34	18.15	

Note: Higher scores indicate more external locus of control.
$p < 0.05$
From Lamontagne, L. L. (1984). Children's locus of control beliefs as predictors of preoperative coping behavior. *Nursing Research, 33* (2), 76–79, 85.

intervention should be appropriate to the child's coping strategy and the situational demands (Lamontagne, 1984, p. 85).

EXERCISES FOR CHAPTER 9

1. In a study on pain control, investigators tried three different methods of pain management: relaxation, therapeutic touch, and laughter. A total of 33 patients with chronic back pain were assigned to one of these conditions. The effect of each intervention was evaluated by the length of time (in hours) patients remained pain free. The following table presents the scores (rounded to nearest hour) obtained by each subject in the groups.

GROUPS

Relaxation	Therapeutic Touch	Laughter
2	7	5
2	6	8
3	4	6
3	5	7
4	3	7
5	3	8
6	5	6
4	6	5
3	5	5
4	3	6
	4	8
		7

Calculate an ANOVA to determine whether or not the groups are different. Display your results in a summary of ANOVA table. Interpret your results (alpha = .05).

2. For the above problem, use the appropriate test to determine which groups are specifically different from one another at the .05 level. Interpret your results.

3. Patients hospitalized with cardiovascular accidents were randomly assigned to one of three different care programs, which varied in the type of neuro-stimulation provided. The treatment protocols were evaluated in terms of length of time measured in days to resumption of weight-bearing ability. These are the results:

Groups	$\bar{X}$s	ns
I	20	15
II	22	15
III	14	15

Summary of ANOVA

Source	SS	df	MS	F	p
Between	496.04				
Within	2155.20				
Total	2351.24				

Complete the ANOVA table and interpret the results (alpha = .05).

4. For the above problem, find the between group differences and interpret the results. Use the appropriate post hoc test and the .05 level of significance.

CHAPTER 10

Differences Among Group Means: Multifactorial Analysis of Variance

Barbara Hazard Munro

OBJECTIVES FOR CHAPTER 10

After reading this chapter and completing the exercises, you should be able to

1. Discuss the advantages of testing for interactions.
2. Calculate a two-way analysis of variance.
3. Report the results of a multifactorial analysis of variance in a summary table.
4. Interpret the output produced by the SAS GLM program.

TWO-WAY ANALYSIS OF VARIANCE

We have been discussing the use of analysis of variance (ANOVA) with one categorical independent variable (with two or more levels) and one continuous dependent variable. Here we extend the number of independent variables to two or more. There is still just one dependent variable. It is possible to extend ANOVA to the use of more than one dependent variable in a given analysis. Such an analysis is usually referred to as MANOVA (multivariate analysis of variance) and allows the researcher to look for relationships among dependent, as well as among independent, variables. For more information on MANOVA, consult a text such as Finn and Mattson's (1978) *Multivariate Analysis in Educational Research*.

There are great advantages in having more than one independent variable in an ANOVA. One advantage is economy: testing many hypotheses for almost the same cost. The other is the ability to test for *interactions*. Although it is interesting and valuable to learn whether a particular approach works better than another, it may be even more important to find out whether the effect of an approach varies depending on the group of subjects. Testing for an interaction allows us to answer the question of whether or not the results of a given treatment vary depending on the groups or conditions in which it is applied.

For example, in one study, we are measuring the effect of relaxation therapy on several outcome measures for a group of post-myocardial infarction (post-MI) patients. The one-way approach would be to have two equivalent groups of post MI patients (one group would practice relaxation, the other group would not). We could then say whether or not those who practiced relaxation "did better" than those who did not. We wondered, however, whether the basic personality style of the subject would be related to the efficacy of relaxation. If Type A people subject themselves to more stress, would relaxation benefit them more than it would benefit a group of more "relaxed" subjects (Type Bs)? See Table 10-1 for a diagram of this study.

If we treated the variables separately, we could run two one-way analyses of variance; that is, we could see whether treatment approach (relaxation vs. no relaxation) had an effect on that dependent variable and whether personality type (A or B) had an effect. By combining the two independent variables into a two-way analysis of variance, we can still answer the first two questions but can also answer a third: Is there an *interaction* between the two independent variables? Then we would be asking whether relaxation had differing effects depending on whether the subject was Type A or B.

The first question, whether relaxation therapy makes a difference, is answered by comparing the *column* means. That is, cells A and C would be considered as a whole group, representing all those who used relaxation therapy, and cells B and D would constitute the nonrelaxation group. The means of those two groups would be compared to answer the research question.

The second question, whether personality type makes a difference, is answered by comparing the *row* means. Cells A and B include the Type A subjects, and cells C and D are the Type Bs. The mean for the Type As is compared with the mean for the Type Bs to answer the second research question.

The third question, about the interaction between the two independent variables, is answered by comparing the diagonals; that is, the combination for cells A and D is compared with the combination of cells B and C.

Table 10-1   Example of a Two-Way Analysis of Variance

Personality	Treatment		Rows
	Relaxation	*No Relaxation*	*Rows*
Type A	A	B	A and B
Type B	C	D	C and D
Columns	*A and C*	*B and D*	

In this example, we test for two *main effects,* that is, the effects of the independent variables, and the *interaction* between the two independent variables. The independent variables are often called *factors,* and, from that, comes the term *factorial analysis of variance.* Our example is a 2×2 factorial design. Such a designation indicates two independent variables with two levels each and, therefore, 2×2, or 4, individual cells. The results of such a study would be displayed in a format such as the one shown in Table 10-2.

COMPUTATION OF TWO-WAY ANALYSES OF VARIANCE

The data for computation of a two-way ANOVA is outlined in Table 10-3. This is a 2×2 design in which we have a treatment variable with two levels, A and B, and a sex variable (male and female).

Our first test is to check for homogeneity of variance. To do this, we must first determine the variance of each cell of our design and then divide the smallest variance into the largest to get the F-ratio necessary to check for homogeneity of variance. We will demonstrate the calculation of the variance for the first cell (males in treatment A) and then give you the variances of the other three groups.

$$s^2 = \frac{\Sigma X^2 - \frac{(\Sigma X)^2}{n}}{n - 1},$$

so, for our first group we have,

$$s^2 = \frac{34 - \frac{(12)^2}{5}}{4} = \frac{34 - 28.8}{4} = 1.3$$

The variances for the four groups are:

Rx A, Males   1.3
Rx B, Males   2.5
Rx A, Females   1.3
Rx B Females   1.7

Table 10-2   Two-Way Analysis of Variance of Outcomes of Rehabilitation Among Post MI Patients

Source	SS	df	MS	F	*p*
Treatment group					
Personality type					
Treatment group × Personality type					
Error					

Table 10-3   Data for Computation of a Two-Way ANOVA

Sex	Treatment A		B		Row Totals	
	X	X^2	X	X^2	X	X^2
Males	1	1	8	64		
	3	9	9	81		
	4	16	10	100		
	2	4	6	36		
	2	4	7	49		
Subtotal	12	34	40	330	52	364
Females	10	100	4	16		
	9	81	2	4		
	9	81	3	9		
	7	49	4	16		
	8	64	1	1		
Subtotal	43	375	14	46	57	421
						Overall Total
Column Totals	*55*	*409*	*54*	*376*	*109*	*785*

Our F ratio is $2.5/1.3 = 1.9$. The degrees of freedom (df) are $n - 1$ (number in group minus 1) for each group, or $5 - 1 = 4$. With 4, 4 df, the critical value at the .01 level (.02 for two-tailed) (see Appendix E) is 15.98. We therefore have met the test for homogeneity of variance and move on to the calculations for a two-way ANOVA.

Sum of Squares

Total Sum of Squares. The total sum of squares is a measure of the total variance in the sample and is calculated as $\Sigma X_{tot}^2 - \dfrac{(\Sigma X_{tot})^2}{n_{tot}}$. Note that adding the total of the row Xs equals 109 (52 + 57), and the sum of the column Xs (55 + 54) also equals 109. In similar fashion, the sum of X^2 for the rows equals 364 plus 421, or 785, and the sum of X^2 for the columns also equals 785 (409 + 376). This is always the case and provides a check on the accuracy of our calculations. For total sum of squares we have

$$785 - \frac{(109)^2}{20} = 785 - 594.05 = 190.95$$

Between Groups Sum of Squares. Since we have two groups (treatment and sex), we will calculate *two* between groups sums of squares. The formula is

$$\Sigma \frac{(\Sigma X_g)^2}{n_g} - \frac{(\Sigma X_{tot})^2}{n_{tot}}$$

First, let us consider the treatment groups, A and B. The column totals represent the totals for these groups. The total of the scores (ΣX) for the A group is 55, and the total score for group B is 54. Substituting these numbers into our formula, we have

$$\text{Treatment Group } SS = \frac{(55)^2}{10} + \frac{(54)^2}{10} - \frac{(109)^2}{20}$$
$$= 302.5 + 291.6 - 594.05$$
$$= .05$$

This represents the portion of the variation attributable to the variable treatment. It is a measure of the difference between the means of treatment groups A and B.

The sum of squares for the second independent variable, sex, is calculated in the same way except that there the row totals are used. The 10 males had a total score of 52, and the 10 females had a total score of 57.

$$\text{Sex group } SS = \frac{(52)^2}{10} + \frac{(57)^2}{10} - \frac{(109)^2}{20}$$
$$= 270.4 + 324.9 - 594.05$$
$$= 1.25$$

or

$$270.4 + 324.9 - 594.05 = 1.25$$

This represents the difference between the means of males and females.

Interaction Sum of Squares. Each cell is included when measuring the interaction. The *first* step is to calculate the sum of squares for each individual cell. The formula is

$$\text{Subgroups } SS = \Sigma \frac{(\Sigma X_{sg})^2}{n_{sg}} - \frac{(\Sigma X_{tot})^2}{n_{tot}}$$
$$= \frac{(12)^2}{5} + \frac{(40)^2}{5} + \frac{(43)^2}{5} + \frac{(14)^2}{5} - \frac{(109)^2}{20}$$
$$= 28.8 + 320 + 369.8 + 39.2 - 594.05$$
$$= 163.75$$

The *second* step is to calculate the interaction sum of squares using the following formula where the between groups sums of squares are subtracted from the subgroup sum of squares. The formula is

$$\text{Interaction } SS = \text{Subgroup } SS - \text{Between } SS$$

For our example,

Interaction $SS = 163.75 - (.05 + 1.25)$
$$= 163.75 - 1.3$$
$$= 162.45$$

This represents the portion of the total sum of squares attributable to the effect of an interaction between the two independent variables on the dependent variable.

Within Groups Sum of Squares. This is the portion of the total sum of squares left over after the between and interaction sums of squares have been accounted for. The formula is

$$\text{Within } SS = \text{Total } SS - (\text{Between } SS + \textit{Interaction})$$

In our example, we had two between SSs; therefore, our formula is

Within $SS = 190.95 - (.05 + 1.25 + 162.45)$
$$= 190.95 - 163.75$$
$$= 27.2$$

Degrees of Freedom

The following formulas are used:

Total Between SS = number of subgroups $- 1$
Factor (independent variable) $SS = k - 1$
Interaction $SS = df$ for first group $\times$ df for second group
Within SS = number in sample $-$ number of groups in first variable $\times$ number of groups in second variable
Total SS = number in sample $- 1$

In our example, we have the following df:

	df
Total Between Groups	$4 - 1 = 3$
Treatment	$2 - 1 = 1$
Sex	$2 - 1 = 1$
Interaction	$1 \times 1 = 1$
Within Groups	$20 - (2 \times 2) = 16$
Total	$20 - 1 = 19$

Note that the df for the between groups, the interaction, and the within groups sums of squares add up to the df for the total ($1 + 1 + 1 + 16 = 19$). See Table 10-4 for the completion of the report of this data. The mean squares are obtained by dividing the sums of squares by their respective df. We then test the two main effects (one for each independent variable) and the interaction effect by calculating three F ratios.

In each case, the *within mean square* is placed in the denominator. Our three F ratios are:

For treatment group:

$$F1, 16 = \frac{.05}{1.70}$$
$$= .029$$

For sex group:

$$F1, 16 = \frac{1.25}{1.70}$$
$$= .735$$

For treatment × sex:

$$F1, 16 = \frac{162.45}{1.70}$$
$$= 95.559$$

Using Appendix E, we see that the Fs for the main effects are both nonsignificant, but the F associated with the interaction far exceeds the tabled value (8.53) for the .01 level.

Table 10-4   Summary Table for Two-Way Analysis of Variance

Source of Variance	SS	df	MS	F	p
Between groups	163.75	3	54.78	32.108	< .01
Treatment	.05	1	.05	.029	ns
Sex	1.25	1	1.25	.735	ns
Treatment × sex	162.45	1	162.45	95.559	< .01
Within groups	27.20	16	1.70		
Total	190.95	19			

Group	Means
A	5.5
B	5.4
Male	5.2
Female	5.7
Group A males	2.4
Group B males	8.0
Group A females	8.6
Group B females	2.8

This contrived example demonstrates the value of moving beyond one-way ANOVA and being able to test for interactions. If we had simply done two one-way ANOVAs, we would have concluded that types of treatment made no difference and that men and women did equally well. Looking at the means for those groups (Table 10-4), we can see that they are almost identical. However, the significant interaction means that the treatments have different effects depending on whether the subject is male or female. In fact, males scored low when exposed to treatment A and high when exposed to treatment B. For females, the pattern was reversed. Thus, the treatment does make a difference when gender is considered. When interpreting the results of ANOVA, interactions should be considered first, before the main effects. As seen in this example, a significant interaction changes the interpretation of the main effects.

THREE-WAY ANALYSIS OF VARIANCE

Let us expand these techniques. Consider the case in which there are three independent variables (A, B, C) and each of these has two or more levels. We would therefore test for three main effects (one for each independent variable). The testing for interactions becomes more complex here. The following tests could be made: $A \times B$, $A \times C$, $B \times C$, and $A \times B \times C$. With three treatments, it becomes somewhat difficult to make sense of the interactions, and moving to four or more independent variables complicates it to the point at which most people would advise ignoring the complex interactions and pooling them as "error." Others would advise using multiple regression. Note, if one wishes to study interactions using multiple regression, the interactions must be coded for entry into the regression equation. See the section on coding in Chapter 6 for a demonstration of how this is done.

An example of a three-way ANOVA would be the relaxation study if we were to add sex as an independent variable (Fig. 10-1). We now have a $2 \times 2 \times 2$ factorial design, or three independent variables with two levels each, and eight individual cells. The summary table is shown in Table 10-5.

As with one-way ANOVA, when the overall Fs are significant, post hoc tests may be used with two- and three-way ANOVA to test for specific group differences.

Hypothesized a priori contrasts were discussed in Chapter 6. Such contrasts may also be tested with the ANOVA approach. Both SPSS and SAS allow the user to specify which contrasts should be tested. The rules for specifying orthogonal contrasts, as presented in Chapter 6, also apply here.

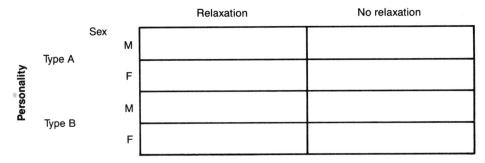

This could also be depicted as follows:

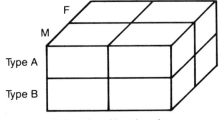

Figure 10-1   An example of a three-way analyses of variance treatment.

Table 10-5   Summary Table for Three-Way Analysis of Variance (n = 80)

Source of Variance	SS	df	MS	F	p
Between Groups		$8 - 1 = 7$			
Treatment		$2 - 1 = 1$			
Personality		$2 - 1 = 1$			
Sex		$2 - 1 = 1$			
Treatment × personality		$1 \times 1 = 1$			
Treatment × sex		$1 \times 1 = 1$			
Personality × sex		$1 \times 1 = 1$			
Treatment × personality × sex		$1 \times 1 \times 1 = 1$			
Within Groups		$80 - (2 \times 2 \times 2) = 72$			
Total		$80 - 1 = 79$			

EXAMPLE OF A COMPUTER PRINTOUT
OF A TWO-WAY ANALYSIS OF VARIANCE

Figure 10-2 contains a two-way ANOVA produced by the GLM procedure in SAS.*
There are two independent variables. "SGENDER" is a two-level variable, indicating the sex of the child, and "CENTER" contains nine levels, each being a
different child care facility. The dependent variable is a measure of intelligence,
"INTELL1." In the "CLASS LEVEL INFORMATION" section, (①), the independent variables are described and the number of subjects are explained.

The ANOVA summary table, (②), is in a slightly different format from the one
we have been describing and may, therefore, be somewhat confusing at first glance.
The overall model with 17 df is first tested for significance. This is analogous to
testing the overall R^2 for significance and then determining where variables are
contributing significantly to the variance explained. Here the overall model is
significant at $p = .0030$. This model accounts for 22.69% of the variance in the
dependent variable (R-SQUARE = .226862).

In the lower portion of the figure are two types of sums of squares, TYPE I and
TYPE III (③). Type I are used with equal cell sizes, and Type III can be used with
unequal cell size. In this example, we should use Type III. SGENDER with 1 df has
a Type III sum of squares equal to .13270150 and is not significant ($p = .4170$). Boys
and girls did not differ on the measure of intelligence. The mean squares are not
printed for these sums of squares, but let us calculate one to demonstrate how the F
value is calculated. CENTER has 8 df, and $SS = 4.93027202$. The mean square for
center = .616284. To calculate the F value, the computer divides the mean square
for center by the mean square for the error term (within mean square). That
calculation is

$$F = \frac{.616284}{.20020437} = 3.078, \text{ or } 3.08,$$

which is significant ($p = .0032$).

In the next section, we see the means for girls and boys (4.0439 and 3.9192).
Because the F value associated with the centers was significant, we need to determine which centers differed significantly from which. In the next section, the
Student-Newman-Keuls test is shown as a post hoc test (④), Although the means for
the centers are printed with double spacing, between the strings of As and Bs are
printed single spaced and that can be confusing. It may be helpful to use a ruler to
determine which means have different letters. Here, Center 58, with a mean of
4.3262, is significantly higher than centers 55 and 53, which had means of 3.7355 and
3.6981, respectively.

The means of the subgroups are given in the next section of the printout (⑤).
There we can see the means for the boys at each center and for the girls at each
center.

* This example was prepared by Susan Grajek of the Yale Computer Center staff.

(*Text continues on page 213*)

Figure 10-2 Two-way analysis of variance produced by SAS.

Procedure Cards

```
PROC GLM;
  CLASS SGENDER CENTER;
  MODEL INTELL1 = SGENDER CENTER SGENDER*CENTER;
  MEANS SGENDER CENTER SGENDER*CENTER/SNK TUKEY;
  TITLE1 EXAMPLE OF PROC GLM FOR ANOVA;
  TITLE2 INTELL1 IS CONTINUOUS DEPENDENT VARIABLE;
  TITLE3 SGENDER AND CENTER ARE CATEGORICAL INDEPENDENT VARIABLES;
  TITLE4 SGENDER AND CENTER MAY INTERACT;
```

Output

```
                    EXAMPLE OF PROC GLM FOR ANOVA
              INTELL1 IS CONTINUOUS DEPENDENT VARIABLE
    SGENDER AND CENTER ARE CATEGORICAL INDEPENDENT VARIABLES
              SGENDER AND CENTER MAY INTERACT

               GENERAL LINEAR MODELS PROCEDURE

                  CLASS LEVEL INFORMATION

①  CLASS          LEVELS         VALUES
   SGENDER          2            1 2
   CENTER -         9            51 52 53 54 55 56 57 58 59

        NUMBER OF OBSERVATIONS IN DATA SET = 167

                    EXAMPLE OF PROC GLM FOR ANOVA
              INTELL1 IS CONTINUOUS DEPENDENT VARIABLE
    SGENDER AND CENTER ARE CATEGORICAL INDEPENDENT VARIABLES
              SGENDER AND CENTER MAY INTERACT

               GENERAL LINEAR MODELS PROCEDURE
```

② DEPENDENT VARIABLE: INTELLI   PARENT RATING CBI INTELLIGENCE

SOURCE	DF	SUM OF SQUARES	MEAN SQUARE	F VALUE	PR > F	R-SQUARE	C.V.
MODEL	17	8.10693530	0.47687855	2.38	0.0030	0.226862	11.2491
ERROR	138	27.62820265	0.20020437		ROOT MSE		INTELLI MEAN
CORRECTED TOTAL	155	35.73513795			0.44744203		3.97758778

SOURCE	DF	③ TYPE I SS	F VALUE	PR > F	DF	③ TYPE III SS	F VALUE	PR > F
SGENDER	1	0.60373042	3.02	0.0847	1	0.13270150	0.66	0.4170
CENTER	8	4.80376374	3.00	0.0039	8	4.93027202	3.08	0.0032
SGENDER*CENTER	8	2.69944114	1.69	0.1071	8	2.69944114	1.69	0.1071

STUDENT-NEWMAN-KEULS TEST FOR VARIABLE: INTELLI
NOTE: THIS TEST COTNROLS THE TYPE I EXPERIMENTWISE ERROR RATE
       UNDER THE COMPLETE NULL HYPOTHESIS BUT NOT UNDER PARTIAL
       NULL HYPOTHESES.

ALPHA = 0.05   DF = 138   MSE = 0.200204

WARNING: CELL SIZES ARE NOT EQUAL.
HARMONIC MEAN OF CELL SIZES = 77.6795

MEANS WITH THE SAME LETTER ARE NOT SIGNIFICANTLY DIFFERENT.

SNK	GROUPING	MEAN	N	SGENDER
	A	4.0439	73	2
	A			
	A	3.9192	83	1

(Continued)

211

Figure 10-2 (continued)

```
STUDENT-NEWMAN-KEULS TEST FOR VARIABLE: INTELL1
NOTE: THIS TEST CONTROLS THE TYPE I EXPERIMENTWISE ERROR RATE
      UNDER THE COMPLETE NULL HYPOTHESIS BUT NOT UNDER PARTIAL
      NULL HYPOTHESES.

ALPHA = 0.05   DF = 138   MSE = 0.200204

WARNING: CELL SIZES ARE NOT EQUAL.
HARMONIC MEAN OF CELL SIZES = 14.5207

MEANS WITH THE SAME LETTER ARE NOT SIGNIFICANTLY DIFFERENT.
```

SNK GROUPING	MEAN	N	CENTER
A	4.3263	12	58
A			
B A	4.1112	20	51
B A			
B A	4.0892	16	56
B A			
B A	4.0843	13	59
B A			
B A	4.0752	23	57
B A			
B A	3.8587	21	54
B A			
B A	3.8520	24	52
B			
B	3.7353	21	55
B			
B	3.6981	6	53

④

MEANS

SGENDER	CENTER	N	INTELL1
1	51	9	4.04568713
1	52	15	3.63146428
1	53	3	3.79824561
1	54	11	3.76231061
1	55	8	3.72057211
1	56	10	3.96518640
1	57	16	4.04448785
1	58	4	4.62865497
1	59	7	4.14160401
2	51	11	4.16473950
2	52	9	4.21949318
2	53	3	3.59795322
2	54	10	3.96476608
2	55	13	3.74471683
2	56	6	4.29580897
2	57	7	4.14531119
2	58	8	4.17490110
2	59	6	4.01744066

⑤

EXAMPLE OF TWO-WAY ANALYSIS OF VARIANCE FROM PUBLISHED RESEARCH

Question Posed

Rice and Johnson, 1984, sought to determine whether self-instructional booklets about postoperative exercises sent to patients before hospital admission would be effective teaching devices.

The following two hypotheses were tested:

1. Patients who receive pre-admission booklets containing specific exercise instructions will achieve higher exercise performance scores during hospitalization than patients who receive the pre-admission booklets containing nonspecific instruction.
2. Teaching time required for patients to demonstrate mastery of the exercises will depend on the type of booklet:

    shortest time—patients who receive the booklets containing specific instructions

    intermediate time—patients who receive booklets containing nonspecific instructions

    longest time—patients who receive no pre-admission instructions (Rice and Johnson, 1984, p. 148)

Data Gathered

Data were gathered from 130 presurgical cholecystectomy and herniorrhaphy patients. Patients were randomly assigned to one of the three levels of pre-admission instruction: specific, nonspecific, and none. "A 3 × 2 factorial design was used with pre-admission exercise instructions as the experimental factor, and type of surgery was used as the second factor." (Rice & Johnson, 1984, p. 148)

The dependent variables were exercise performance and teaching time. On admission, patients were asked to perform the exercises and were given a score based on the number they performed. They were then taught the exercises they did not know until they could perform all the exercises. The total time spent with the patient constituted the teaching time.

Tabular Presentation of Results

Tables 10-6 through 10-9 contain the tables from the study. Table 10-6 contains a two-way ANOVA. There was a significant difference among the experimental groups, but there was no difference between the two surgical groups, and no interaction.

Table 10-6   Analysis of Variance for Behaviors Common to Both Booklets

Source	df	MS	F	p
Experimental groups	1	158.98	9.03	.001
Type of surgery	1	40.06	2.27	ns
Experimental group × type of surgery	1	1.96	.11	ns
Error	97	17.60		

From Rice, V. H., & Johnson, J. E. (1984). Pre-admission self-instruction booklets, post-admission exercise performance, and teaching time. *Nursing Research, 33*(3), 147–151.

Table 10-7   Mean Number of Behaviors Performed by Experimental Groups and Type of Surgery

Experimental Groups		Cholecystectomy	Herniorrhaphy	Totals
Specific booklet	$\overline{X}$	13.23	12.90	13.07
	SD	4.15	4.71	4.30
	n	26	21	47
Nonspecific booklet	$\overline{X}$	11.48	9.69	10.57
	SD	4.19	3.78	4.01
	n	27	27	54
Type of surgery	$\overline{X}$	12.33	11.08	
	SD	4.17	4.25	
Total	n	*53*	*48*	

Note: The possible range of scores was 0 to 20.
From Rice, V. H., & Johnson, J. E. (1984). Pre-admission self-instruction booklets, post-admission exercise performance, and teaching time. *Nursing Research, 33*(3), 147–151.

Table 10-7 contains the means and standard deviations. There we see that the mean for the specific booklet group (13.07) was higher than the mean for the nonspecific booklet group (10.57). The means for the two surgical groups were quite similar (12.33 and 11.08).

Table 10-8 also contains a two-way ANOVA with a significant main effect for experimental group. In Table 10-9, we can see that the no pre-admission booklet group had the highest score in teaching-time (12.72), the nonspecific booklet group came next (9.70), and the specific group had the lowest teaching time (8.70).

Description of Results

The results from testing hypothesis I are presented in Tables 10-6 and 10-7. There, just the two groups who did receive pre-admission booklets are being compared in the number of exercises they knew how to do on admission. (The specific booklet group knew more exercises than did the nonspecific booklet group (13.07 vs. 10.57).

Table 10-8   Analysis of Variance for Amount of Teaching Time

Source	df	MS	F	p
Experimental group	2	133.84	11.39	.001
Type of surgery	1	28.72	1.44	ns
Experimental group × type of surgery	2	6.63	.56	ns
Error	124	11.75		

From Rice, V. H., & Johnson, J. E. (1984). Pre-admission self-instruction booklets, post-admission exercise performance, and teaching time. *Nursing Research, 33* (3), 147–151.

Table 10-9   Means of Minutes of Teaching Time by Experimental Group and Type of Surgery

Experimental Groups		Cholecystectomy	Herniorrhaphy	Totals*
Specific booklet	$\overline{X}$	9.58	8.24	8.70
	SD	2.64	2.79	2.71
	n	26	21	47
Nonspecific booklet	$\overline{X}$	10.48	9.29	9.70
	SD	2.55	3.14	2.86
	n	27	27	54
No pre-admission booklet	$\overline{X}$	12.43	13.00	12.72
	SD	3.30	4.48	3.89
	n	14	15	29
Type of surgery	$\overline{X}$	10.39	11.22	
	SD	2.83	3.47	
Totals	n	67	63	

* Comparison of Specific vs nonspecific = $t(124) = 1.46$, p = ns
  Comparison of Specific vs no booklet = $t(124) = 4.97$, $p = .001$
  Comparison of Nonspecific vs no booklet = $t(124) = 3.83$, $p = .001$
From Rice, V. H., & Johnson, J. E. (1984). Pre-admission self-instruction booklets, post-admission exercise performance, and teaching time. *Nursing Research, 33* (3), 147–151.

The results related to hypothesis II are presented in Tables 10-8 and 10-9. The comparisons related to the significant *F* for the experimental groups are given in the footnote to Table 10-9. We see that both of the groups that received pre-admission booklets required less teaching time than the group who received no booklet before admission. The two groups who received information did not differ significantly, however.

Conclusions

The patients in this study were able to learn exercises prior to admission, and specific instructions facilitated their learning. Having information prior to admission decreased the staff time spent in teaching the exercises after admission. With shorter hospital stays, such savings in time are particularly relevant.

SUMMARY

Analysis of variance is a powerful, "robust" test that allows us to test for relationships between categorical independent variables and a continuous dependent variable. Testing for interactions between the independent variables is a particularly useful technique when we want to determine whether or not the effects of some intervention will be the same for all types of people or conditions. ANOVA may be extended to the use of more than one dependent variable in a given analysis. This analysis is usually referred to as MANOVA (multiple analysis of variance) and allows the researcher to look for relationships among dependent, as well as many independent variables.

EXERCISES FOR CHAPTER 10

1. To investigate the efficacy of various methods for preparing patients for discharge, a 2×2 factorial design is used. Patients are randomly assigned to one of four conditions outlined in the diagram. Four weeks after discharge, subjects are tested on their knowledge of information provided in tapes. Their scores are given in the diagram. State and list the three research questions. Write the summary table.

Type of Follow-Up Discussion	Type of Teaching	
	Audio Tape	*Audio Visual Tape*
One-on-one with nurse	6	9
	5	8
	3	7
	4	5
	2	6
	4	6
	5	7
	3	5
	6	8
	4	8
With group of patients led by nurse	8	10
	7	9
	4	8
	6	7
	4	8
	5	9
	4	6
	5	7
	6	8
	7	10

2. You have the following independent variables: treatment group (4 levels), marital status (single, married, divorced), and race (Black, Caucasian, Oriental). There are 800 subjects in the study. Write the summary table for the analysis, including the source of variation and the degrees of freedom.

CHAPTER 11
Analysis of Covariance

Madelon A. Visintainer and Barbara Hazard Munro

OBJECTIVES FOR CHAPTER 11

After reading this chapter and completing the exercises, you should be able to

1. Determine when analysis of covariance is the appropriate technique to use.
2. Explain the relationship between analysis of variance and regression.
3. Discuss the assumptions, interpretations, and limitations of analysis of covariance.

In the preceding chapters, the statistical methods of analysis of variance (ANOVA)—one-way and complex—were described as techniques to investigate differences among group means. Those tests were used either when more than two groups were involved or when we were interested in the effects of several categorical (independent) variables on a continuous (dependent) measure.

In this chapter, we present another ANOVA technique: the analysis of covariance, or ANCOVA. This technique combines the ANOVA with regression to measure the differences among group means. The advantages that ANCOVA holds over other techniques are in its ability to reduce the error variance in the outcome measure, and to measure group differences after allowing for other differences between subjects. The error variance is reduced by controlling for variation in the dependent measure that comes from separate measurable variables that influence all the groups being compared. Such a separate variable is considered to be neither "independent" nor "dependent" in the ANOVA. However, it contributes to the variation and reduces the magnitude of the differences among groups. In ANCOVA, the variation from this variable is measured and extracted from the within (or error) variation. The net effect is the reduction of error variance and, therefore, an increase in the power of the analysis. Recall that power is the *likelihood of correctly rejecting the null hypothesis*. With ANCOVA, the control of the extraneous variation will provide a more accurate estimate of the real difference among groups.

In this chapter, examples of research in which ANCOVA is the correct statistical analysis will be presented together with the underlying assumptions that must be met in order to have valid results.

STATISTICAL QUESTIONS FOR ANCOVA

In general, ANCOVA answers the same research questions that ANOVA addresses: Do the experimental groups differ to a greater degree than we would expect by chance alone? However, with ANOVA, two sets of variables were involved in the analysis: the independent variables and the dependent variable. In ANCOVA, a third type of variable is included. It is the *covariate*.

Consider the following example: An investigator is interested in the effects of three different methods—lecture, instruction manual, and programmed instruction manual—designed to teach student nurses to use the computer. The investigator randomly assigns 30 students to these three methods and then, after the instruction is complete, measures their competency by a test. The research question is the following: Which method of teaching produces a greater mastery of the material (*i.e.,* higher test scores)?

The investigator prepares to measure the differences among the three groups, but she knows from previous research that general mathematical ability influences a person's readiness to master computers. Those students who have a stronger aptitude for mathematics tend to have greater facility with computers. In this study, the mathematical aptitude of students will influence their learning. This influence has the potential to add variation to the scores and, thus, increase the "error variance."

Since the investigator has the Scholastic Aptitude Test (SAT) scores for mathematics for each student, she decides to control for this variation by using ANCOVA for her analysis. In the example, the teaching method is the independent variable (experimental variable). The class computer score is the dependent variable (outcome variable). These are the two variables that would be included in the usual ANOVA. But here the math SAT score is the *covariate*. This is the unique addition to the ANCOVA analysis. It is called the covariate because it *varies along with the outcome measure.*

By adding the covariate, the SAT math score, to the analysis, the investigator hopes to reduce the variability assigned to the error term and thus increase the power of her analysis. Such an approach is typical of the original purpose for using ANCOVA. Since then, the technique has been used in other ways as well. Frequently, it has been used to "equate" groups. In quasi-experimental designs, individuals have not been randomly assigned to groups, and intact groups are often used. A typical example is using already established classes in a school to test different teaching methods. Because the subjects are not randomly assigned, there may be differences among groups. In classroom situations, the major concern would be that the groups might differ in intelligence. In a hospital situation, one might be concerned that patients in one unit were "sicker" than those in another unit. If the groups are found to be different, ANCOVA is often used to "equate" them; that is, in the classroom example, IQ would be the covariate and the effect of intelligence would be "removed" before the means of the groups on the dependent variable were compared. In the hospital example, degree of illness might be used as a covariate.

ANCOVA has also been used when random assignment has not "worked." Especially with small samples, an investigator may find that even after random assignment, the groups differ on some important variable. ANCOVA might then be used to statistically equate the groups.

Also, in nonexperimental studies, there is no manipulation of the independent variable, but groups may be compared. In a study that looked at the impact of a husband's chronic obstructive pulmonary disease (COPD) on his spouse's life (Sexton & Munro, 1985), the investigators recruited a comparison group of wives whose husbands did not have a chronic disease. Although efforts were made to recruit women who were similar to the wives of COPD patients, when the data were analyzed it was discovered that the COPD wives were older and of lower socioeconomic status (SES) than the comparison wives. If those variables had been related to the outcome measures (they were not), the comparison of the two groups would have been hard to interpret. In that case, ANCOVA could have been used in such a situation to statistically control age and SES.

Although ANCOVA has been widely used for such statistical "equalization" of groups, it is not a cure-all and should be used with caution. Some authors condemn its use for anything but the intent to remove another source of variation from the dependent variable. They do not believe that it should be used to equate groups. To use ANCOVA with dissimilar groups, one would have to be able to assert that the groups were essentially equivalent except for the variable(s) being used as covariate(s). This equivalence is virtually impossible to know for certain.

TYPE OF DATA REQUIRED

As with ANOVA, we have one or more categorical variables as independent variables and a continuous measure for the dependent variable. In addition, the covariate should be at the interval or ratio level. This is discussed in further detail in the following section.

ASSUMPTIONS

To ensure a valid interpretation of ANCOVA results, several assumptions should be met. These assumptions are based on requirements necessary for the validity of both the regression and the ANOVA components of the test. The first four assumptions are those associated with ANOVA:

1. The groups should be mutually exclusive.
2. The variances of the groups should be equivalent (homogeneity of variance).
3. Continuous data should be used for the dependent variable.
4. The dependent variable should be normally distributed.

In addition,

5. The covariate should be measured at the interval or ratio level. As previously discussed, it may be possible to treat ordinal data as though it were interval data if there is good rationale for such treatment. If a variable is at the nominal level, it cannot be used as a covariate. (But a nominal variable may be included as an additional independent variable in ANOVA, rather than as a covariate.)
6. The covariate and the dependent variable must show a linear relationship. When this assumption is violated, the analysis will have little benefit, because there will be little reduction in error variance. The test is most effective when that relationship lies above $r = .30$. The stronger the relationship, the more effective the ANCOVA analysis will be; that is, the more the two variables are related, the greater is the reduction in the error variance by controlling for the covariate. In cases in which the relationship between the covariate and dependent variable is not linear, one appropriate test would be the complex ANOVA, with the levels of the covariate as another independent variable. Another possibility would be mathematical transformation of the variables to achieve a linear relationship. The transformed variables could then be used in ANCOVA.

Consider an example that demonstrates a violation of this assumption. Suppose that we wished to study the effects of two different patient teaching methods on diabetic patients' performances in insulin administration (scored on a 20-point scale). Suppose also that the investigator wished to control for the effects of anxiety. However, ANCOVA analysis with level of anxiety as a covariate would violate the assumption of a linear correlation between the covariate and the outcome variable. Previous research implies that there is a "U"-shaped relationship between anxiety and performance and on learning; that is, performance and learning seem to be enhanced by moderate levels of anxiety. However, at both high and low levels, learning and performance are hampered. This relation is depicted graphically in Figure 11-1.

One appropriate analysis in this case would be a complex ANOVA with three levels of anxiety as one main effect variable and types of teaching as a second main effect. Another approach would be to use curvilinear regression analysis, in which case the anxiety scores could be treated as continuous, rather than categorical, data. For further information on curvilinear regression, see Pedhazur (1982, Chapter 11).

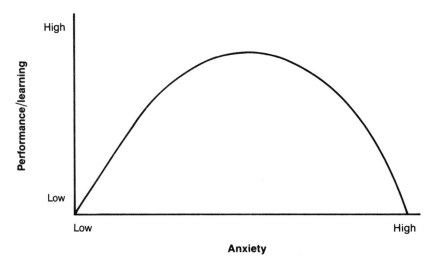

Figure 11-1   Possible relationship between performance and anxiety.

7. The direction and strength of the relationship between the covariate and dependent variable must be similar in each group. We call this requirement *homogeneity of regression across groups.* When this assumption is violated, the chance of a Type 1 error is increased. This assumption can be expressed in another way: that the independent variable should not have an effect on *the relationship between the covariate and the dependent variable.*

Consider the following example of a violation of this assumption. Suppose that an investigator is evaluating ways of reducing upset in hospitalized children. There is strong evidence that manifest upset is related to the age of the child: Younger children express more upset than older children. In the analysis, the investigator includes age as a covariate when measuring the effectiveness of three pediatric nursing interventions. The first intervention is a videotape about the hospital, which is available to children in their hospital room throughout their stay. The second intervention is primary nursing care, and the third intervention is a liberal rooming-in policy, which encourages parents to stay with their children. In this analysis of the results, the investigator finds a lack of homogeneity of regression across the three interventions (see Fig. 11-2).

The relationship between age and manifest upset is affected by the interventions. In the videotape intervention, there is a strong inverse relationship between upset and age (the younger the child, the greater the upset). However, in the other two groups, the relationships are weaker: The interventions affected the relationship. Theoretically, we can hypothesize that because much of the upset that younger children express is related to separation anxiety, any intervention that works through a stable relationship

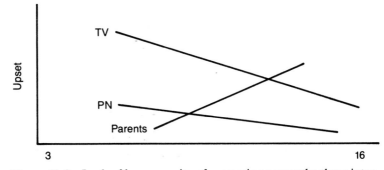

Figure 11-2   Lack of homogeneity of regression across the three interventions.

(primary nursing) will produce more reduction in anxiety for the younger child. Moreover, an intervention that increases the time with parents will produce more reduction in anxiety for the younger child, while potentially increasing some upset for the young adolescent.

ANCOVA used in this example will increase the chance of a Type 1 error. An appropriate analysis would be a complex ANOVA with the children's ages categorized into age groups. The complex ANOVA would provide information on the interaction between age group and intervention.

One further note on this assumption calls attention to the graph in Figure 11-2. When there is homogeneity of regression, the regression lines will be parallel. In the example given, the lines are not parallel, indicating that the interventions affected the covariate-dependent relationship differentially.

RELATIONSHIP OF ANOVA
AND REGRESSION TO ANCOVA

To understand the rationale behind the mathematical operations involved in ANCOVA, it is necessary to understand the concept of "residual." This notion is well explained in Kerlinger and Pedhazur (1973), and the following explanation relies heavily on their work.

In Chapter 5, we explained that squaring the correlation coefficient results in a quantity, r^2, known as a *coefficient of determination*. This coefficient is often used as a measure of the meaningfulness of r, because it is a measure of the variance shared by the two variables. To calculate the proportion of variance that is *not shared* by the two variables, we would subtract r^2 from 1.00. For example, if the correlation between two variables is .50, $r^2 = .25$, and $1 - r^2 = .75$. We could then state that 25% of the variance was shared by the two variables and 75% was not shared. This 75% is called the *variance of the residual*. The residual variance is not due to the relationship between the two variables. In regression analysis, we talk about the regression sum of squares and the residual sum of squares. In ANOVA, the within sum of squares, or error term, is analogous to the residual sum of squares. Thus, the residual variance is that variation not explained by the variables in the study. In ANCOVA, we use the residuals to determine whether or not groups differ *after* the effect of some other variable has been removed.

Let us return to the first example, where we had three methods of teaching students to use the computer and wished to remove the effect of mathematical ability from the test scores in the computer course. The SAT math scores can be used to predict final examination scores; that is, final examination scores are regressed on math ability, and a prediction equation is developed. The prediction equation can then be applied to a group of students. Given their SAT math scores, we predict their final examination scores. We could then give the final examination and calculate the difference between an individual's actual score, Y, and his predicted score, Y'. The difference between those two scores, $Y - Y'$, is the *residual*. It is the error, or unexplained part of the variation. The residual score for each individual would have no correlation with mathematical ability. If we had groups of students taught by three different methods, we could then calculate mean residual scores for each group. Comparing those scores would tell us whether or not the groups differed *after* the effect of mathematical ability was removed.

An example of such an analysis follows.

EXAMPLE OF ANCOVA

Table 11-1 gives the final examination scores for the students in each group. Also presented are the SAT math scores. Each student has two data entries for analysis: a computer test score (the dependent measure result), and the SAT math score (the covariate measure).

Three sources of variation are accounted for in this analysis. *First,* the variation due to the relationship between mathematical ability (SAT scores) and final examination scores is removed. There are also two other sources of variation in the scores: variation due to the teaching method (between variance), and variation not due to the teaching methods or mathematical aptitude (within variance). Because the variation associated with mathematical ability comes out of the "within variance," the within variance is reduced. There is now a more focused emphasis on the statistical difference between the groups. The results of this ANCOVA are presented in Table 11-2. The terms and presentation common to all forms of ANOVA are given in this table. The partitioning of variance is also shown. In addition to the familiar entries of Main Effects and Within (Error) Variances, we have added the variance from the covariate. In the presentation of data, the covariate information is listed first, followed by information about the main effects and error variation. A second column of information that is familiar in all ANOVAs contains the degrees

Table 11-1   Example of ANCOVA

Teaching Method

| | Lecture | | | Programmed Instruction | | | Instruction Manual | |
Subject	Computer Exam	SAT Score	Subject	Computer Exam	SAT Score	Subject	Computer Exam	SAT Score
1	20	180	11	27	130	21	33	140
2	24	340	12	49	190	22	43	200
3	51	300	13	44	170	23	35	300
4	46	350	14	35	270	24	37	300
5	50	400	15	53	350	25	36	340
6	43	440	16	47	390	26	48	420
7	60	420	17	44	210	27	63	400
8	61	470	18	74	380	28	57	380
9	55	420	19	70	310	29	56	540
10	54	540	20	67	510	30	78	560

Table 11-2   Analysis of Covariance on Test Data Across Teaching Methods

Source	SS	df	MS	F	p
Covariate-Aptitude	1147.36	1	1147.36	17.75	.01
Main Effects-Teaching	707.99	2	354.00	5.48	.05
Within (Error)	1680.65	26	64.64		
Total	3536.00	29			

of freedom (df) for each category of variance. The df for each covariate included in an analysis is 1. In the above example, there is one covariate—mathematical aptitude; therefore, there is 1 df.

The df for main effects in ANCOVA is the same as in ANOVA:

$$k - 1$$

where k = number of groups. In this example, there are three teaching groups; so, the df for main effects equal

$$3 - 1 = 2$$

For the within or error variance in ANCOVA, df equal

$$n - k - 1$$

where

$$n = \text{the total sample}$$
$$k = \text{the number of groups}$$

In this example, the df for the residual variance equals $30 - 3 - 1$, or 26. The df for the total variance is equal to the total number of subjects less 1, or, in this example, 29.

Interpretation of ANCOVA

The information provided by ANCOVA is primarily about the *difference between groups* with the variation associated with the covariate accounted for. Once the sums of squares are calculated, the interpretation proceeds in the same way as in ANOVA. The sums of squares are divided by the appropriate df to give the mean squares. The F test is then calculated for the covariate and main effects. The F table gives the probability level reached for each F calculated.

In our example, the F values for the covariate of aptitude and the main effects of teaching method are calculated by dividing the respective means squares of 1147.36 and 354.00 by the mean square for the error of 64.64. We reach an F of 17.75 for the covariate and an F of 5.48 for the main effects.

To find the probability reached by these F values, we consult the F table (Appendix E). For the significance of the F for the covariate, we use $df\ 1, 26$. We see from the table, that for a p value of .01, we need an F value of 7.72. With a value of 17.75, we reject the null hypothesis that there is no relationship between the final examination scores and the mathematical aptitude. Moving to the F value obtained for the main effects 5.48, we consult the F table with $df\ 2, 26$. On the table we see that for a p value of .05, we need an F value of 3.37. The main effects F value of 5.48 is larger than this but smaller than the value needed for the .01 level (5.53). We reject the null hypothesis that the differences in the group mean happened by chance alone.

This ANCOVA provides two pieces of information: first, that there is a correlation between mathematical ability and final examination scores in a computer course. Second, that teaching methods had an effect on the students' performances on the test. To find out which groups differ from each other, secondary analysis using a multiple comparison technique, as discussed in Chapter 9, would be necessary.

COMPUTATION—ANCOVA

Although we present the calculation of an ANCOVA with one independent variable, in actual practice you would use the computer. Going through the calculations should help solidify your understanding of the relationship of ANCOVA to ANOVA and regression and enhance your appreciation of computer analysis. The calculations are not difficult, but they are tedious. In presenting the explanation of ANCOVA, we described the analysis of residuals on measuring the difference between each individual's predicted score and actual score $(Y - Y')$. Fortunately, we do not actually have to calculate these residuals but can use the formulas for sum of squares. This is analogous to our discussion of standard deviation where we first used a formula that included each score's deviation from the mean $(\chi = X - \overline{X})$ for purposes of clarifying your understanding of this measure of variation. We then demonstrated that an equivalent formula could be used where we squared the raw scores, rather than calculating all the deviations from the mean.

Example for Computation

First, let us suppose that we wanted to test two nursing interventions designed to improve post-hospital adjustment. We will call the interventions A and B. There are two medical units in our hospital, so we randomly assign intervention A to one unit and intervention B to the other. The post-hospital adjustment scale measures physical, psychological, and social adjustment and has a potential range of scores of 1 to 20. Table 11-3 contains the results from this study. The means of the two groups are quite similar, 8.5 and 8.0. Applying the pooled t-test to these data results in a t value of $-.273$, which is nonsignificant. We could, therefore, conclude that there is no difference between interventions A and B in relation to post-hospital adjustment.

However, suppose that the two units are not really equivalent, that the unit assigned the A intervention has much sicker patients than the other unit. Degree of illness would be expected to be related to post-hospital adjustment. We rate all the

Table 11-3   Comparison of the Effect of Two Nursing Interventions on Post-Hospital Adjustment

Treatment Groups	
A **Adjustment Scores**	**B** **Adjustment Scores**
3	10
5	7
14	7
8	3
7	3
10	12
6	14
15	9
13	4
4	11
85	80
$\overline{X}s$ 8.5	8.0

Table 11-4   Comparison of Illness Scores for Two Units

Treatment Groups

A		B	
Illness Scale	Adjustment Score	Illness Scale	Adjustment Score
10	3	3	10
9	5	4	7
6	14	4	7
8	8	6	3
8	7	5	3
7	10	2	12
9	6	1	14
6	15	3	9
7	13	5	4
10	4	2	11
80	85	35	80
$\bar{X}s$ 8.0	8.5	3.5	8.0

subjects on their degree of illness (on a scale ranging from 0 to 10, with 10 being the sickest) and present the additional data in Table 11-4. Now we see that the patients exposed to treatment A had a much higher mean illness score (8.0) than the patients exposed to B (3.5). To adjust for this difference between the groups, we use ANCOVA with one independent variable, treatment group; one covariate, illness score; and one dependent variable, post-hospital adjustment score. The data are displayed in Table 11-5, where X is used as a symbol for the covariate and Y as a symbol for the dependent variable.

Homogeneity of Regression Coefficients

To adjust for a covariate, the difference between the score of an individual on the covariate and the grand mean of the covariate is weighted by what is called a *common* regression coefficient (b). Use of such a common regression coefficient is based on the assumption that there is no interaction between the covariate and the independent variable. If such an interaction exists, ANCOVA should *not* be used. Alternate approaches were discussed under the assumptions for ANCOVA.

Rather than do the calculations necessary for the testing of this assumption and run the risk of losing all our readers, we will simply demonstrate how the computer can generate the necessary statistics. Table 11-6 contains the data necessary to obtain this analysis. There we have the scores on the dependent variable, Y, and on the covariate, X. We have used dummy coding to enter treatment groups. Individu-

Table 11-5 Data for One-Way Analysis of Covariance

Groups	Illness Score (Covariate)		Adjustment Score		
	X	X²	Y	Y²	XY
	10	100	3	9	30
	9	81	5	25	45
	6	36	14	196	84
	8	64	8	64	64
A	8	64	7	49	56
	7	49	10	100	70
	9	81	6	36	54
	6	36	15	225	90
	7	49	13	169	91
	10	100	4	16	40
	80	660	85	889	624
	3	9	10	100	30
	4	16	7	49	28
	4	16	7	49	28
	6	36	3	9	18
B	5	25	3	9	15
	2	4	12	144	24
	1	1	14	196	14
	3	9	9	81	27
	5	25	4	16	20
	2	4	11	121	22
	35	145	80	774	226
Overall	*115*	*805*	*165*	*1663*	*850*

als in Group *A* are entered as 1s and those in group *B* as 0s. We labeled that vector *T*. An interaction vector is created by multiplying the score on the covariate by the code for the treatment group. That vector is labeled, *I*. If the interaction vector adds significantly to the variance accounted for, ANCOVA would not be the appropriate technique to use.

Remember with regression that we could determine not only the overall R^2 but how much, if any, variance was accounted for by each independent variable. Here we want to know whether the interaction vector (labeled *I*) will contribute significantly to the variance. To find that out, we need to calculate two R^2s. *Y* (the adjustment scores) is regressed on *X* (the covariate, illness scores) and *T* (the treatment groups) to determine how much variance is accounted for by group membership and the covariate. *Y* is also regressed on *X, T,* and *I* (the interaction

Table 11-6 Testing the Homogeneity of Regression Assumption

Groups	Adjustment Score Y	Illness Covariate X	Treatment Groups (Dummy Coding) T	Interaction (X × T) I
A	3	10	1	10
	5	9	1	9
	14	6	1	6
	8	8	1	8
	7	8	1	8
	10	7	1	7
	6	9	1	9
	15	6	1	6
	13	7	1	7
	4	10	1	10
B	10	3	0	0
	7	4	0	0
	7	4	0	0
	3	6	0	0
	3	5	0	0
	12	2	0	0
	14	1	0	0
	9	3	0	0
	4	5	0	0
	11	2	0	0

term). If the R^2 that contains the interaction vector is significantly larger than the R^2 that does not contain that vector, there would be a significant interaction between covariate and treatment group. Let us look at the formula for testing this difference.

$$F = \frac{(R^2 Y.XTI - R^2 Y.XT)/(k_1 - k_2)}{(1 - R^2 Y.XTI)/(n - k - 1)}$$

In the numerator, we measure the difference between two R^2s—one that contains the interaction vector $(R^2 Y.XTI)$, and one that does not $(R^2 Y.XT)$. Those R^2s are divided by their df. The df for the R^2s are equal to the number of independent variables. Therefore, $k_1 = 3$ and $k_2 = 2$. The denominator contains the residual variance $(1 - R^2)$ and is divided by its df $(n - k - 1)$. Here, $n = 20$ and $k = 3$, so $n - k - 1 = 20 - 3 - 1 = 16$.

The regression of Y on X and T yields an R^2 of .94766. The regression of Y on X, T, and I yields an R^2 of .95327. Our formula is therefore

$$F = \frac{(.95327 - .94766)/3 - 2}{(1 - .95327)/20 - 3 - 1}$$

$$= \frac{.00561/1}{.04673/16}$$

$$= \frac{.00561}{.00292062}$$

$$= 1.92$$

An F of 1.92 with 1, 16 df is not significant. Therefore, there is no significant interaction between the covariate and the independent variable. The data have met the assumption of homogeneity of variance and we may proceed with the calculation of ANCOVA.

Calculation of Sums of Squares

We must now calculate the sums of squares necessary for this analysis. These include *total* and *within* values for Σy^2, Σx^2, Σxy. The calculations are shown in Table 11-7. A summary of the calculations is given in Table 11-8. The sum of squares of the residuals must now be computed for total and within. The formula and calculations are given in Table 11-9.

Because *between* plus *within* residual sum of squares equals *total* sum of squares, we may subtract the *within* sum of squares of the residuals from the *total* sum of squares of the residuals to solve for the *between* residual sum of squares. The between residual sum of squares represents the amount of the variance due to differences between (or among) group means after adjusting for the covariate. In this example, it represents the difference between the means of groups A and B on post-hospital adjustment *after* equalizing the groups on level of illness (the covariate).

Total SS of residual − within SS of residual = Between SS of residuals.

In our example,

$$233.91 - 15.79 = 218.12$$

In analysis of covariance, 1 df is removed for each covariate. For the total df, the formula is $n - 1$ − number of covariates. In our example, that would be $20 - 1 - 1$, or 18 df.

The df for between groups sums of squares are calculated in the same way as for regular ANOVA, that is, number of groups − 1. The df for the within SS equals the total df minus the df for between.

Table 11-7   Calculation of Sums of Squares for ANCOVA

Σy^2 total

$$\Sigma y^2 = \Sigma Y_{tot}^2 - \frac{(\Sigma Y_{tot})^2}{n_{tot}}$$

$$= 1663 - \frac{(165)^2}{20}$$

$$= 1663 - 1361.25$$

$$= 301.75$$

Σy^2 within (A and B indicate the two treatment groups)

$$\Sigma y^2 = \Sigma Y_{tot}^2 - \left[\frac{(\Sigma Y_A)^2}{n_A} + \frac{(\Sigma Y_B)^2}{n_B}\right]$$

$$= 1663 - \left[\frac{(85)^2}{10} + \frac{(80)^2}{10}\right]$$

$$= 1663 - [722.5 + 640]$$

$$= 1663 - 1362.5$$

$$= 300.5$$

Σx^2 total

$$\Sigma x^2 = \Sigma X^2 - \frac{(\Sigma X)^2}{n}$$

$$= 805 - \frac{(115)^2}{20}$$

$$= 143.75$$

Σx^2 within

$$\Sigma x^2 = \Sigma X^2 - \left[\frac{(\Sigma X_A)^2}{n_A} + \frac{(\Sigma X_B)^2}{n_B}\right]$$

$$= 805 - \left[\frac{(80)^2}{10} + \frac{(35)^2}{10}\right]$$

$$= 805 - 762.5$$

$$= 42.5$$

Σxy total

$$\Sigma xy = \Sigma XY - \frac{(\Sigma X)(\Sigma Y)}{n}$$

$$= 850 - \frac{(115)(165)}{20}$$

$$= 850 - 948.75$$

$$= 98.75$$

Σxy within

$$\Sigma xy = \Sigma XY - \left[\frac{(\Sigma X_A)(\Sigma Y_A)}{n_A} + \frac{(\Sigma X_B)(\Sigma Y_B)}{n_B}\right]$$

$$= 850 - \left[\frac{(80)(85)}{10} + \frac{(35)(80)}{10}\right]$$

$$= 850 - [680 + 280]$$

$$= 850 - 960$$

$$= -110$$

In our sample,

Source	df
Total	$20 - 1 - 1 = 18$
Between	$2 - 1 = 1$
Within	$18 - 1 = 17$

The summary table would be written as in Table 11-10. We see that the groups really are different on their post-hospital adjustment scores. The final step is to adjust the groups means on the dependent variable; that is, we can see what the means are after the influence of the covariate is removed. In this case, we want to see what the means of the post-hospital adjustment scores for the two groups would be if they had been equal in their degree of illness.

Table 11-8   Summary of Calculation of Sums of Squares

Sums of Squares	Total	Within
Σy^2	301.75	300.5
$\Sigma \chi^2$	143.75	42.5
$\Sigma \chi y$	-98.75	-110.0

Table 11-9   Calculation of Residual Sums of Squares for ANCOVA

Residual SS $= \Sigma y^2 - [(\Sigma \chi y)^2 / \Sigma \chi^2]$

Total residual SS

Residual SS $= 301.75 - [(-98.75)^2 / 143.75]$

$= 301.75 - 67.84$

$= 233.91$

Within residual SS

Residual SS $= 300.5 - [(-110)^2 / 42.5]$

$= 300.5 - 284.71$

$= 15.79$

Table 11-10   Summary Table for Analysis of Covariance Example

Source of Variation	SS	df	MS	F	p
Between	218.12	1	218.12	234.54	$< .01$
Within	15.79	17	.93		
Total	233.91	18			

Adjustment of Means

We use this technique to see what the outcome means would have been if the groups had been equal at the beginning. The formula is

$$\overline{Y}_{adj} = \overline{Y}_{group} - b(\overline{X}_{group} - \overline{X})$$

$\overline{Y}_{group}$ — mean of group — before adjustment
$\overline{X}_{group}$ — mean of covariate for a group
$\overline{X}$ — grand mean of covariate
b — is the within regression coefficient

The formula for b is

$$b = \frac{\Sigma \chi y}{\Sigma \chi^2}$$

Here we use the within sums of squares (See Table 11-8 for the figures):

$$b = \frac{-110}{42.5}$$
$$= -2.59$$

Table 11-11 contains the means of the groups on the dependent variable and the covariate and the grand mean of the variable. These numbers are derived from Table 11-4.

Adjusted Mean for Group A

$\overline{Y}\,adj = \overline{Y}\,group - b(\overline{X}\,group - \overline{X})$
$= 8.5 - (-2.59)(8 - 5.75)$
$= 8.5 - (-2.59)(2.25)$
$= 8.5 - (-5.8275)$
$= 14.3275$

Adjusted Mean for Group B

$\overline{Y} = 8.0 - (-2.59)(3.5 - 5.75)$
$= 8.0 - (-2.59)(-2.25)$
$= 8.0 - 5.8275$
$= 2.1725$

Table 11-11   Group Means and Grand Mean of Covariate

Groups	Adjustment ($\overline{Y}$)	Wellness ($\overline{X}$)
A	8.5	8.0
B	8.0	3.5
	Grand mean 5.75	

Thus, we have

Groups	Original Means	Adjusted Means
A	8.5	14.3275
B	8.0	2.1725

Although the original means were almost equal, adjusting for the difference in wellness of the two groups changes the means dramatically. We see that individuals in group A had significantly higher (14.3275) adjustment scores than individuals in group B (2.1725). The use of ANCOVA has allowed us to compare our two nursing interventions as though they were applied to groups who were equivalent in terms of wellness.

SUMMARY

ANCOVA is an extension of ANOVA that allows us to remove additional sources of variation from the error term, thus enhancing the power of our analysis. This technique is not a cure-all for difficulties with unequal groups and should be used only after careful consideration is given to meeting the underlying assumptions. It is especially important to check for homogeneity of regression, because if that assumption is violated, ANCOVA can lead to improper interpretation of results.

EXAMPLE OF A COMPUTER PRINTOUT

Figure 11-3 contains an example of an analysis of covariance produced by the PROC GLM program in SAS.*

In this example, subjects at nine different child care centers were compared on a measure of hyperactivity (HYPER2). A pretest of hyperactivity, measured before the children started at the child care centers (HYPER1) is used as the covariate.

The overall model with an F value of 5.61 is significant at the .0001 level (①). In the lower portion (②) of the table, note the 8 df for center (there were 9 centers) and an F value (associated with Type III SS because there were unequal ns) of 5.55, which is significant at the .0001 level. The covariate, HYPER1, with 1 df, is also significant ($p = .0025$). In the next table (③), the unadjusted means for the dependent variable and covariate are given for each of nine centers. Center 53 had the highest pre-test score (1.85) and Center 59 had the lowest (1.57). On the post-test scores, Center 57 had the highest mean score (2.261) and Center 58 had the lowest (1.571).

* This example was prepared by Susan Grajek for a class in the use of the computer given to Yale School of Nursing students.

(*Text continues on page 238*)

Figure 11-3 Example of ANCOVA produced by SAS's PROC GLM program.

Procedure Cards

```
PROC GLM;
  CLASS CENTER;
  MODEL HYPER2 = CENTER HYPER1;
  MEANS CENTER;
  LSMEANS CENTER/STDERR PDIFF;
TITLE1 EXAMPLE OF PROC GLM FOR ANCOVA;
TITLE2 HYPER2 IS CONTINUOUS DEPENDENT VARIABLE;
TITLE3 HYPER1 IS CONTINUOUS COVARIATE;
TITLE4 CENTER IS CATEGORICAL INDEPENDENT VARIABLE;
```

Output

```
                        EXAMPLE OF PROC GLM FOR ANCOVA
                 HYPER2 IS CONTINUOUS DEPENDENT VARAIBLE
                      HYPER1 IS CONTINUOUS COVARIATE
                 CENTER IS CATEGORICAL INDEPENDENT VARIABLE

                      GENERAL LINEAR MODELS PROCEDURE
```

DEPENDENT VARIABLE: HYPER2   TEACHER RATING PBQ HYPER DISTRACT

SOURCE	DF	SUM OF SQUARES	MEAN SQUARE	F VALUE	① PR > F
MODEL	9	9.98193553	1.10910395	5.61	0.0001
ERROR	138	27.30422954	0.19785674		ROOT MSE
CORRECTED TOTAL	147	37.28616507			0.44481090

R-SQUARE	C.V.
0.267712	22.6974
	HYPER2 MEAN
	1.95974099

SOURCE	DF	TYPE I SS	F VALUE	PR > F
CENTER	8	8.09756113	5.12	0.0001
HYPER1	1	1.88437440	9.52	0.0025

SOURCE	DF	TYPE III SS	F VALUE	PR > F
CENTER	8 ②	8.79178164	5.55	0.0001
HYPER1	1	1.88437440	9.52	0.0025

[Unadjusted] MEANS

CENTER	N	HYPER2	HYPER1
51	20	2.12500000	1.59583333
52	21	2.15674603	1.78571429
53 ③	5	1.87500000	1.85000000
54	21	1.98809524	1.66269841
55	17	1.73529412	1.82352941
56	16	1.63281250	1.83333333
57	22	2.26136364	1.64772727
58	14	1.57142857	1.58035714
59	12	1.97916667	1.56770833

[Adjusted] LEAST SQUARES MEANS

CENTER	HYPER2 LSMEAN	STD ERR LSMEAN	PROB >|T| H0:LSMEAN=0	I/J	1	2	3	4	5 ⑤	6	7	8	9
51	2.15838713	0.10004938	0.0001	1	.	0.8249	0.1381	0.2551	0.0022	0.0002	0.3877	0.0005	0.4022
52	2.12725076	0.09753510	0.0001	2	0.8249	.	0.1734	0.3553	0.0033	0.0004	0.2728	0.0011	0.5181
53	1.82421538	0.19960498	0.0001	3	0.1381	0.1734	.	0.4321	0.5638	0.3009	0.0425	0.3605	0.4091
54	1.99933883	0.09713405	0.0001	4	0.2551	0.3553	0.4321	.	0.0381	0.0064	0.0422	0.0124	0.8891
55	1.69327570	0.10873827	0.0001	5	0.0022	0.0033	0.5638	0.0381	.	0.4961	0.0001	0.6092	0.0552
56	1.58754734	0.11216587	0.0001	6	0.0002	0.0004	0.3009	0.0064	0.4961	.	0.0001	0.8923	0.0128
57	2.27756518	0.09497920	0.0001	7	0.3877	0.2728	0.0425	0.0422	0.0001	0.0001	.	0.0001	0.1120
58	1.60094092	0.11953392	0.0001	8	0.0005	0.0011	0.3605	0.0124	0.6092	0.8923	0.0001	.	0.0200
59 ④	2.02186789	0.12914920	0.0001	9	0.4022	0.5181	0.4091	0.8891	0.0552	0.0128	0.1120	0.0200	.

NOTE: TO ENSURE OVERALL PROTECTION LEVEL, ONLY PROBABILITIES ASSOCIATED WITH PRE-PLANNED COMPARISONS SHOULD BE USED.

237

In the next table (④) are the adjusted means. After adjusting for the pre-test scores, Center 57 still had the highest mean score (2.277), and Center 56 (rather than 58) had the lowest.

All possible comparisons between groups are given in the right side of the table (⑤). The numbers for the centers are shortened to one digit, so Center 51 is designated 1, Center 52, 2, and so on. Because Centers 57 and 56 differed the most on their adjusted post-test scores, we would expect those means to differ significantly. In the table, we see the probability for that difference is .0001. Note that the bottom triangle of numbers is simply a mirror image of the top. Starting with Center 51 (and reading horizontally), we see that Center 51 differed significantly from Centers 55, 56, and 58. Center 51 with an adjusted mean score of 2.158 scored significantly higher than Centers 55, 56 and 58, which were the three centers with the lowest adjusted post-test scores.

EXAMPLE FROM PUBLISHED RESEARCH

ANCOVA was used to test the effects of progressive relaxation training for participants in a cardiac exercise program (Bohachick, 1984).

Hypotheses

The post-test means of selected psychological variables will be lower in the group of participants taught progressive relaxation than in a control group.

Data Gathered

Thirty-seven individuals involved in a cardiac exercise program served as subjects in this study. During a 3-week period, 18 of them were taught to use progressive relaxation. The other 19 subjects served as controls. All subjects were measured pre- and post-treatment on state anxiety and on a symptom checklist designed to measure psychological symptoms. Six dimensions of the symptom checklist were used.

Tabular Presentation and Display of Results

The results of the study are displayed in Tables 11-12 through 11-16. To check on the comparability of the experimental and control group, independent t-tests were used to compare the groups on their pretest scores on the anxiety scale and the six dimensions of the symptom checklist. There were no significant differences between the two groups on any of these measures, thus indicating that these groups were equivalent in relation to the variables of interest in the study (see Table 11-12).

Next, ANCOVA was used to compare the experimental and control groups on the post-test measures. The pre-test measures were used as covariates. "This analy-

Table 11-12   Means, Standard Deviations, and *t* Tests on PreTreatment Stress Measures for the Experimental and Control Group

Variable	Experimental (N = 18) Mean	SD	Control (N = 19) Mean	SD	t Value
State anxiety	33.17	8.47	30.37	8.06	1.03
Somatization	5.67	3.91	4.84	3.91	.64
Depression	6.72	3.75	5.89	3.96	.65
Anxiety	4.33	3.36	2.95	2.82	1.36
Interpersonal sensitivity	4.11	3.07	3.95	2.53	.18
Obsessive compulsive	8.06	4.98	6.58	5.10	.89
Hostility	3.11	2.30	2.53	1.95	.84

From Bohachick, P. (1984). Progressive relaxation training in cardiac rehabilitation: effect on psychological variables. *Nursing Research, 33*(5), 283–287.

Table 11-13   Pre-, Post- and Adjusted Post-test Means for Anxiety State Scores

Group	Pre-	Post-	Adjusted Post
Experimental	33.17	29.06	28.17
Control	30.37	31.58	32.42

From Bohachick, P. (1984). Progressive relaxation training in cardiac rehabilitation: effect on psychological variables. *Nursing Research, 33*(5), 283–287.

sis enabled a comparison of post-treatment psychologic distress scores in both groups by statistically controlling for any differences in the pre-treatment scores that were present but not significant." (Bohachick, 1984, p. 285)

Table 11-13 contains the pre- and post-means and the adjusted post-mean on the state anxiety scores. Although the groups were not significantly different on the pre-test, the experimental group did have a higher mean score (33.17) than the control group (30.37). Thus, when the post-test scores are adjusted for the pre-test score, we see that the experimental group's mean is adjusted downward (from 29.06 to 28.17), and the control group's mean is adjusted upward (from 31.58 to 32.42). These adjustments have the net result of making the means of the two groups farther apart. This is a good example of the usefulness of ANCOVA. In Table 11-14, we see that the adjusted means were significantly different ($p < .05$).

Tables 11-15 and 11-16 report the results of the comparison of the two groups on the six dimensions of the symptom scores. In each case, although the differences were not significant, the experimental group scored higher than the control group

Table 11-14   Summary of ANVOCAs for Anxiety State Scale

Adjusted MS Between	Adjusted MS Within	$F(1, 34)$
162.11	21.97	7.38*

* $p < .05$

From Bohachick, P. (1984). Progressive relaxation training in cardiac rehabilitation: effect on psychological variables. *Nursing Research, 33*(5), 283–287.

Table 11-15   Pre-, Post-, and Adjusted Post-test Means for SCL-90-R Symptom Scores

Scale		Pre	Post	Adjusted Post
Somatization	Experimental	5.67	2.67	2.46
	Control	4.84	4.52	4.72
Depression	Experimental	6.72	3.61	3.41
	Control	5.89	5.26	5.45
Anxiety	Experimental	4.33	1.78	1.42
	Control	2.95	2.74	3.08
Interpersonal	Experimental	4.11	1.94	1.89
sensitivity	Control	3.95	3.74	3.79
Obsessive-	Experimental	8.06	6.06	5.55
compulsive	Control	6.58	5.47	5.95
Hostility	Experimental	3.11	2.44	2.21
	Control	2.53	1.89	2.12

From Bohachick, P. (1984). Progressive relaxation training in cardiac rehabilitation: effect on psychological variables. *Nursing Research, 33*(5), 283–287.

on the pre-test. As with the anxiety measure, the experimental group's post-test means are adjusted upward and the control group's are adjusted downward. On four of the dimensions, the experimental group scored significantly lower than the control group.

The investigators demonstrated that it is feasible to incorporate relaxation training into a cardiac exercise program and that compared to a control group, cardiac patients trained in relaxation techniques demonstrated significant improvement in psychological distress measures. The findings of this study indicate that multiple dependent variables are required to sufficiently evaluate the effects of a relaxation training program (Bohachick, 1984, p. 287).

Table 11-16   Summary of ANCOVAs for SCL-90-R Symptom Measures

Scale	Adjusted Means Between	Adjusted Means Within	$F(1, 34)$
Somatization	46.73	3.93	11.88†
Depression	38.25	5.69	6.72*
Anxiety	24.15	3.04	7.94*
Interpersonal sensitivity	33.36	3.12	10.68†
Obsessive-compulsive	1.39	5.73	0.24
Hostility	0.08	2.09	0.04

*$p < .05$
†$p < .01$
From Bohachick, P. (1984). Progressive relaxation training in cardiac rehabilitation: effect on psychological variables. *Nursing Research, 33*(5), 283–287.

EXERCISES FOR CHAPTER 11

1. What is the main function of analysis of covariance (ANCOVA)?
2. Suppose you wanted to compare men and women on their ability to follow written instructions. Because you know that women usually have higher verbal ability than men, you decide to use ANCOVA to control for that difference. Would that be an acceptable use of ANCOVA?
3. What does homogeneity of regression, as an assumption for ANCOVA, mean?
4. Y = dependent variable
   X = covariate
   T = treatment variable
   I = interaction variable
   $RY.XTI = .620$
   $RY.XT = .504$
   $n = 104$

   Test for homogeneity of variance. What action would you take based on these results?
5. The homogeneity of regression assumption has been met for the following data. Subjects have been randomly assigned to the two treatment groups. A high score on the covariate indicates high anxiety. A high score on the dependent variable indicates a high level of adjustment. Calculate ANCOVA. Interpret the results.

Groups	Covariate (Pre-test) Anxiety Level	Psychological Adjustment
Practice relaxation:	20	10
	18	11
	8	17
	6	19
	10	16
	12	15
	14	14
	4	20
	16	12
	13	15
Do not practice relaxation:	4	10
	7	8
	19	2
	15	4
	7	9
	3	12
	18	3
	11	7
	18	4
	17	6

CHAPTER 12
Repeated Measures

Barbara Hazard Munro

OBJECTIVES FOR CHAPTER 12

After reading this chapter and completing the exercises, you should be able to

1. Describe the two major ways in which repeated measures ANOVA is used.
2. Explain the assumption of compound symmetry.
3. Interpret a repeated measures ANOVA summary table.
4. Discuss difficulties that may arise with the use of this technique.
5. Demonstrate the application of the Greenhouse-Geisser procedure.

Repeated measures analysis of variance (ANOVA) is an approach that helps us deal with individual differences. Those differences are usually part of the error term. Because they increase the error term, they decrease the likelihood of finding a significant result. While individual differences reflect actual differences among individuals, they also reflect the individual's particular state when the instrument was administered (*e.g.,* tired, bored, angry), environmental factors (*e.g.,* noise, heat, cold) and response styles (*e.g.,* unwillingness to check extreme value). With repeated measures ANOVA, we may be able to measure, and thus control, some of this variation.

There are two main types of repeated measures designs (also called within subjects designs). One type involves taking repeated measures of the same variable(s) over time on a group or groups of subjects. For example, if we were studying hypertension, we would probably want more than one blood pressure reading on our subjects.

The other main type of repeated measures design involves exposing the same subjects to all levels of the treatment. Suppose we wanted to see whether therapeutic touch or practicing meditation reduced pain any more than the standard treatment. We could randomly assign individuals experiencing pain to one of the following three conditions: touch, meditation, or control. However, if our subjects varied widely in the amount of pain they reported, the within subject variability would be very large. Because the F statistic is based on the ratio of between group variance to within group variance, there would have to be a very large between group difference to attain a significant result; that is, the large variability among the subjects could obscure any real differences between the groups. This would be especially true if the groups were small. One way to remove these individual differences would be to assign each subject to all treatments. Each subject would be exposed to touch, meditation, and regular treatment. Thus, each subject would serve as his or her own control, and the within or error variance would be decreased. This would result in a more powerful test and would decrease the number of subjects needed for the study.

TYPE OF DATA REQUIRED

The requirements are the same as those for the usual ANOVA. The independent variable(s) are categorical, and the dependent variable is continuous.

ASSUMPTIONS

The basic assumptions for the t-test and ANOVA are also necessary here. The dependent variable should be normally distributed, and the homogeneity of variance requirement should be met.

There is one major difference, however. In ANOVA, the observations are independent of each other. This is achieved by having subjects randomly assigned to mutually exclusive groups. With repeated measures, however, there is correlation between the measures, because they are from the same people. It is necessary, therefore, to meet another assumption. This is called the assumption of *compound symmetry*.

There are two parts to this assumption. The first part is the assumption that the correlations across the measurements are the same. Suppose you measured a variable three times. You could then calculate the correlation between the first measure and the second, between the first and the third, and between the second and the third. All three of these correlations should be about the same, or $r_{12} = r_{13} = r_{23}$.

The second part of the assumption is that the variances should be equal across measurements. With three measurements, we would need $s_1^2 = s_2^2 = s_3^2$. This second assumption is critical. The general robustness of the ANOVA model does not withstand much violation of this assumption. This will be discussed further under "Problems With Use of Repeated Measures."

REPEATED MEASURES OVER TIME

The simplest example of such an analysis was presented in Chapter 8 where we discussed the use of the correlated t-test to compare the means of a pre-test and a post-test administered to the same people. Because the same people took both tests, their scores should be correlated. The correlated *t*-test removes this relationship and thus increases the power of the comparison of the two means. We can extend this concept to situations in which there is more than one group and to situations in which subjects are measured several times on the same variable.

Suppose that instead of one group measured pre- and post-treatment, we had a true experimental design with subjects assigned randomly to an experimental group and a control group. If we measured these subjects pre- and post-experiment, we could no longer use the correlated *t*-test. We would now have two groups that were measured twice. This is called a *mixed design* because we have both between and within subjects measures. First, we have two different groups, the experimental and the control group. These two groups constitute the between group measure. Comparing them answers the question of whether or not the experimental condition had an effect on outcomes. The *second* part of the design, or the within group component, consists of the fact that each group is measured twice on the same variable. The question answered here is whether or not there is a difference between the pre- and post-test measures.

Another example is represented in Figure 12-1. We wish to study the effectiveness of various treatment modalities on hypertension, and we want to examine the effects over time. We randomly assign individuals with hypertension to one of three groups: drug therapy, relaxation therapy, or control. Each subject is in one, and only one, group. All subjects' blood pressure is measured before treatment and at the following intervals during 1 year of treatment: 4 weeks, 3 months, 6 months, and 1 year. The pre-test could be used to determine whether randomization worked. There should, of course, be no significant difference among the groups before treatment. The measures of interest are the measures after treatment began.

Treatment group

Time	Drug therapy (DT) n = 10	Relaxation therapy (RT) n = 10	Control (C) n = 10	**Row** **X̄s**
Pretest	$\bar{X}_{DT}$, Pre	$\bar{X}_{RT}$, Pre	$\bar{X}_{C}$, Pre	$\bar{X}$ Pre
4 weeks	$\bar{X}_{DT}$, 4 weeks	$\bar{X}_{RT}$, 4 weeks	$\bar{X}_{C}$, 4 weeks	$\bar{X}$ 4 weeks
3 months	$\bar{X}_{DT}$, 3 months	$\bar{X}_{RT}$, 3 months	$\bar{X}_{C}$, 3 months	$\bar{X}$ 3 months
6 months	$\bar{X}_{DT}$, 6 months	$\bar{X}_{RT}$, 6 months	$\bar{X}_{C}$, 6 months	$\bar{X}$ 6 months
1 year	$\bar{X}_{DT}$, 1 year	$\bar{X}_{RT}$, 1 year	$\bar{X}_{C}$, 1 year	$\bar{X}$ 1 year
Column **X̄s**	$\bar{X}_{DT}$	$\bar{X}_{RT}$	$\bar{X}_{C}$	

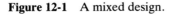

Figure 12-1   A mixed design.

If we were to use regular one-way ANOVA to analyze these data, we would have to calculate five ANOVAs, one for each time the blood pressure was measured. The individual differences would be part of the error term.

If we use repeated measure ANOVA, we have two independent variables (rather than one independent variable measured against five different measures of the same variable). One independent variable is treatment group, with three levels. The other independent variable is time, with five levels. With the repeated measures approach, we can answer three main questions.

1. Do the three groups have significantly different blood pressures after treatment? All blood pressure recordings would be included here; that is, the time component is ignored, and the question is answered by comparing the three column means, $\overline{X}_{DT}$, $\overline{X}_{RT}$, and $\overline{X}_C$ (see Fig. 12-1). If the overall F is significant, post-hoc tests would be used to find differences between pairs of scores.
2. Are there significant differences in blood pressure across the five time periods? Treatment group is ignored here, and the mean blood pressure is calculated for each of the time periods. In our example, the row means would be compared.
3. Is there an interaction between treatment type and time? Fifteen means would be compared to answer this question (three levels of first independent variable times five levels of second). In Figure 12-1, those means are shown in the cells. This would tell us whether different approaches worked better at one point in time than at another.

Tables 12-1 and 12-2 contain the summary tables for such an analysis. Table 12-1 contains the formulas, and Table 12-2 shows the calculations involved. The

Table 12-1   Summary Table for Repeated Measures Over Time—Formulas

Source of Variation	SS	df	MS	F	p
Between subjects		$n_c k - 1$		$\dfrac{\text{MS treatment}}{\text{MS within groups}}$	
Treatment		$k - 1$			
Within groups (error)		$k(n_c - 1)$			
Within subjects		$n_c k(t - 1)$			
Time		$t - 1$		$\dfrac{\text{MS time}}{\text{MS time} \times \text{within groups}}$	
Treatment × Time		$(k - 1)(t - 1)$		$\dfrac{\text{MS treatment} \times \text{time}}{\text{MS time} \times \text{within groups}}$	
Time × Within groups (error)		$k(n_c - 1)(t - 1)$			

n_c = number of subjects in each cell
k = number of levels in between fctor
t = number of repeated measures

Table 12-2   Summary Table for Repeated Measured Over Time—Calculations

Source of Variation	SS	df	MS	F	p
Between subjects	4630	$(10)(3) - 1 = 29$			
Treatment	1120	$3 - 1 = 2$	560	4.31	$< .05$
Within groups (error)	3510	$3(10 - 1) = 27$	130		
Within subjects	19864	$(10)(3)(5 - 1) = 120$			
Time	3520	$5 - 1 = 4$	880	6.38	$< .01$
Treatment × Time	1440	$(3 - 1)(5 - 1) = 8$	180	1.30	ns
Time × Within groups (error)	14904	$3(10 - 1)(5 - 1) = 108$	138		

n_c = number of subjects in each cell (in our example, 10 in each group)
k = number of levels in between factor (in our example, 3 treatment groups)
t = number of repeated measures (in our example, 5, pre-test to 1 year)

variation is divided into *between subjects* and *within subjects* components. Between subjects variation contains the usual elements from ANOVA. There is the between groups variation and the error term, which consists of the variability within the groups. The degrees of freedom (*df*) are calculated differently from ANOVA, however. Here we use n_c, the number of subjects per cell in the design, and *k*, the number of levels in the between group factor. In our example, we have 10 subjects in each cell of the design, and there are three treatment groups, so $n_c = 10$ and $k = 3$. For the total between group variation, the *df* are $(10)(3) - 1 = 29$. Note that the *df* for treatment plus the *df* for the error term equal the total *df* for the between groups variation $(2 + 27 = 29)$. This provides a check on your calculations. The sums of squares are divided by their *df* to calculate the mean squares. Dividing the mean square for the treatment by the mean square for the associated error term results in an *F* ratio, which tests for significant differences among the three treatment groups. In this example, 560/130 equals an *F* of 4.31. With 2, 27 *df,* this is significant at $< .05$ (see Appendix E).

The within subjects variation contains variance due to measures across time, the interaction between treatment and time, and the error term. The error term consists of the interaction between time and the within groups variability. In the formulas for *df,* *t* indicates the number of levels in the repeated factor. In our example, that is the time factor, so $t = 5$. The calculations of the *df* for the within subjects variations are given in Table 12-2. The error term used in calculating *F* ratios for within subjects variation is time × within groups. In our example, two within subjects *F* ratios are tested. The first *F* ratio tests whether there is a significant difference between the time periods. The mean square for time, 880, is divided by the mean square for the error term, 138, resulting in an *F* of 6.38. With 4,108 *df,* this is significant at $< .01$.

The second *F* ratio tests the interaction between treatment and time. The *F* ratio for that test is $180/138 = 1.30$. With 8,108 *df,* this is not significant. In this analysis, there was a significant difference among the three treatment groups and a significant difference over time. Post-hoc tests would be necessary to determine where these differences lie.

SUBJECTS EXPOSED TO
ALL TREATMENT LEVELS

An example is given in Figure 12-2. Ten subjects are each exposed to four different methods of pain control. The dependent variable is a rating by the patient of his perceived level of pain. This rating is taken four times, once after each treatment. Note that each cell contains only one score. Subject A's rating of perceived pain after exposure to drug therapy is the only score in the upper left cell. Because there is only one score in each cell, there is no variability within the cells of this design.

The total variation consists of *between subjects variation* and *within subjects*

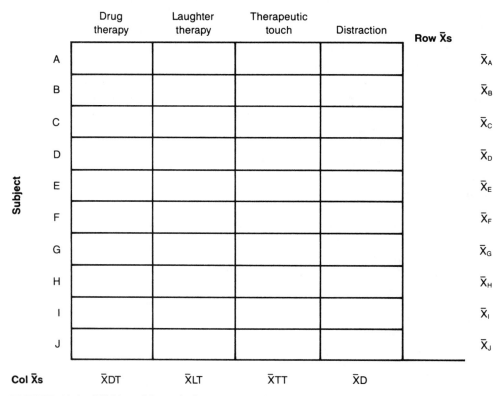

FIGURE 12-2 Within subjects design.

variation. Between subjects variation consists of the differences among the 10 subjects in this design. Testing the significance of that amount of variation would tell us whether or not the row means differed significantly from each other. That is not what we are really interested in, of course. What we want to know is whether or not there were differences among the treatments. By calculating the between people variation, however, we are able to remove that source of variation from the error term. If the variability among subjects is large, this would mean a substantial reduction in the error term.

The second main source of variation is the within subject variation. This measures how much each subject's scores varied across the treatment levels. This is what we are interested in. Do the subjects have lower ratings of pain with some treatments than with others? There are two components to this within people variation. One is due to the effect of treatment, and the other is due to uncontrolled factors that influence how a subject rates his pain at a given point in time.

Tables 12-3 and 12-4 contain the summary tables for such an analysis. The formulas are shown in Table 12-3; the calculations are shown in Table 12-4. For the between subjects variation, the row means are being compared. There is one mean for each subject, so the *df* are $n - 1$. In our example, there are 10 subjects. Therefore, the *df* for between subjects would be $10 - 1 = 9$.

For the within subjects variation, divided into *Treatments* and *Residual,* we are

Table 12-3 Summary Table for Subjects Exposed to All Treatment Levels—Formulas for *dfs*

Source of Variation	SS	*df*	MS	F	*p*
Between Subjects		$n - 1$			
Within Subjects		$n(k - 1)$			
Treatment		$k - 1$			
Residual (Error)		$(n - 1)(k - 1)$			
Total		*kn - 1*			

Table 12-4 Summary Table for Subjects Exposed to All Treatment Levels—Calculations

Source of Variation	SS	*df*	MS	F	*p*
Between Subjects		$10 - 1 = 9$			
Within Subjects	6060	$10(4 - 1) = 30$			
Treatment	2280	$4 - 1 = 3$	760	5.43	< .01
Residual (Error)	3780	$(10 - 1)(4 - 1) = 27$	140		
Total		$(4)(10) - 1 = 39$			

comparing each subject's rating for each treatment. The df for treatments are the number of treatments (k) minus one. In our example, there are four treatments, so the df are $4 - 1 = 3$. The residual df are calculated as $(n - 1)(k - 1)$, or $(10 - 1)(4 - 1) = 27$. The total within subject variation is based on all the subjects in the study and is therefore $n(k - 1)$. In our example, this would be $10(4 - 1) = 30$. For the total variation the df are $kn - 1$ or $(4)(10) - 1 = 39$.

Although the F ratio associated with between subjects may be tested for significance, that is not the source of variation that we are interested in. Here, we test the variation due to the treatments. The F ratio consists of the mean square for treatments, 760, divided by the mean square for the residual, 140. The resulting F is 5.43, and with 3,27 df, it is significant at $< .01$. Post-hoc tests would be necessary to determine which treatment means were significantly different.

PROBLEMS WITH USE
OF REPEATED MEASURES

Because subjects are measured repeatedly, there may be difficulties with such things as sensitization to the instruments. Scores on an anxiety scale may vary due to repeated exposure to the scale, rather than to real changes in anxiety. Even physiological measures may reflect this. For example, vital signs may increase with a new situation, then decrease with repeated measures. Practice with previous tests may increase scores on later tests. Subjects may be bored by repeated measures and be careless with later tests.

When subjects are exposed to more than one treatment, we need to consider that previous treatments may still be having an effect. In cases in which you expect carry-over effects, you should not use repeated measures ANOVA. As Winer (1962, p. 301) states:

> A strong word of warning is required in connection with order (or sequence) effects. Practice, fatigue, transfer of training, the effects of an immediately preceding success or failure illustrate what fall in the latter category. If such effects exist, randomizing or counterbalancing does not remove them; rather, such procedures completely entangle the latter with treatment effects. . . . In experiments . . . when the sequence effects are likely to be marked and where primary interest lies in evaluating the effect of individual treatments in the absence of possible sequence effects, a repeated measures design is to be avoided.

If such sequence effects are relatively small, repeated measures designs can be used. Randomizing the order in which the subjects are exposed to the treatments tends to spread the sequence effects over all the treatment levels and prevents them from being a confounding influence on only certain levels (Winer, 1962, p. 301).

The most important problem is that of meeting the criterion for compound symmetry. This should be tested before performing repeated measures ANOVA.

The MANOVA program in SPSS, the *BMDP* Program (Dixon, 1983), and the MULTIVARIANCE program (Finn & Mattsson, 1978) all have tests for compound symmetry. This assumption is often violated, leading to improper interpretation of results. According to Finn and Mattsson (1978, p. 83), "In practice, behavioral data rarely meet the assumption of compound symmetry." They also state, "It is a critical assumption in the univariate analysis of repeated measures data, and it is one that is not required by the corresponding *multivariate* analysis." (p. 82)

By "multivariate," Finn and Mattsson (1978) are referring to the use of more than one dependent variable in an analysis. Let us use an example to explain the differences in these approaches.

In our example of repeated measures over time (see Fig. 12-1), we used time as the second independent variable. We thus had two independent variables, and the dependent variable was a measure of blood pressure.

With a multivariate approach, the analysis would be treated as including only one independent variable, treatment group. It would also include five dependent variables. These would be the measures of blood pressure at the five time intervals. This sounds like the separate ANOVAs we said might be used. However, here the analysis does not take each ANOVA separately, but rather examines the relationships among the levels of the dependent variable, as well as the relationship between the independent variable and each dependent variable. This multivariate approach is more robust and can, therefore, handle the failure to meet the compound symmetry requirement. According to Finn and Mattsson (1978, p. 111), "The multivariate approach to the analysis of repeated measures is not only less restrictive, but usually more realistic. Especially in longitudinal data, we expect the correlations will not be uniform." If, however, the assumptions of the univariate model are met, the univariate analysis should be used, because it is more powerful and requires fewer subjects (p. 80).

Although Finn and Mattsson strongly advocate the use of the multivariate approach when the assumption of compound symmetry is not met, there is another approach that might be taken. It is called the Greenhouse-Geisser (1959) procedure. If the assumption of compound symmetry is not met, we are more likely to make a Type 1 error, that is, find a significant result when none exists. To avoid that, a more stringent, or "corrected," *F* can be used. To do this, the *df* in both the numerator and denominator are decreased. The original *df* for both the numerator and the denominator are divided by the *df* associated with the repeated factor. These new *df* can be used to give a more conservative estimate of the significance level.

Let us demonstrate this process with the summary data in Table 12-2. If the assumption for compound symmetry could not be met, we could apply the Greenhouse-Geisser procedure to decrease the *df* for testing the significance of the associated *F*s.

Because the *F* for treatment is related only to a between group sum of squares, no adjustment in *df* would be made. That *F* would still be tested by 2, 27 *df*.

The other two *F*s both involve repeated, or within subjects, measures; therefore, both need to be adjusted. The *df* associated with the *F* test for time are 4, 108. These *df* must each be divided by the *df* associated with time (4); so, for the numerator, we have

$$\frac{4}{4} = 1$$

and, for the denominator, we have,

$$\frac{108}{4} = 27$$

We would now test that *F* that equaled 6.38, with 1, 27 *df*. It would now be significant at the .05 level but not at the .01 level.

The *F* associated with the treatment × time interaction was tested by 8, 108 *df*. Applying the Greenhouse-Geisser procedure, for the numerator, we have

$$\frac{8}{4} = 2,$$

and, for the denominator, we have

$$\frac{108}{4} = 27$$

The *F* of 1.30 would be tested with 2, 27 *df* instead of 8, 108. Because it was not significant before, it will not be significant now.

The major difficulty with this correction is that it tends to overcorrect, thus increasing the likelihood of a Type II error (Keppel, 1973, p. 466). A determination of the relative importance of making a Type I or Type II error in a given analysis should be considered.

As must be evident by now, this is an area of complexity, and, for further clarification, the interested reader is advised to consult references mentioned in this chapter.

EXAMPLES OF COMPUTER PRINTOUTS

Figures 12-3 and 12-4 contain examples of repeated measures ANOVA produced by the BMDP, P2V program. A mixed design is presented in Figure 12-3 (the data are fictitious). Twenty subjects are randomly assigned to one of two groups, experimental or control, and all subjects are measured three times: before treatment, immediately after treatment, and 3 months after treatment. The dependent variable is a measure of distress, with a high score indicating high distress. Scores range from 0 to 20. In the computer analysis, the between subjects factor is termed GROUP, and the within subjects factor is known as TIME. The time periods in the within subjects factor are labeled PRETEST, POSTTEST, and FOLLOWUP.

The BMDP program tests the symmetry of orthogonal components rather than compound symmetry. The tests are similar, but according to Dixon (1983, p. 379), "Compound symmetry is a sufficient but not necessary condition. The symmetry test of P2V is a sufficient and necessary condition; it is less restrictive than compound symmetry." On the printout, the test is labeled *Sphericity Test Applied to Orthogonal Components* (①). In this example, the probability associated with the test is .2367, not significant. The data have, therefore, met this assumption.

The cell means and standard deviations are shown next on the printout (②). We can see that both groups scored about the same on the pre-test, with means of 17.4 and 17.2, respectively. On the post-test, the experimental group (group 1) had lower distress scores ($\overline{X} = 11.2$) than the control group (group 2, $\overline{X} = 16.8$). At the time of follow-up, the experimental group had still lower distress scores ($\overline{X} = 5.0$). The control groups still had fairly high scores ($\overline{X} = 16.2$).

In the summary table (③), the grand mean (MEAN) is tested for significance, but that is not of interest in this analysis. Because there were two groups (experimental and control), there is 1 *df* associated with the between subject factor ($k - 1$). The *F* associated with the GROUP variable is testing whether or not the two groups differed significantly on their distress scores. It asks, therefore, whether there is a significant difference between the overall distress score of 11.2 for the experimental group and 16.73 for the control group (see the marginals in the cell means portion of printout). The *F* is significant at the 0.0000 level; that is, the experimental group had significantly lower distress scores. "Tail probability" in BMDP means that the probability is appropriate if the data meet the criteria of normal distribution and homogeneity of variance. The *df* associated with the between error term are $k(n_c - 1)$. In this example, we have $2(10 - 1) = 18$.

There are three levels within the Time factor, so the *df* are $3 - 1 = 2(t - 1)$. TG represents the interaction between Time and Group. The *df* for the interaction are $(k - 1)(t - 1)$, or $(2 - 1)(3 - 1) = 2$. For the error term, the *df* are $k(n_c - 1)(t - 1)$, or $2(10 - 1)(3 - 1) = 36$. Both the time and interaction factors are significant, $p = 0.0000$. Because the assumption of symmetry was met, we do not need the Greenhouse-Geisser correction. The Huynh Feld probability is another type of correction that could be applied if the assumption of symmetry was not met.

The significant result for the Time factor tells us that 17.3, 14.0, and 10.6 are not equal (see marginals in cell means table). To test for significant differences between the pairs of means ($17.3 - 14.0$, $17.3 - 10.6$, and $14.0 - 10.6$), we would need to apply post-hoc tests. We can see that the means decreased from pre-test to follow-up.

The significant interaction tells us that the cell means differ significantly. Again, post-hoc tests would need to be applied to test for differences between pairs of means. We can see, by looking at the means, that they all decreased over time, but there was very little decrease for the control groups, and a great deal of decrease for the experimental group.

The second example of a computer generated repeated measures ANOVA is

(*Text continues on page 258*)

Figure 12-3 Repeated measures ANOVA for a mixed design produced by BMDP-P2V.

Procedure Cards

```
/ PROBLEM      TITLE IS 'REPEATED MEASURES, MIXED DESIGN'.
/ INPUT        VARIABLES ARE 4.
               FORMAT IS FREE.
/ VARIABLE     NAMES ARE GROUP, PRETEST, POSTTEST, FOLLOWUP.
/ DESIGN       DEPENDENT ARE 2 TO 4.
               LEVEL IS 3.
               GROUPING IS GROUP.
               NAME IS TIME.
               SYMMETRY.

/ END
```

Output

GROUP STRUCTURE

GROUP	COUNT
*1.00000	10.
*2.00000	10.

SUMS OF SQUARES AND CORRELATION MATRIX OF THE ORTHOGONAL COMPONENTS POOLED FOR ERROR 2 IN ANOVA TABLE BELOW

```
      12.20000     1.000
       5.93333     0.204     1.000
```

① SPHERICITY TEST APPLIED TO ORTHOGONAL COMPONENTS - TAIL PROBABILITY   0.2367

CELL MEANS FOR 1-ST DEPENDENT VARIABLE

		GROUP =	*1.00000	*2.00000	MARGINAL
	TIME				
PRETEST	1		17.40000	17.20000	17.30000
② POSTTEST	2		11.20000	16.80000	14.00000
FOLLOWUP	3		5.00000	16.20000	10.60000

MARGINAL   11.20000   16.73333   13.96667

COUNT   10   10   20

STANDARD DEVIATIONS FOR 1-ST DEPENDENT VARIABLE

GROUP   =   *1.00000   *2.00000
TIME

PRETEST   1   1.71270   1.75119
POSTTEST   2   2.29976   1.39841
FOLLOWUP   3   2.58199   1.81353

ANALYSIS OF VARIANCE FOR 1-ST
DEPENDENT VARIABLE - PRETEST POSTTEST FOLLOWUP

	SOURCE	SUM OF SQUARES	DEGREES OF FREEDOM	MEAN SQUARE	F	TAIL PROB.	GREENHOUSE GEISSER PROB.	HUYNH FELDT PROB.
	MEAN	11704.06667	1	11704.06667	1104.93	0.0000		
	GROUP	459.26667	1	459.26667	43.36	0.0000		
③ 1	ERROR	190.66667	18	10.59259				
	TIME	448.93333	2	224.46667	445.63	0.0000	0.0	0.0
	TG	324.93333	2	162.46667	322.54	0.0000	0.0	0.0
2	ERROR	18.13333	36	0.50370				

ERROR
TERM   EPSILON FACTORS FOR DEGREES OF FREEDOM ADJUSTMENT

                     GREENHOUSE-GEISSER   HUYNH-FELDT
2   0.8651   1.0000

NUMBER OF INTEGER WORDS OF STORAGE USED IN PRECEDING PROBLEM   1011
CPU TIME USED   1.130 SECONDS

255

Figure 12-4 Repeated measures ANOVA for a within-subjects design produced by BMDP-P2V.

Procedure Cards

```
/ PROBLEM      TITLE IS 'WITHIN SUBJECTS DESIGN'.
/ INPUT        VARIABLES ARE 3.
               FORMAT IS FREE.
/ VARIABLE     NAMES ARE EXP1, EXP2, CONTROL.
/ DESIGN       DEPENDENT ARE 1 TO 3.
               LEVELS ARE 3.
               NAMES ARE RX.
               SYMMETRY.
/ END
```

Output

SUMS OF SQUARES AND CORRELATION MATRIX OF THE ORTHOGONAL COMPONENTS POOLED FOR ERROR 2 IN ANOVA TABLE BELOW

```
28.90000      1.000
14.30000     -0.537     1.000
```

① SPHERICITY TEST APPLIED TO ORTHOGONAL COMPONENTS - TAIL PROBABILITY   0.0158

CELL MEANS FOR 1-ST DEPENDENT VARIABLE

```
         RX                    MARGINAL

EXP1      1      42.85000      42.85000
EXP2      2      28.35000      28.35000
CONTROL   3      11.75000      11.75000

       MARGINAL  27.65000      27.65000

       COUNT     20            20
```

STANDARD DEVIATIONS FOR 1-ST DEPENDENT VARIABLE

```
           RX

    EXP1      1      4.34408
②   EXP2      2      4.31978
    CONTROL   3      4.83273
```

ANALYSIS OF VARIANCE FOR 1-ST
DEPENDENT VARIABLE - EXP1   EXP2   CONTROL

	SOURCE	SUM OF SQUARES	DEGREES OF FREEDOM	MEAN SQUARE	F	TAIL PROB.	GREENHOUSE GEISSER PROB.	HUYNH FELDT PROB.
1	MEAN	45871.35000	1	45871.35000	782.61	0.0000		
	ERROR	1113.65000	19	58.61316				
③	RX	9686.80000	2	4843.40000	4260.39	0.0000	0.0	0.0
2	ERROR	43.20000	38	1.13684				

ERROR
TERM   EPSILON FACTORS FOR DEGREES OF FREEDOM ADJUSTMENT

              GREENHOUSE-GEISSER   HUYNH-FELDT
    2   0.7302   0.7757

257

shown in Figure 12-4. There is no grouping factor in this example; it is a within subjects design. There are 20 subjects, and they are all exposed to three different treatments. Each subject is, therefore, his own control. There are two experimental (EXP1 and EXP2), and one control condition. After exposure to the treatment, the subject is measured on an adjustment scale, which ranges from a low of 1 to a high of 50. (The data are fictitious.) Each subject is, therefore, measured three times, once after each treatment.

In this example, the criterion of symmetry (①) is *not* met, $p = 0.0158$; therefore, the Greenhouse-Geisser of Huynh Feld probabilities should be used. The highest adjustment scores occurred after exposure to the first experimental condition (②); $(\overline{X} = 42.85)$. After EXP2, the mean score was 28.35, and, after the control condition, it was 11.75.

The different treatments are labeled RX in the summary table (③). The *df* associated with RX are $k - 1$, or $3 - 1 = 2$. For the error, the *df* are $(n - 1)(k - 1)$, or $(20 - 1)(3 - 1) = 38$. There is a significant difference among the means for the treatment groups, with the Greenhouse-Geisser probability equal to 0.0. Although post-hoc tests could be applied to the pairs of means, it appears that subjects had very high adjustment after EXP1, moderate adjustment after EXP2, and low adjustment after the control condition.

EXAMPLE FROM PUBLISHED RESEARCH

Research Problem

Repeated measures ANOVA was used in a study designed to investigate the effect of nursing interventions on the malnutrition that results from cancer (Dixon, 1984).

Data Gathered

Eighty-eight individuals who were at risk nutritionally due to cancer were recruited into the study, and 55 subjects completed the 4-month intervention period. Subjects were randomly assigned to one of five groups, four experimental condition and one control group. The four experimental conditions in which subjects were visited every other week by a nurse included

1. Nutritional supplementation
2. Relaxation training
3. Nutritional supplementation and relaxation training
4. Nurse visits only

The dependent variables were measures of nutritional and performance status.

Results

Table 12-5 contains the results of this study. The significant main effect for time indicates that the groups changed significantly over time. On the triceps skinfold

Table 12-5 Means and Repeated Measures Analysis Results of Initial and Postintervention Values

| | | Group | | | | | Analysis of Variance Results | | |
| | | Supplement/ Relaxation ($n = 14$) | Relaxation ($n = 13$) | Supplement ($n = 9$) | Visits Only ($n = 9$) | Control ($n = 10$) | Significant Effects | F | p |
Measure	Time								
Weight[a]	pre	96.7	102.6	98.0	101.8	98.9	Group × time	3.0	$p < .05$
	post	95.9	106.6	99.3	102.6	94.0			
Arm muscle circumference[b]	pre	99.9	98.3	98.0	95.1	93.5	Time	8.4	$p < .001$
	post	97.9	104.5	96.9	90.2	86.1	Group × time	2.7	$p < .05$
Triceps skinfold[b]	pre	98.7	96.9	105.6	82.6	91.3	Time	6.9	$p < .05$
	post	95.3	96.1	87.4	79.1	76.4			
Karnofsky Performance Status	pre	7.5	7.5	7.6	7.4	7.1	Group × time[c]	2.2	$p < .10$
	post	7.1	8.3	7.3	6.7	6.1			

[a] Mean weight values are in terms of percentage of desirable weight for each individual, calculated as follows: $\dfrac{\text{measured weight}}{\text{ideal weight}} \times 100$

[b] Mean arm muscle circumference and triceps skinfold values are in terms of percentage of standard, calculated as follows: $\dfrac{\text{measured value}}{\text{standard value}} \times 100$

[c] F value would occur by change less than 10 times in 100, but greater than 5 times in 100.
From Dixon, J. (1984). Effect of nursing interventions on nutritional and performance status in cancer patients. *Nursing Research, 33* (6), 330–335.

measure, we see that all groups had lower post-study scores than pre-study scores. On arm muscle circumference, we see similar results, but the significant interaction indicates that not all groups responded in the same way. Inspection of the means shows that the relaxation group had higher post-study scores and all the other groups had lower scores. The control group had the lowest score, and the next lowest score was the visit only group. On the weight measure, some groups gained weight and some lost; therefore, overall, there was no main effect for time. The highest gain was for the relaxation group, and the greatest loss was for the control group.

Conclusions

On three of the four outcome measures, the relaxation group gained the most and the control group lost the most. "These findings suggest that the cachexia of cancer may be slowed or reversed through noninvasive nursing interventions" (Dixon, 1984, p. 330).

SUMMARY

Repeated measures ANOVA is a particularly interesting technique for us because we tend to take repeated measures on our patients, and it often makes sense to do so with our research subjects as well. There are stringent requirements for this analysis, however. If the requirements cannot be met and if we have enough subjects, it is possible to use a multivariate approach, or we might use the Greenhouse-Geisser procedure. The reader is advised to consult other sources for a thorough description of all these techniques.

EXERCISES FOR CHAPTER 12

1. What two criteria are part of the assumption of compound symmetry?
2. Fifteen subjects each are randomly assigned to one of four treatment groups. All subjects are measured three times. Complete the following summary table. Interpret the results. Would you do post-hoc tests? If so, for what?

SUMMARY TABLE

Source of Variation	SS	df	MS	F	p
Between Subjects					
Treatment	804.75				
Within Treatment (Error)	2970.50				
Within Subjects					
Time	982.60				
Treatment × Time	498.00				
Time × Within Groups	9170.90				

3. Twenty subjects are each exposed to three different treatment groups. Complete the following summary table. Interpret the results. Are post-hoc tests necessary?

SUMMARY TABLE

Source of Variation	SS	df	MS	F	p
Between Subjects	507.4				
Within Subjects					
Treatments	106.8				
Residual	1094.4				
Total	1708.6				

4. If you expect strong carry-over effects from one treatment to the next, should you use a repeated measures design on those subjects who serve as their own controls?

5. What approaches might you take if the data in a repeated measures design fail to meet the criterion of compound symmetry?

6. The degrees of freedom associated with the repeated factor equal 3. Perform the Greenhouse-Geisser procedure on the following *df*.

    a. 3, 27

    b. 6, 81

    c. 9, 300

SECTION 4
Extensions of Correlational Techniques

CHAPTER 13
Grouping Techniques

Jane Dixon

Researchers in the health fields often focus their attention on multiple variables. This is a direct result of the nature of the problems we study, which, in the real world of patient care, are indeed complex. For example, with regard to major causes of illness and death in the developed world (*e.g.,* cancer, heart disease, stroke, diabetes, accidents), we have learned to speak of "risk factors," rather than one single "cause." In some cases, a particular disease may exist only with a particular agent (*e.g.,* clinical mononucleosis with the Epstein-Barr virus). Even then, variables such as person and environment are crucial in influencing the course of the illness or even whether symptoms occur. Also, multiple issues affect such nursing concerns as recuperation following surgery and compliance with health care recommendations. In other chapters of this book, we have discussed how multivariate strategies can be used to understand the way multiple causes may lead to a single event.

This chapter treats a related problem—that of understanding *concepts*. Often, in labeling variables, a single word or phrase is used to represent something with multiple parts. Then our language may be overly general, blending the multiple aspects of the phenomenon of interest. Consider, for example, the term *satisfaction with care*. Superficially, it seems logical to measure this with a single rating. ("Rate your satisfaction with the care you received.") But with thought, we realize that such a rating might involve opinions on a variety of matters, such as knowledge and competence of caregivers, and convenience and appearance of the environment. (As an exercise, think of at least two other aspects that might affect satisfaction. Also, consider personal prejudices about the caregiver's race, sex, or age.) It is hard to know which of these influences are reflected in a subject's satisfaction rating and what such a rating really means. Instead of a global rating, should each aspect be measured separately? There are so many potentially important variables, we may feel at a loss to decide which should be measured and which should not.

The amount of information on which our minds can focus simultaneously is limited. As a convenience, we may concentrate on those factors thought to be primary. This will reduce the "data burden." In some research endeavors, however, simplicity of questionnaire may not be necessary, because we have techniques for organizing such data. Grouping techniques serve the purpose of *data reduction*. A large set of variables may be reduced by such techniques, much in the manner that we calculate means, variances, or correlation coefficients to reduce the individual scores on one or two values. In this chapter, two grouping techniques are introduced: *factor analysis* and *cluster analysis*. In factor analysis, a large number of variables are grouped into a smaller number of "factors;" with cluster analysis, subjects are grouped into subsets or "clusters." Since factor analysis is more used in patient care research, it is given primary emphasis.

OBJECTIVES FOR CHAPTER 13

Factor analysis is the most complex statistical technique usually used by clinical researchers.

After reading this chapter and completing the exercises, you should be able to

1. Identify situations in which factor analysis or cluster analysis would be appropriate.
2. Describe the steps involved in carrying out a factor analysis or cluster analysis procedure.
3. Interpret factor and cluster results from a computer printout or published study.

For further information regarding these techniques, the reader may consult Rummel (1970) on factor analysis or Tryon and Bailey (1970) on cluster analysis.

EXAMPLE OF A FACTOR ANALYSIS

A hypothetical example of a factor analytic situation may be helpful. Suppose a researcher measures six variables within a sample of adult male participants in a Health Maintenance Organization. Three of these variables are aspects of body size: height, arm length, and leg length. Three are derived from a health history in which the subject is asked to report the number of specific episodes occurring over the past year. These variables are number of sore throats, number of headaches, and number of earaches. In a matrix of correlations for these six variables, we will probably see that the three size variables have high intercorrelations and that the three history variables also have high intercorrelations; that is, a man with longer than average legs, may also have longer than average arms. He is also likely to be taller than average. A person reporting frequent sore throats may report other discomforts, too. On the other hand, it would be surprising if the size variables and the history variables were highly related.

A correlation matrix is shown in Table 13-1. If such a matrix is factor analyzed, a factor matrix defining the two groups of variables would be derived, as shown in Table 13-2. Each column in this table reflects one of the variable groupings. The "size" variables have high values in one column, and the "history" variables have high values in the other column. This table, indicating the presence of two distinct groups of variables, summarizes the information contained in the larger correlation matrix. It reduces the data.

You may object that such groupings were already apparent from the cor-

Table 13-1   Six by Six Correlation Matrix: Size and History Variables

	Height	Arm Length	Leg Length	Number of Sore Throats	Number of Headaches	Number of Earaches
Height	—	hi	hi	lo	lo	lo
Arm length		—	hi	lo	lo	lo
Leg length			—	lo	lo	lo
Number of sore throats				—	hi	hi
Number of headaches					—	hi
Number of earaches						—

"Hi" means correlation of high magnitude, regardless of direction (approaching +1.00 or approaching −1.00)
"Lo" means correlation of low magnitude (near zero)

Table 13-2   Abbreviated Factor Matrix: Size and History Variables

Variables	Factors I	II
Height	hi	lo
Arm length	hi	lo
Leg length	hi	lo
Number of sore throats	lo	hi
Number of headaches	lo	hi
Number of earaches	lo	hi

"Hi" means an absolute value of .40 or above.
"Lo" means an absolute value of less than .40.

relation table. This is true, but it will not be the usual case. Suppose that we had a 20×20 correlation matrix with widely ranging correlation coefficients and the groupings among the variables were subtle. The variables would appear in random order, rather than neatly arranged according to grouping. Then patterns will not be obvious. A careful inspection of the correlation matrix in Figure 5-6 (see Chapter 5) should validate this assertion. Factor analysis is a tool through which we may study variables in groupings that are *not* obvious.

USE OF FACTOR ANALYSIS

The practical purpose of factor analysis is to reduce a set of data so that it may be easily described and used. But there are two other purposes that may be served by such data reduction. These are *instrument development* (as implied in the chapter introduction) and *theory construction.*

Instrument Development

Factor analysis may be a vital part of creating a new measurement tool. It is a method for organizing the items into *factors.* A factor is a group of items that may be said to "go together." A person who scores high on one item is likely to score above average on others, and vice versa. Such an item has high correlations with other items of the same factor and low correlations with items of different factors. This principle provides the mathematical basis for assignment of items to factors through the statistical technique of factor analysis.

Factor analysis is often used to test the validity of ideas about item types in order to decide which items should be included. Such factors justify our use of *summated scales* (sets of items summed into a single scale score). For instance, such a method was used to develop a student evaluation of classroom teaching in nursing (Dixon & Koerner, 1976). Based on preliminary work, it was anticipated that student ratings would be based on four separate considerations; thus, four factors were expected. However, in factor analysis of the new instrument, only two factors were obtained. This indicated that the instrument should be revised, so as to contain only two scales. (Such discrepancies are common in the real world of instrument development but are not often described in the published literature.) Factor analysis is the most important statistical tool for validating the structure of our instruments.

Theory Development

The building of theory is a principal purpose of research, perhaps even *the* principal purpose. In 1968, James Dickoff, Patricia James, and Ernestine Wiedenbach described various types of theory applicable to the practice discipline of nursing. Donna Diers (1979) identified related types of study design, among them "factor searching" and "relation searching." It is at these exploratory levels of research that factor analysis may have its greatest role, provided that we have sufficient and appropriate measures. For example, Coffman (1979) used factor analysis to identify the crucial aspects of coping in graduate students. Factor analysis can identify constructs that unite a set of elements, build systems of classification, explore relationships, and test hypotheses. All these are theory-building functions.

Data Reduction for Subsequent Analysis

Sometimes factor analysis is used solely for data reduction, because such reduction may be needed for subsequent analysis. One goal of scientific inquiry is *parsimony,* simplicity of explanation; that is, it is preferable to use one variable, rather than many, to explain a phenomenon. Factor analysis provides a means for creating a single composite variable out of many variables. Often, it is used to identify several composite variables, which, taken together, summarize the sources of variance contained in all (or most) variables included in a study (or, at least, of those variables of a particular type). These composite variables are mathematically constructed through combination of the measured variables. Then, the several composite variables, rather than the larger number of measured variables, are used in subsequent data analysis. Data reduction of this sort may serve a highly pragmatic function. The researcher may collect a large amount of data, "reduce" the data through factor analysis, and conduct other analyses (such as regression or analysis of variance) on the reduced data. In these subsequent analyses, the number of variables relative to the number of subjects is kept within reasonable bounds, reliability is augmented, and, provided that the meanings of factors are clearly defined and communicated, interpretation of the analysis may be simplified. An example of this usage of factor analysis is provided by Stitt, Frane, and Frane (1977), who studied the effects of medication on mood changes in rheumatoid arthritics. Based on factor analysis of baseline values of 65 mood scale adjectives from the Profile of Mood States, seven composite variables were derived. These seven variables, considered to represent fatigue, hostility, friendliness, vigor, depression, tension, and confusion, were used as the dependent variables in a longitudinal experiment. More about this study later.

TYPE OF DATA REQUIRED AND ASSUMPTIONS

You are already familiar with the correlation matrix, the beginnings of many of our statistical treatments. In such a matrix (as in Figure 5-6 of Chapter 5), the two halves are identical; that is, the correlation of X with Y is the same as the correlation of Y with X. We call such a matrix *symmetrical.* Factor analysis may be performed with any symmetrical matrix of correlations. There are no special assumptions or requirements beyond those applicable to the calculation or interpretation of correlation, or both. It should be remembered, however, that a curvilinear relationship between two variables cannot be detected using the Pearson product–moment correlation.

In addition, although factor analysis is especially appropriate to situations in which there is a large amount of data, the number of variables that may be included in a factor analysis procedure is limited. It is tied to sample size. Certainly, the number of cases should always exceed the number of variables. A ratio of at least five subjects for each variable is desirable if one wishes to generalize from the sample to a wider population. With smaller ratios, the influence of relationships based on random patterns within the data is pronounced.

SIX MATRICES

The mathematics of factor analysis is complex. It is based on *matrix algebra*—that branch of mathematics that deals with the manipulation of matrices (plural of matrix). However, matrix algebra is beyond the scope of this book, and one does not need an understanding of matrix algebra to conduct a factor analysis. All mathematics can be done by computer.

The process of conducting a factor analysis, as experienced by the clinical researcher working within the structure of a "packaged" statistical program for the computer such as *SPSS,* will now be presented. This process involves six matrices. Each matrix is derived from the previous one through the computer program. But the researcher should still *understand* each matrix.

Raw Data Matrix

This is the data that the researcher collects about the study subjects. It is entered into the computer by the researcher in the form of data lines, each containing information about one subject. In such a matrix, each row represents a single subject, and each column represents a variable. The reader is already familiar with this sort of matrix; it is the beginning of any data analysis. Table 5-1 (see Chapter 5) provides an example of the structure of a raw data matrix. A raw data matrix to be factor analyzed would, by definition, contain many variables.

Correlation Matrix

The reader is also familiar with the correlation matrix. When fully depicted, the correlation matrix is a square, symmetrical matrix in which the number of rows and the number of columns each equal the number of variables. Because the correlation matrix is symmetrical (therefore containing much duplication), it is often depicted in one of several abbreviated forms. The table from the Mahon study (Table 5-6, Chapter 5) is one example. The correlation matrix summarizes information in the raw data matrix. It is smaller, with fewer rows and elements than the raw data matrix. This is a beginning of the data reduction process.

Factor Matrix, Unrotated

Based on the correlation matrix, the first of two factor matrices is calculated. In a factor matrix (Table 13-3), each row represents one variable included in the factor analysis. There are fewer columns, each column representing one factor. In the unrotated factor matrix, the elements within the matrix are the unrotated *factor loadings*—numbers ranging between -1.00 and $+1.00$, which may be thought of as "correlations" of the variable with the factor. The square of a factor loading represents the proportion of variance that the item and the factor have in common, or, to say it another way, this is the proportion of item variance explained by the factor. For example, in Table 13-3, illustrating an unrotated factor matrix, the first variable (1) has a loading of .85 on Factor I; approximately 72% of variance is accounted for by this loading $((.85)^2 = .7225)$. If one adds the squared loadings across a row, one arrives at the item communality (h^2). This is the portion of item variance accounted for by the various factors. For Variable 1 of Table 13-3, the squared factor loadings are totaled as follows: $.85^2 + .22^2 + .03^2 = .72 + .05 + .00 = .77$. The item communality is .77; that is, 77% of item variance is "explained" by the three factors.

Likewise, one may add the squared loadings contained in a single column to obtain the *eigenvalue* for the factor. The eigenvalue represents the total amount of variance explained by a factor. The average of the squared loadings in a column is obtained by dividing the eigenvalue by the number of items in the column (eigenvalue/n). This average represents the percent of interitem variance accounted for by the factor. For the first factor in Table 13-3, the eigenvalue is calculated as follows: $.85^2 + .15^2 + .51^2 + .83^2 + .26^2 = .72 + .02 + .26 + .69 + .07 = 1.76$. This eigenvalue of 1.76 is divided by 5 (because there are 5 variables), yielding .352. Thus, approximately 35% of total item variance is accounted for by the first factor.

Table 13-3   Factor Loading Matrix

		Factors			
		I	II	III	h^2
	1	.85	.22	.03	.77
	2	.15	•	•	•
Variables	3	.51	•	•	•
	4	.83	•	•	•
	5	.26	•	•	•
Eigenvalues		*1.76*			
% of variance		*.35*			

Adding up the percent of variance accounted for by each factor tells us how much variance was explained by all the factors.

Factor eigenvalues and variance accounted for are the most important figures contained in the unrotated factor matrix. One may be especially interested in how much variance is accounted for altogether by the important factors; this is simply the sum of variance accounted for by individual factors. Either factor eigenvalues or the variance accounted for by factors may be used to determine the number of potentially interpretable factors contained in the data. Typically, researchers wish to interpret the number of factors that each account for at least 5% of variance, or, similarly, that number of factors for which the eigenvalue is 1.00 or greater. Determination of the appropriate number of factors paves the way for the next matrix of the factor analysis process.

Factor Matrix, Rotated

The unrotated factors are created (based on the correlations between variables), such that the amount of variance accounted for by each successive factor is maximized. This means that factors may (in geometric terms) run between independent groups of related variables, rather than accurately reflecting the meaning of one group of variables or another. The consequence of this fact is that unrotated factors can rarely be meaningfully interpreted. However, just as one may alter an algebraic equation by performing the same operation on both sides, one may transform or *"rotate"* a factor matrix into any one of an infinite number of mathematically equivalent matrices. If factor rotation is conducted according to the criteria of *simple structure* as described by Thurstone in 1947, the result is a set of factors that are distinct from one another and that, in most situations, can be meaningfully and creatively interpreted by the researcher. In simple structure, factors are set so as to maximize the number of loadings of great magnitude (near +1.00 and −1.00) and loadings of small magnitude (near 0.00) for each factor; that is, a distinct pattern emerges in the factor matrix, such that each factor has certain variables that "go with" it, while other variables do not. Likewise, as simple structure is approached, each variable is identified with *one* and *only one* factor. According to Thurstone (1947), in a factor matrix:

1. Each row should have at least one loading close to zero.
2. Each column should have about as many variables with near-zero loadings as there are factors.
3. For pairs of columns (factors), there should be several variables that load on one and not on the other.

The essence of interpreting factor analytic results is the process of identifying, from the rotated factor matrix, which variables go with a factor, then naming the factor based on whatever meanings these variables with high loadings have in common. The criteria for considering a loading "high" varies from study to study, with some researchers using cutoff points as low as .35; others use cutoff points as high as .55.

In naming and describing factors, the researcher uses not only knowledge of the statistical technique and how it works but also an understanding of the subject matter under study, and especially an ability to construct new understandings of that subject matter. By facilitating the organization of individual variables into variable groupings, factor analysis opens the door to new conceptualizations and new ways of thinking, provided that the researcher is ready to discover these in the data. More than any other statistical technique, factor analysis requires the full exercise of one's creative potential.

Factor Score Matrix

Based on the rotated factor matrix, a score for each subject on each factor may be computed. To calculate such *factor scores,* an individual's score on each variable included in a factor is multiplied times the factor loading for the particular variable. The sum of these products is the individual's factor score. The general formula is:

$$\text{Factor Score} = \text{Sum of} \begin{pmatrix} \text{individual's} \\ \text{score on} \\ \text{variable} \end{pmatrix} \times \begin{pmatrix} \text{factor loading} \\ \text{of variable} \\ \text{on factor} \end{pmatrix}$$

Factor scores can be calculated automatically within factor analysis procedures in statistical packages for the computer such as SPSS. Let's consider an individual included in the data of Table 13-3 who received scores as follows:

Variable	Scores
1	2
2	4
3	1
4	5
5	2

This person's factor score on Factor 1 would be calculated this way: $(.85)(2) + (.15)(4) + (.51)(1) + (.83)(5) + (.26)(2) = 1.7 + .6 + .51 + 4.15 + .52 = 7.48$. This factor score, based on the strength of the correlation of each variable with the factor, could be used instead of the individual's raw score on the factor. The factor score is based on the relative "importance" of each variable as indicated by that correlation. This individual's raw score would be the sum of the scores on the five variables $(2 + 4 + 1 + 5 + 2 = 14)$.

The factor score matrix has as many rows as there are subjects, with each column representing one factor. The structure of such a matrix is illustrated in Table 13-4. The factor score matrix is smaller than the raw data matrix. The data have been reduced.

Table 13-4   Factor Score Matrix

		Factors			
		I	II	•	•
Subjects	1	7.48	•	•	•
	2	•			
	•	•			
	•	•			
	•	•			
	n	•			

Factor Correlation Matrix

Factor Rotation. Factor rotation is often *orthogonal,* with factors uncorrelated with each other. This is usually desirable for instrument development, in which the researcher seeks to determine subscales that are independent of one another. Alternatively, factor rotation may also be *oblique,* with factors that are not totally unrelated to each other. Advocates of oblique rotation assert that, in the real world, important factors are likely to be correlated; thus, searching for unrelated factors is unrealistic. Novice factor analysts should probably plan to use an orthogonal, rather than oblique, rotation, because it is easier to interpret. The *Varimax* ("variance maximized") method, available on all widely used computer packages, is recommended for orthogonal rotation.

With orthogonal rotation, one factor loading matrix is produced. It represents both regression weights (called a *pattern matrix*) and correlation coefficients (called a *structure matrix*). Because the solution is orthogonal, the regression weights are equal to the correlation coefficients. The loadings are interpreted as were those in the unrotated factor matrix. A squared loading represents the variance accounted for in a variable by a particular factor. The squared loadings may be added up across a row to determine total variance accounted for in a variable by all the factors, and so on.

Since with oblique rotation there is correlation among the factors, the *factor pattern matrix* (the regression weights) and the *factor structure matrix* (containing correlation coefficients) are not the same. The two matrices are produced and interpreted differently. According to Nie and associates (1975, p. 476), the factor pattern matrix "delineates more clearly the grouping or clustering of variables than [does] the [factor] structure matrix." The square of a loading in a factor pattern matrix represents the variance accounted for by a particular variable, but because other factors may share some of this variance (due to intercorrelation among factors in an oblique solution), the total variance in an item accounted for by all the factors *cannot* be determined by adding up the squared loadings in a row (h^2).

Table 13-5   Factor Correlation Matrix

	Factor 1	Factor 2	Factor 3
Factor 1	1.00	0.65	0.30
Factor 2		1.00	0.45
Factor 3			1.00

Factor Correlations. In orthogonal rotation, because there is no correlation among the factors, no factor correlation matrix is produced. In oblique rotation, a matrix displaying the correlation of each factor with every other factor is displayed in a factor correlation matrix. The structure of such a matrix is displayed in Table 13-5.

STEPS OF A FACTOR ANALYTIC STUDY

The steps of a factor analytic study are as follows:

1. Formulate research question or hypothesis. If factor analysis is the appropriate statistical technique for answering research questions or testing the hypothesis, proceed with the following steps.
2. Collect data of interest.
3. Calculate and examine univariate data on a variable by variable basis, identifying those variables that should not be included in the factor analysis because of failure to meet initial assumptions or criteria.
4. Calculate and examine bivariate relationship data—again with an eye toward identifying those variables and those relationships that should not be included in the factor analysis.
5. "Run" factor analysis. Unless you have some good reason to do otherwise, use Varimax rotation. If you have predicted certain factors, specify in the computer program how many factors you expect; otherwise, let the computer determine the number of factors in the course of the factor analysis. Note the total proportion of interitem variance accounted for by the factor solution and the number of factors involved.
6. Name and interpret factors from the rotated factor loading matrix. (Sometimes researchers experiment with several factor solutions in order to choose the one that can be most meaningfully interpreted.)
7. If subsequent analyses are planned, use factor analysis results to decide how to combine variables; calculate these new or combined variables for each subject. (Usually, factor scores can be easily calculated on the computer.) Then conduct the subsequent analyses.
8. Relate findings to the existing literature and disseminate results through presentation and publication. If appropriate, repeat the analysis with other available populations.

COMBINING FACTOR ANALYSIS
WITH OTHER APPROACHES

When used for its data reduction purpose, factor analysis is often an early stage of a multi-stage analysis, as indicated by Steps 7 and 8 above. Subsequent analyses may also be conducted in studies involving an instrument development process. For example, Matthews, Glass, Rosenman, and Bortner (1977) factor analyzed data from interviews used to assess tendency toward Type A behavior, a behavior pattern associated with increased risk of coronary heart disease. They obtained five factors. Then, to compare individuals who developed clinical coronary heart disease over the first 4½ years of follow-up with matched controls who did not, the researchers conducted *t*-tests on factor scores for each of the five factors. The groups were significantly different from each other on only two of the five factors. Thus, a substantial portion of the Type A assessment interview did not, in fact, predict clinical coronary disease over this time period; only selected aspects of the interview were predictive. Such findings have important instrument development implications. Generally, factor analysis tends to be most useful when combined with other analyses within a single study.

EXAMPLE OF A COMPUTER PRINTOUT

Examples of sections of a computer printout of a factor analysis are shown in Figures 13-1 through 13-5. The data analyzed are from a 28-item rating scale of nursing behaviors relative to care of persons with cancer. One hundred and four nurses were rated by a clinical specialist in oncology. Typical items of the rating scale are as follows:

Expresses respect for dignity of patient, including the disfigured and dying.
Responds appropriately to emergency situations such as obstruction of neck
    stoma.
Assesses physiologic strengths and weaknesses of the cancer patient.

Based on review of univariate characteristics of the 28 items and their bivariate relationships, 10 items were excluded prior to factor analysis. The major reason for exclusion was that the data for a given item were not normally distributed. Eighteen items remained. The 18×18 correlation matrix was submitted to factor analysis with Varimax rotation using the SPSS computer package.

The factor loadings of the unrotated factor matrix were not requested as part of the output; these were not needed. Figure 13-1 contains the information needed relative to general characteristics of the unrotated factors. Note that 18 factors are listed. This is because the number of unrotated factors obtainable equals the number of variables included in a factor analysis. The purpose of this part of the analysis is, however, to determine how many of the 18 items should be rotated for concep-

Procedure Cards

```
1              16
FACTOR         VARIABLES = SPEC1 TO SPEC4, SPEC6, SPEC8 TO SPEC10, SPEC12, SPEC16,
               SPEC17, SPEC19 TO SPEC21, SPEC24 TO SPEC26, SPEC28/
STATISTICS     4, 6
```

Output

FACTOR	EIGENVALUE	PCT OF VAR	CUM PCT
1	8.24434	45.8	45.8
2	1.54871	8.6	54.4
3	1.18889	6.6	61.0
4	1.08630	6.0	67.0
5	0.91621	5.1	72.1
6	0.85721	4.8	76.9
7	0.71778	4.0	80.9
8	0.60134	3.3	84.2
9	0.48889	2.7	86.9
10	0.42782	2.4	89.3
11	0.40065	2.2	91.5
12	0.30294	1.7	93.2
13	0.28335	1.6	94.8
14	0.25080	1.4	96.2
15	0.22611	1.3	97.5
16	0.17126	1.0	98.4
17	0.15116	0.8	99.2
18	0.13622	0.8	100.0

Figure 13-1   Characteristics of factors before rotation as shown on SPSS printout.

tual interpretation. Eigenvalues and percent of variance accounted for are given. The first four factors each have an eigenvalue greater than 1 (default on SPSS), and each of these account for 6% of variance or more. The righthand column gives cumulative percent of variance accounted for; the four factors together account for 67.0% of the interitem variance.

The four factors with eigenvalues greater than 1 are rotated, and the rotated factor loadings are displayed in Figure 13-2. In order to name and describe the factors obtained, the researcher should identify (perhaps by underlining on the printout using a colored pen) the high loadings. Most often, .30, .35, or .40 is used as the cutoff that separates high loadings from those that are not so high. In this example, .40 is used as the cutoff point. In Figure 13-2, underline or highlight all items loading .40 or above. Note that all the items loaded on at least one factor. Also note that four items (4, 6, 12, 17) loaded on two factors.

The next step is to list the items loading .40 or above on a factor from highest to lowest loading. Figure 13-3 contains the result of such grouping. This grouping

	FACTOR 1	FACTOR 2	FACTOR 3	FACTOR 4
SPEC1	0.48283	0.35259	0.05976	0.26956
SPEC2	0.31426	0.64214	-0.08898	0.23214
SPEC3	0.06877	0.58051	0.20693	0.26660
SPEC4	0.43727	0.46446	0.29827	0.27991
SPEC6	0.48133	0.67956	0.08745	0.11387
SPEC8	0.39108	0.43389	0.38768	0.05521
SPEC9	0.07195	0.78288	0.28268	0.01849
SPEC10	0.63465	0.27093	0.10448	0.22341
SPEC12	0.26248	0.50228	0.41547	-0.03427
SPEC16	0.20456	0.17726	0.24914	0.81024
SPEC17	0.45102	0.15908	0.23988	0.62722
SPEC19	0.72082	0.09747	0.29946	0.12765
SPEC20	0.58837	0.13629	0.27261	0.06512
SPEC21	0.68958	0.19150	0.25510	0.30075
SPEC24	0.60660	0.30791	0.31569	0.18455
SPEC25	0.30490	0.38282	0.55875	0.28337
SPEC26	0.19579	0.06032	0.56898	0.16413
SPEC28	0.33053	0.25024	0.61849	0.29851

Figure 13-2   Loadings of variables on factors after rotation as shown on SPSS printout.

allows us to see clearly which items load at a substantial level on a given factor and which of those items have the highest loadings, and thus are most highly related to the factor.

After looking at the items that load on a factor and at their respective weights, the investigator gives each factor an appropriate name. In this example, Factor 1 might be labeled, "emotional support." Factor 2 is knowledge of cancer and its treatment. Factor 3 is less clear, but it might be labeled as assistance with patient problem solving. Factor 4 is knowledge of the psychological aspects of cancer. Nurses could receive a score for each of these factors.

Figure 13-4 shows summary information about the rotated factors. The reader should note that eigenvalues and percentage of variance accounted for are different from those of the first four unrotated factors. In this figure, the righthand column, labeled "CUM PCT," refers to cumulative percentage of variance accounted for relative to that part of the interitem variance accounted for by the four-factor solution. Thus, the four factors together account for 100% of the variance accounted for in the solution. Remember, however (see Fig. 13-1), that the four factors accounted for 67% of the total variance. Thus, the first factor accounts for about 50% of the *total* variance (75% of the 67% of explained variance). The second factor accounts for 7.5% of the total variance ($.112 \times .67 = .075$). The third factor accounts for about 5%, and the fourth factor accounts for 4%.

Figure 13-5 displays item communalities. For the item labeled SPEC1, the four factors account for 43% of the variance in that item (.43368). The researcher who wishes to include a tabular presentation of a factor analysis in a research thesis or

Factor 1

Items	Item Stems	Loading
19	Involves patient and family in planning	.72
21	Withholds judgmental response to patient behavior or statement of feelings	.69
10	Allows patient to react to diagnosis of cancer	.63
24	Gives appropriate support to patients in crises	.61
20	Maintains supportive relationships with other staff members	.59
1	Elicits feelings	.48
6	Looks for subtle physiological changes	.48
17	Assesses patient's ability to cope with diagnosis of cancer	.45
4	Teaches patient	.44

Factor 2

9	Knows basic principles related to cancer treatments and potential complications	.78
6	Looks for subtle physiological changes	.68
2	Assesses physiological strengths and weaknesses	.64
3	Knows basic principles related to cancer epidemiology and etiology	.58
12	Anticipates potential problems	.50
4	Teaches patient	.46
8	Takes initiative in sharing information with physician	.43

Factor 3

28	Notes subtle changes in emotional reaction	.62
26	Knows what community resources are available	.57
25	Assists patient with decision making	.56
12	Anticipates potential problems	.42

Factor 4

16	Knows basic principles related to psychological aspects	.81
17	Assesses patient's ability to cope with diagnosis of cancer	.63

Figure 13-3 Grouping of items on factors according to strength of loading.

FACTOR	EIGENVALUE	PCT OF VAR	CUM PCT
1	7.83864	75.0	75.0
2	1.16653	11.2	86.1
3	0.75897	7.3	93.4
4	0.69340	6.6	100.0

Figure 13-4 Characteristics of four factors after rotation as shown on SPSS printout.

VARIABLE	COMMUNALITY
SPEC1	0.43368
SPEC2	0.57292
SPEC3	0.45561
SPEC4	0.57425
SPEC6	0.71409
SPEC8	0.49454
SPEC9	0.69833
SPEC10	0.53701
SPEC12	0.49498
SPEC16	0.79182
SPEC17	0.67968
SPEC19	0.63505
SPEC20	0.44332
SPEC21	0.66772
SPEC24	0.59649
SPEC25	0.63202
SPEC26	0.39265
SPEC28	0.64350

Figure 13-5   Item communalities after rotation as shown on SPSS printout.

article must select information from printout tables (such as Figs. 13-1 through 13-5) and rearrange it into one of several easily readable formats. An example follows.

EXAMPLE FROM PUBLISHED RESEARCH

The study by Stitt, Frane, and Frane (1977) entitled "Mood Change in Rheumatoid Arthritis" was mentioned earlier in this chapter. The authors of that article reasoned that in evaluating the efficacy of a new medication for treating rheumatoid arthritis, one should measure its analgesic and mood effects separately from its anti-inflammatory effects. They used the Profile of Mood States (POMS), which contains 65 adjectives describing mood, to record mood changes associated with placebo treatment; these data were reduced with factor analysis, and factor scores were used in subsequent analysis.

Data Gathered

One hundred and eighty-one persons with rheumatoid arthritis completed the POMS at three points in time. The baseline measure was taken before the research intervention was begun. Usual medication was then discontinued, and the subject was given placebo treatment for up to 2 weeks. At the end of the placebo period, the POMS was again completed. Then, the patient received aspirin treatment for 2 weeks, after which the subject completed the POMS for the third time. It was anticipated that exacerbation of disease during the placebo period would be reflected in poorer mood ratings at the second measurement. Factor analysis was conducted, and factor scores were derived. Change over time was then assessed using repeated measures analysis of variance.

Tabular Presentation of Results

Table 13-6 contains the factor matrix presented in the article. Note that this table contains 65 variables and seven factors, plus an additional column reflecting item communalities. Yet, in contrast to Figure 13-2, it is easy to read; patterns of item groupings can be immediately grasped. To accomplish this, the authors considerably rearranged information derived from their computer printouts. They reorganized the variables listed along the lefthand column in two ways: First, they grouped items loading on the same factor together, leaving an extra space between groupings; second, they organized items within each grouping such that items are ordered from highest loading to lowest loading. Also, the authors succeeded in accenting the important information to be conveyed by leaving out information that was not relevant. Only loadings of + .25 or above are included. In addition, the authors labeled the columns with factor names that they assigned after reviewing the printout. More extensive verbal descriptions of the factors are provided elsewhere in the article. One additional step that may be taken to enhance communication is to round each loading to only two digits and drop the leftmost 0 and decimal point. Thus, .892 becomes 89. Its meaning is the same provided that the table is footnoted with a comment that loadings have been multiplied by 100.

Seven repeated measures ANOVA were performed using the seven factor scores from the seven factors as the dependent variables. For five of these seven analyses (fatigue, friendliness, vigor, tension, and depression), significant differences were obtained, with values at the conclusion of the placebo period distinct from values obtained at the other two times. This is displayed graphically in Figure 13-6.

Conclusions

Stitt and colleagues summarize their conclusions with this statement. "The POMS seems to be a useful test both for assessing the mood of patients with rheumatoid arthritis, and for determining mood changes brought about by medication used to relieve the symptoms of arthritis." Do you agree? Think about how such findings might be applied in future clinical studies; then decide whether the factor analysis itself was useful.

THE CLUSTER ANALYSIS QUESTION

Although factor analysis is the technique of choice for summarizing a correlation matrix in order to determine how the study variables tend to group together, cluster analysis is the technique of choice for obtaining empirical groupings of subjects based on the subjects' values on selected variables. Cluster analysis is used to identify homogeneous subsets of subjects or patients. Individuals within each of such subsets are more similar to each other than they are to individuals in other subsets. In nursing research, this offers the possibility of developing clinical inter-

(*Text continues on page 285*)

Table 13-6 Sorted Rotated Factor Loadings (Pattern)

Item	Fatigue	Hostility	Friendliness	Vigor	Depression	Tension	Confusion	Communalities
Fatigued	0.907							0.7364
Exhausted	0.891							0.8131
Bushed	0.980							0.7586
Wornout	0.688							0.6312
Weary	0.684							0.5948
Sluggish	0.607			−0.275				0.6278
Listless	0.537							0.4837
Miserable	0.328				0.260			0.5707
Helpless	0.259			−0.252				0.4486
Furious		0.739						0.6012
Rebellious		0.712						0.5875
Bad-tempered		0.614						0.5953
Ready to fight		0.607						0.3486
Spiteful		0.591						0.5242
Resentful		0.545			0.323			0.6180
Peeved		0.507						0.5685
Annoyed		0.481						0.5981
Angry		0.475					−0.251	0.5500
Guilty		0.304					0.260	0.3379
Good-natured			0.737					0.5850
Considerate			0.709					0.5123
Trusting			0.561					0.4058
Sympathetic			0.557					0.3353
Friendly			0.549					0.3973
Alert			0.533					0.4905
Cheerful			0.467	0.321				0.6010
Helpful			0.467	0.334				0.4672
Clear-headed			0.415				−0.332	0.2806
Carefree			0.376					0.2996
Energetic				0.790				0.6517
Active				0.751				0.6011
Vigorous				0.695				0.5169

							h²
Full of pep	0.645						0.6471
Lively	0.614						0.5147
Efficient	0.436					0.305	0.4552
Sad		0.615					0.6205
Unhappy		0.577					0.6584
Blue		0.571					0.6314
Discouraged		0.476					0.5795
Bitter		0.456		0.437			0.5760
Desperate		0.433		0.397			0.5334
Hopeless		0.429					0.3480
Gloomy		0.366					0.6455
Unworthy		0.315					0.3274
Lonely		0.302			0.254		0.3008
Worthless		0.285					0.3517
Terrified		0.278		0.276			0.3627
Nervous			0.615				0.5538
Tense			0.580				0.5063
On Edge			0.554				0.6355
Shaky			0.464		0.279		0.4880
Uneasy			0.411				0.5881
Restless			0.409				0.4357
Grouchy			0.344	0.309		0.253	0.5163
Relaxed			-0.344			0.322	0.4420
Forgetful					0.539		0.3550
Muddled					0.538		0.6335
Bewildered					0.510		0.5655
Unable to concentrate					0.461		0.3094
Uncertain about things					0.363		0.4032
Panicky					0.305		0.4085
Confused			0.267		0.283		0.3852
Anxious							0.2193
Deceived							0.3110
Sorry for things done							0.2097

From Stitt, F. W., Frane, M., Frane, J. W. (1977). Mood change in rheumatoid arthritis: factor analysis as a tool in clinical research. *Journal of Chronic Diseases, 30,* 135–145. By permission of Pergamon Press, Ltd.

Factor score
means

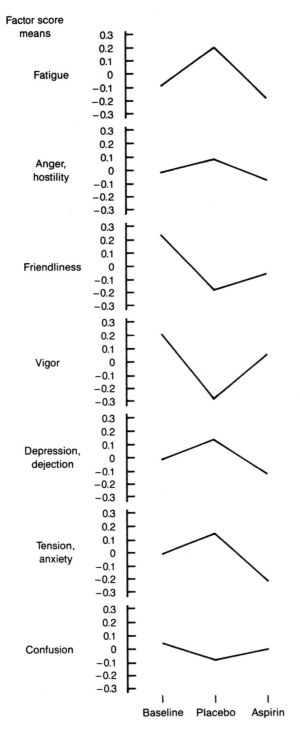

Figure 13-6 Change in factor score means over the course of the trial. (Factor score means [181 patients] for each of three visits: baseline, after placebo administration, and after 2 weeks of aspirin treatment. Note that the length of placebo treatment varied for different patients [see Methods].) (From: Stitt, F.W., Frane, M., Frane, J.W. [1977]. Mood change in rheumatoid arthritis: factor analysis as a tool in clinical research. *Journal of Chronic Diseases, 30,* 135–145. By permission of Pergamon Press, Ltd.)

ventions specific to the needs of a particular group. Because individuals within a homogeneous subset or cluster may respond to a particular nursing intervention differently from individuals in other clusters, cluster analysis may also be a useful first step in any evaluative study; the way individuals cluster into groups may help to explain variance between individuals in response to treatment. In fact, the very process of diagnosis, whether within the realm of medicine or of nursing, is a clustering process. Based on observable indicators, an individual is classified as a member of a group made up of persons who are similar, but probably not identical, on certain characteristics. To the extent that this grouping helps us to understand the individual or to predict future events and responses of the individual, the grouping may be considered useful. Cluster analysis is simply an empirical method of arriving at such groupings or diagnoses. Although it is much less commonly used than factor analysis, cluster analysis is applicable to many problems studied by health care researchers. In an age of diagnostic-related groups and cost containment efforts, one can expect cluster analysis methodology to be used with increasing frequency.

CLUSTER ANALYSIS PROCEDURE

Cluster analysis is based on the premise that a valid measure of similarity between any two individuals can be obtained. Thus, one can construct a square, symmetrical matrix in which study subjects are represented by rows and by columns; the elements of the matrix are indices of similarity of each subject with each other subject. This similarity index may take any one of several forms. It may take the form of a correlation; that is, one may compute the Pearson product–moment correlation between two individuals across a variety of variables by using the standard formula, by simply considering one person's values on all measures to represent the X variable, while the other person's values on all measures represent the Y variable. However, because it emphasizes the pattern that emerges, not actual magnitude of values, correlation is flawed as a measure of similarity between individuals. For example, in Figure 13-7, because Mary and Alice each did best on Test 2 and worst on Test 3, a high correlation between these individuals would be obtained even though, overall, Mary scored much higher than did Alice. In contrast, although Mary's scores and Sue's scores on each test are close in magnitude, these individuals followed differing patterns, such that Mary's best test is Sue's worst and vice versa; a high correlation between these individuals would not be obtained. These problems can be solved by using Euclidean distance as the measure of similarity between individuals. With this measure, similarity is determined by how far apart two individuals are on each test; the distance between Mary and Sue would be small, and the distance between Mary and Alice would be large.

Unfortunately, not all packaged statistical programs contain a cluster analysis program. The remainder of this section describes the cluster analysis approach available on Biomedical Computer Programs (Dixon, 1983). Based on distance

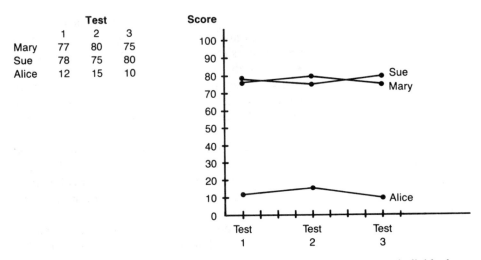

Figure 13-7   Three sets of test scores for determining distances between individuals.

between each set of two individuals in the sample, clustering proceeds in steps. Initially, each subject represents an independent cluster. At the final step, all subjects are joined together into one great, inclusive cluster. At each intermediate step, whichever two clusters are most similar (as indicated, for example, by the smallest Euclidean distance) are joined together. Then means are computed to describe the new cluster. All together, the amalgamation process consists of one fewer step than there are cases.

The computer printout obtained consists of details concerning the amalgamation process with a description of the new cluster formed at each step and a vertically depicted tree diagram for visual interpretation. Using this information, the researcher decides what step in the amalgamation process represents the most valid cluster solution, taking into consideration both conceptual meaningfulness of interpretation and empirical similarities and differences within and between clusters.

Implementing the cluster analysis procedure on a set of data requires that three decisions be made.

1. Cluster analysis should be based on a small number of variables; this may require selecting variables from a larger number of measures included in the data. With too many variables, it is difficult, if not impossible, to find clinically relevant meaning in the results. The author of this chapter has made a point of clustering data on not more than five or six key variables, even when 100 or more subjects are involved. Variables should be interval or ratio level.
2. The researcher must decide whether Euclidean distance or some other measure will be used as the gauge of difference between individuals. As indicated above, this may affect the results in profound ways.

3. If Euclidean distance is chosen as the measure by which similarity and differences between individuals are gauged, the researcher should consider standardizing the data before distances are computed. Standardization involves transforming raw scores into standard scores or z-scores (see Chapter 3), such that, on these standard scores, the mean for the variable is equal to 0, and the standard deviation is equal to 1. (In computation of Pearson product–moment correlation and many other statistics, standardization occurs automatically, because it is built into the computational formulas.) The advantage of standardization is that it prevents distortion due to score differences between variables; otherwise, a variable with a wide range and large variance would, in essence, be most heavily weighted in the cluster analysis. The disadvantage of standardization is that any transformation of data may obscure meanings of the variables and lead to confusions in interpretation.

A BRIEF EXAMPLE OF CLUSTER ANALYSIS

As part of an evaluation study of a graduate nursing program, 106 employed graduates submitted information about their current roles. Data included the percentage of working time spent in a variety of activities, including clinical duties, teaching, administration, research, and consultation. Cluster analysis was based on these time variables.

A three-cluster solution comprising all but one of the employed respondents emerged. Within each of these main clusters, at least one subcluster could be identified; and two sets of second level subclusters were also discovered. A brief verbal description of the primary clusters was constructed as follows:

> Cluster I was characterized by a usually high administrative emphasis ($\overline{X} = 53\%$). The 18 individuals falling into this cluster spent more of their other working time on teaching ($\overline{X} = 22\%$) than on clinical activities ($\overline{X} = 8\%$), and more time on consultation ($\overline{X} = 11\%$) than on research ($\overline{X} = 6\%$).
>
> Cluster II individuals were involved predominantly in activities of a clinical nature ($\overline{X} = 66\%$). Teaching occupied only 11% of the time of these individuals, followed by administration (6%), consultation (4%), and research (3%). With 57 subjects, this was the largest of the main clusters.
>
> Cluster III was characterized primarily by teaching activity ($\overline{X} = 84\%$). Clinical activity occupied only 7% of the time of respondents classified into this cluster, followed by administration ($\overline{X} = 5\%$), research ($\overline{X} = 2\%$), and consultation ($\overline{X} < 1\%$).

The fact that alumni of a graduate program in nursing would fall into three categories based on whether one's primary emphasis is on clinical practice, teaching, or administration should not surprise any observer of the nursing profession. It is, however, always gratifying to find that data analysis results confirm our most common assumptions. They also provide a basis for further research using these clusters.

In interpreting cluster analytic results, as with factor analysis, it is important to keep in mind that the structure that emerges is based on relationships between variables within the sample, not on differences between this sample and other potential samples. Neither cluster nor factor analysis can ever be considered in isolation; instead, both must be considered in relation to what is already known about the sample and about the variables under study.

VALIDITY OF A CLUSTER STRUCTURE

In discussing factor analysis, we pointed out that a primary value of that technique was its use in creating factor scores for use in subsequent analyses. In both the Stitt, Frane, and Frane (1977) study and the Matthews and colleagues (1977) study, factors scores did, in fact, prove useful in the examination of other substantive issues. In dealing with cluster analysis, this concern about validity of results may be taken yet a step further. In 1980, Blashfield identified more than 100 articles that involved cluster analysis and that dealt with the topic of psychopathology. He pointed out that any set of data, including random numbers, can be cluster analyzed; therefore, adequate evidence of the validity of a cluster structure should be obtained before publication. One way to do this is, as with any statistical technique, by replicating one's results using a different sample. More simply, validity of a cluster structure may be supported by showing that the groups obtained are significantly differrent from each other on a variable not involved in the clustering.

Like factor analysis, cluster analysis may be most useful as a method of grouping subjects for subsequent analysis. Additionally, in the health professions, many studies focus on the process of developing and evaluating clinical interventions oriented to particular patient situations. Cluster analysis may help to identify subgroups that should be considered separately in such research.

EXERCISES FOR CHAPTER 13

1. For each of the following situations, state whether factor analysis (by variables), cluster analysis (by cases), or neither is appropriate. Also consider the possibility of subsequent analysis.

   a. A researcher constructs a scale to measure fear of surgery. She has developed 25 Likert-type items and believes that the item responses will fall into three categories, measuring different special aspects of pre-surgery fears.

   b. A researcher wishes to determine whether school-aged males and females differ in number of absences from school due to illness.

   c. A researcher–clinician finds that the relaxation protocol she has developed for use in late pregnancy works wonders in reducing perceived stress for about one third of her patients. For the others, it seems to have no effect. She wants to learn how to predict for which women it will be effective.

d. In a study examining the uniqueness of human infants, 197 infants are examined relative to 31 characteristics. The researcher wishes to reduce and summarize the data on the infants, and then to relate infant characteristics to type of birth (unmedicated vaginal delivery, medicated vaginal delivery, Caesarean section).

2. In a study of activity following occurrence of stroke, degree of resumption of usual activities is measured using a 5-point scale (1 = not at all; 5 = complete resumption). The following matrix of factor loadings (rotated) is obtained:

	I	II
Walking from room to room	.75	.15
Bathing	.09	.87
Dressing	.19	.82
Eating	.36	.32
Climbing stairs	.72	.08
Walking in the neighborhood	.81	.13
Shopping and marketing	.68	.21
Care of hair	.12	.73

a. To what extent has simple structure been approached?
b. Reorganize the items as they should be listed in a factor loading matrix within a research report, and insert the loadings as appropriate.
c. Name the factors.
d. Compute the eigenvalue and variance accounted for by the first factor.
e. Compute the communality for the item "walking from room to room." What does that figure indicate?

3. In an unrotated matrix, a researcher obtains the following variance accounted for in the first six factors: I, 21.5%; II, 11.6%; III, 8.2%; IV, 6.7%; V, 2.1%; VI, 1.9%.
a. How many factors should be rotated? Why?
b. What percent of variance will be accounted for by the rotated factor solution?
c. Suppose that after rotation, the first factor accounted for 80% of that variance. What would the *total* variance accounted for by Factor I equal?

CHAPTER 14
Path Models of Cause

Ellis Batten Page

As individuals, we are constantly concerned about the causes of events affecting us. Will thorns hurt us? If so, we avoid them. Will a certain book reward us? If so, we seek it out. Will study advance our careers? If so, we are willing, perhaps eager, to study seriously. Will good training help us to help others? If so, we may undergo intensive training. Even our sacrifices may be done with some model of cause, with the idea that our loss may lead to more important gain for others. We could hardly make decisions without thinking about what effects those decisions will probably produce.

A great deal of human scholarship has been devoted to the study of causality. Why does the sun rise in the morning and set half a day later? Why do some berries poison us and others do not? Why does washing often keep people healthier? Why do children, lambs, and tigers act so much like their parents? In such apparently simple questions, we can open up some great themes of religion, philosophy, and science.

The first step toward understanding has typically been description, and statistics began as a way of describing things and events. Following description, statistics have been used to show relationships. And once relationships are established, science has been concerned with causes. We ask, which frequencies are dependent on which others? Or, which measurements are cause, and which are effect? Or, which correlations are caused by unseen, hidden variables we have not considered?

Ultimately, scientists use the growing knowledge of cause to try to control events. We predict weather to ensure an adequate food supply. We seek to understand monetary supply in order to curb inflation. The history of science, then, has been from description, to relations, to causes, to decisions. But before such decisions are made, all of us must be concerned with causes.

The world of science has two principal methods of approaching the problem of cause. One method is the use of experiments; the other method is the use of observational models. In so-called true experiments, subjects are assigned randomly to treatments, and the effects of these treatments are then observed. These subjects may be bacteria, and the treatments might be different antibiotics. Or, the subjects may be student nurses, and the treatments might be types of audio-visual instruction, with the goal of improving the training in some procedure. Experiments are a magnificent method for discovering important causes, and experimental design, the study of arranging experiments for the greatest information, is a major branch of applied statistics. For the statistical procedures, the usual way of analyzing experiments has been analysis of variance (ANOVA), as described in Chapters 9 and 10.

Such advanced experimental methods are, like most of modern science, very new. The father of such complex experimental designs, which answer many questions at once, was the late R. A. Fisher, whose great work was *The Design of Experiments* (1935).

Unfortunately, there are countless important questions that cannot be readily explored by experiments. Many events cannot be controlled (such as travel of the planets, or the evolution of species) or would be too dangerous to apply (pollution in drinking water) or too expensive (large experiments in hospital administration). Thus, we seek more practical methods for studying causes. We wish for some techniques that would manage to imitate experiments, so that we may study the events we are curious about, without actually controlling them.

PATH MODELS

Like experimental design, path analysis is very new, having begun with the writing of a geneticist, Sewall Wright (1921). Paths have been heavily used in economics, sociology, and now other social sciences, and they are often the favored method of explanation wherever we have large data sets available for analysis and where we seek out causal connections. For researchers, paths provide a wonderful method for organizing our data, for "making sense" out of variables that might otherwise confuse and overwhelm us.

This chapter will first present path analysis as a set of simple diagrams and as a way to think about research. But along with these diagrams, some special vocabulary required for path analysis will be presented. Further, we will show how we may use ordinary correlation or regression to "solve" these path models. Finally, we will learn how we may use path models to revise our hypotheses and to improve our causal theories.

OBJECTIVES FOR CHAPTER 14

After reading this chapter and completing the exercises, you should be able to

1. Draw a path model of a problem, of the recurisve sort, with appropriate arrows or curved lines.

2. Use multiple regression to find the path coefficients for each arrow.
3. Set up a decomposition table for the path analysis, calculating the direct and indirect cause from one variable to another.
4. Reduce the path model according to some decision rule, eliminating the unimportant paths.
5. Draw nonrecursive path models for some simple relationships and be able to seek further knowledge for these where necessary.
6. Discuss the possible strengths and weaknesses of LISREL and other programs for covariance-structure analysis.

ELEMENTS OF PATH ANALYSIS

Correlated Variables

By now, we are very familiar with the idea of one variable correlating with another, and we know how to find such a correlation. Suppose, for the following examples, that we are interested in the achievement of student nurses and have certain background information on a group of such students. In the data set, there is a positive relation ($r = .40$) between student achievement (grades) and the student's family income. In path analysis, this relation is represented as in Figure 14-1. Each part of this simple diagram has a meaning. The square variables mean that these variables are "measured," with some scores or numbers for these in our data set. (Later we will note variables that are drawn in circles, implying that such variables are "unmeasured.") Note that the line is curved (not straight) and that there is no arrow point at either end. We have simply the correlation here, no causal path. And we are agnostic about which is cause, Family Income or Student Achievement, and which is effect.

The problem with such a diagram is that we cannot draw any important conclusions from it. And, in general, to draw benefits from statistical analysis, we must build in some assumptions.

Simplest Path Diagram

By adding some assumptions, such a diagram of correlation can be transformed into the simplest possible model of cause. See Figure 14-2, in which these very important changes in the model are explained.

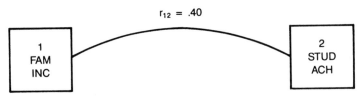

Figure 14-1   Correlated variables.

First, we ask ourselves a question about the "weak causal ordering" of these two variables, the income of the parents, and the achievement of the student nurse. By saying "weak," we are denying that we know one to be an influence on the other. Rather, we are answering the question, "If one is the cause of the other, which would it be?" When the question is so put, virtually everyone will agree that the arrow must be drawn from Family Income to Student Achievement, not the other way around. Why? One major consideration is temporal order, when these events took place, because causality must work forward in time, not backward. Clearly, Family Income was pretty much established before the student went into the nursing education program, ruling out a reversed arrow.

Notice that the decision about "weak causal ordering" is a very important decision in the design and analysis of cause, but it is not a statistical decision. Rather, it depends on reason, logic, and some background knowledge of the variables. Making such decisions is largely a matter of consensus, very close to using persuasion, rather than any inexorable technical conclusion. But such agreements are very easy to find in most of the situations that we study. And when they are not logically obvious, it often will make little difference to the outcome of interest (because they are embedded in the diagram, and because the outcome variables of greatest interest are not much affected by the arrow direction). Having drawn the arrow in this simplest path diagram, some new vocabulary is required, and some new possibilities for analysis emerge.

Exogenous vs. Endogenous Variables

Variable 1, Family Income, has now become the "origin" of the causal model (see Fig. 14-2). And because it has an arrow coming from it, but no arrow leading to it, it is termed an *exogenous* variable. We are stating that any of the causes of Family Income must come from outside the model. On the other hand, Student Achievement has an arrow pointing to it; thus, some of its variance is explained by a variable in the model. Such "internal" variables are called *endogenous* variables.

Path Coefficients

Note that in Figure 14-1, there was a curved line for the equation, $r_{12} = .40$. For Figure 14-2, the correlation between these variables has not changed, but instead of $r = .40$, we have $p_{21} = .40$. Because there are no other influences in the model, the correlation has simply been transformed into the path coefficient. Note that the

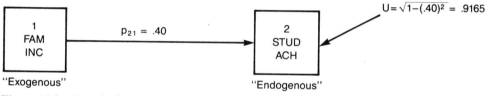

$$U = \sqrt{1-(.40)^2} = .9165$$

1
FAM
INC

$p_{21} = .40$

2
STUD
ACH

"Exogenous"   "Endogenous"

Figure 14-2 A path diagram.

order of the subscripts is changed, because path coefficients are traditionally expressed with the effect variable first, and the cause variable second. Hence, p_{21} expresses the direct influence of Family Income (1) on Student Achievement (2).

What does a path of .40 mean? All the numbers are based on correlations, so they should be thought of in terms of standard scores. Thus, a path of .40 means that if Family Income is changed one standard deviation, Student Achievement will change .40 of a standard deviation.

There is one more addition in the transformation to a path model. We have added another arrow bearing on the endogenous variable—this arrow coming from "U" outside the model. The "U" may be thought of as Unexplained or Unknown influences that are pooled together and computed as the influences *not* explained by the paths leading to Student Achievement. (Some authors use "R" instead of "U.") In this example, with only two variables, U is solved for as

$$U = \sqrt{1 - r^2} \quad \text{or} \quad U = \sqrt{1 - (.40)^2} = .9165$$

So, almost 92% of the variance in Student Achievement is *not* explained by Family Income. Note that $(.9165)^2$ plus $(.40)^2$ is equal to 1.00, accounting for 100% of the variance in Student Achievement. Since the U expression does not add new information, why do we bother ever putting it in our model? Sometimes we do not, but here it serves the following purpose: Since there is no line connecting U with Variable 1, we are indicating that this "Unexplained" (or "Disturbance") variable is uncorrelated with any causes of Student Achievement in the model. Later on, these assumptions will be made clearer.

A Three-Variable Model

The power of path analysis becomes much more important when the problem is expanded to three variables. In Figure 14-3, Parent Education is added to the other two variables. The straight arrows are indicators of causal direction. The origin of the model is now Parent Education. Why? Because Parent Education is ordinarily prior to Family Income and may be thought of as contributing to it. Both of these background variables, Parent Education and Family Income, are possible causes of Student Achievement, and we are therefore granting the "weak causal ordering." In this model, Parent Education (1) is an exogenous variable, whereas Family Income (2) and Student Achievement (3) are endogenous.

A Recursive Model

The path model in Figure 14-3 is called "recursive," because it may be analyzed in the same way as each new variable is added. Note that there are no loops in it. Flow is from left to right, with no doubling back. This particular model is called *complete recursive*, because there are no paths omitted from the diagram. (We shall see later that often a goal of path analysis is to reduce the number of paths.) Some nonrecursive models will be discussed later.

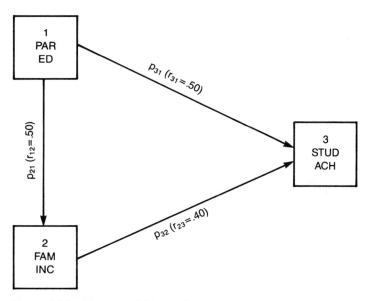

Figure 14-3   Three-variable model.

The Logic of Causal Models

In Figure 14-3, the coefficient for the path between variables 1 and 2 (p_{21}) will equal the correlation between these two variables (r_{12}). This is true because no other causes in the model influence this correlation between the first and second variables. Therefore, since $r_{12} = .50$, $p_{21} = .50$.

The other two paths in Figure 14-3, leading to Student Achievement, are not so simple, because there must be some adjustment made for the confusion of the two causes of Student Achievement and their own correlation with each other.

In the logic of path analysis, the correlation of any two variables is explained by the tracing rule:

> A correlation between variables is the sum of the products of all path tracings from one variable to the other (except that there may be no entering the same variable twice on a tracing and no entering *and* leaving a variable through arrowheads).

In Figure 14-3, we see that for the path between 1 and 2, p_{21}, we count a tracing from 1 to 2 directly. We may not count the tracing 1 to 3 to 2, because that would require entering and leaving 3 through arrowheads. Thus, as already shown, $p_{21} = .50$ and represents r_{12}. The correlation between 1 and 3, however, consists of the direct path (1 to 3) and the indirect path (1 to 2 to 3). The direct path is p_{31}. Indirect paths are calculated as the product of the paths contained within them; so, here, the indirect path from 1 to 3 is the product of $p_{21} \times p_{32}$, or $p_{21} p_{32}$.

The correlation between 2 and 3, r_{23}, consists of the direct path from 2 to 3, p_{32}, and the two-step tracing from 2 to 1 to 3, or $p_{21}p_{31}$. This indirect tracing is not immediately clear from looking at the model, because moving from 2 to 1 seems to be contrary to the arrow on that path. But such a tracing is included under the tracing rule above, because no variable is entered twice; and although $p_{21}p_{31}$ enters and leaves 1, it does not both enter *and* leave 2 through an arrowhead. This noncausal tracing helps us to understand the *correlation* between 2 and 3, since part of this correlation is caused by the fact that 1 has a common impact on both 2 and 3 (Asher, 1976, p. 33). (For another method of determining which paths to include in the indirect path, see Pedhazur, 1982, pp. 583–588.) In path analysis, then, we decompose, or break down, the correlations into direct causal, indirect causal, and noncausal components. And note: all *causal* paths must follow the arrows. From the example, we can write:

	Direct Causal		Indirect Causal		Noncausal
$r_{12} =$	p_{21}	+	—	+	0
$r_{13} =$	p_{31}	+	$p_{21}p_{32}$	+	0
$r_{23} =$	p_{32}	+	0	+	$p_{21}p_{31}$

The path coefficients are calculated by using multiple regression analysis where each endogenous variable is regressed on those variables that are prior to it in the model and assumed to have a causal effect on it, as indicated by the arrows in the model. The standardized or beta weight is the value most commonly used for the path coefficients (although some researchers use the unstandardized or b-weights). In this example, two regressions would be run. Family Income (2) would be regressed on Parent Education (1), and Student Achievement (3) would be regressed on both Family Income (2) and Parent Education (1). The results of these regressions are given in Table 14-1. Substituting those path values in our equation, we can determine the direct, indirect, and total causal effects as presented in Table 14-2.

Direct and Indirect Paths

In Table 14-2, examine the decomposition of r_{13}, and note that Variable 1 has two ways of influencing Variable 3. It influences Variable 3 directly, with a path of .40. It also influences Variable 3 indirectly, with a path of .10, through influencing Variable 2, which in turn influences Variable 3. The total influence of Variable 1 on Variable 3 is .40 + .10, or .50, which is, in fact, the original correlation between

Table 14-1   Regressions Used to Compute Path Coefficients

Regression	Dependent Variable	Independent Variable(s)	Betas
1	Family Income (2)	Parent Education (1)	.50 (p_{21})
2	Student Achievement (3)	Parent Education (1)	.40 (p_{31})
		Family Income (2)	.20 (p_{32})

Variables 1 and 3. The tracing rule is thus demonstrated—that a correlation between two variables is the sum of the products of the tracings, subject to certain
exceptions.

In this simple example, the other causal and noncausal covariation is also
shown. The path analysis allows calculation of both causal and noncausal
components. If there is a difference between the total causal effect and the original
correlation, that indicates that a portion of the original correlation was noncausal or
"spurious." For example, the original correlation between Variables 2 and 3 is 40,
the total causal influences are .20, the noncausal component of the correlation
equals $.40 - .20 = .20$. Path analysis, then, gives us the direct, indirect, and
noncausal components of correlation coefficients.

Importance of Indirect Paths

Often, in path models, the indirect paths may be more important than the direct
paths. The total causal influence of a variable is also likely to be of great interest
to us. Thus, the way we draw some of the arrows in a diagram can be very central to
the apparent findings. It is important that the model be based on reasonable
deductions.

In Figure 14-4, a very frequent event is diagrammed. The investigators do not
declare the priority of the causal variables, preferring to show a curved, two-headed
arrow pointing between them. This is essentially an "agnostic" diagram, as far as
this relation is concerned. There is causal influence acknowledged, but no clear
preference of one direction over the other, and no willingness to exclude either
influence.

In the published literature, this may be the most usual position. Often, researchers are concentrating on the criterion or outcome variable and do not want to
quibble about the causal variables and their relation to each other. Often, too, they
may be principally interested in the direct causal influence on the outcome variable,
and, rightly or not, less interested in the indirect influence.

Such a position is understandable, but we should realize what we lose: any
possibility of recovering the indirect influences, some of which may frequently be
larger than the direct influences. Just as drawing paths allows far more interpretation than plain correlations, so one-directional arrows allow more interpretation
than two-headed, ambiguous arrows.

Table 14-2 Calculation of Direct, Indirect, and Total Causal Effects

r	Direct Effect	Indirect Effect	Total Causal Effect (Direct + Indirect)	Noncausal Covariation
$r_{12} = 50$	$p_{21} = .50$	—	.50	.00
$r_{13} = .50$	$p_{31} = .40$	$p_{21} p_{32} = (.50)(.20) = .10$	.50	.00
$r_{23} = .40$	$p_{32} = .20$	0	.20	.20

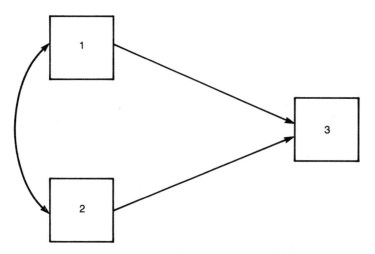

Figure 14-4   Lack of causal ordering between variables 1 and 2.

For these reasons, we strongly encourage students to try, whenever possible, to draw one-directional arrows. Our own research experience supports this. For example, in studying the effects of origins of leadership, the importance of intelligence was operating mostly indirectly, through high school grades. Without a willingness to declare intelligence prior to grades, this influence would have been buried.

In general, how may such arrows be validated? First, we recognize that we are dealing here with matters of logic, background knowledge, and persuasion through evidence. Thus, for one solution, we may declare the directions that appear most wise to us and see whether there is any objection. Or, we may ask some knowledgeable people their own opinions, and take majority opinion as support. Often enough, there is background literature, or published opinion, to support one direction or another. If these efforts still fail to satisfy us, we may calculate it both ways (one trial with the arrow pointing from *A* to *B,* and the other with the arrow reversed). Sometimes, there will be no important differences in results, and the direction will therefore be unimportant. Other times, both results may be published, and the decision is left to the informed reader.

Later in this chapter, we will consider some methods that are nonrecursive, which will permit another kind of consideration where we are actively interested in mutual influences. But for most applications, we will probably wish to stay within the recursive framework.

THEORY TESTING FROM A PATH MODEL

One of the overriding purposes of research, as noted, is the development of theory. Even simple path models, like the three-variable model we have been studying, may help us clarify the causal influences of one variable on another. Before proceeding to more complicated models, let's consider such a case.

As a profession, nursing has invested much time and effort in developing theories to guide practice. One researcher pointed out that "As nursing science evolves, the need for theory becomes more obvious and more crucial" (Fawcett, 1978, p. 17). A recent example of such research is a study of the effect on a wife of a husband's chronic obstructive pulmonary disease (COPD). Data gathered in that study were used to illustrate path analysis (Munro & Sexton, 1984). See Figure 14-5 for the hypothesized relationships among three variables: the severity of illness of the husband (1), the level of stress reported by the wife (2), and a measure of the wife's life satisfaction (3). There is probably little quarrel with such a diagram. We expect that the health problem of the husband will cause stress for the wife, and we are interested in the influence of these factors on the wife's general satisfaction with life. We may predict that all three of the paths will be substantial.

In this study, as with other path models, we may start with the correlation matrix, as shown in Table 14-3. From this table, we might infer that both predictor variables have a direct influence on the wife's satisfaction with life. However, we perform a multiple regression analysis, with the results shown in Table 14-4. There we note that the direct path from illness to satisfaction has now gone to zero, as shown by p_{31}. This suggests that we may redraw the path model as shown in Figure 14-6. There we see that the effect of the severity of the illness of the husband has only an indirect effect on life satisfacton, through its effect on stress.

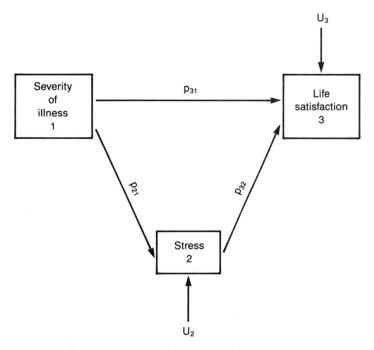

Figure 14-5 Path diagram of postulated relationship between severity of illness and life satisfaction.

Table 14-3   Correlations of Variables for COPD and Stress

Variables	1	2	3
1. Severity of illness	1.00	.27	−.31
2. Wife's stress		1.00	−.67
3. Life satisfaction			1.00

Table 14-4   Regressions Used to Compute Path Coefficients for Model

Regression	Dependent Variable	Independent Variable	Correlation (r)	Beta	R^2
1	Stress (2)	Severity of Illness (1)	$r_{12} =$ .27	.27 (p_{21})	.07
2	Life Satisfaction (3)	Severity of Illness (1)	$r_{13} = -.31$	.00 (p_{31})	.45
		Stress (2)	$r_{23} = -.67$	−.67 (p_{32})	

Trimming a Causal Model

The comparison of Figures 14-5 and 14-6 shows a principal use of path models in making theories more elegant and useful. We remember the general virtue, in science, of parsimony—the reduction of explanations to the simplest forms possible, while retaining as much comprehensive power as we can. Because a two-path model is simpler than a three-path model, and in this case can be shown to be more faithful to the analytic results, we prefer Figure 14-6.

Rules for Simplifying

In this study, it has been easy to erase the chosen path, because it was zero. Naturally, we will seldom find paths that are exactly zero, and, even when we do, we may suspect that the "true" path is at least slightly different (because of sampling error, measurement error, and so on).

What rules may be used to reduce such diagrams? One way is to use statistical significance, and the other way is to use the actual size of the path, or what we may call its meaningfulness. With very large *n*s, such as we have with some available data bases, even small paths are still "significant," although their "meaningfulness" may be trivial. On the other hand, with small numbers of subjects, even substantial paths may still be rather questionable, and we might find it quite difficult to reject the null hypothesis that the "true path" is zero.

For various reasons, then, most researchers lean toward the use of meaningfulness, rather than statistical significance, in deciding which paths to trim. This is done because large samples are usually required for multiple regression, and even

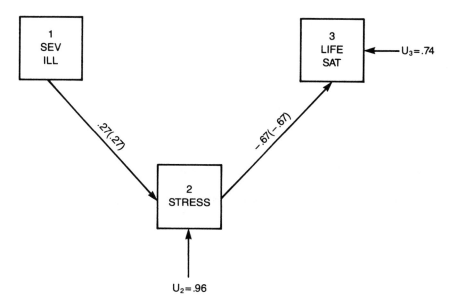

Figure 14-6 Path analysis for COPD study. (Values in parentheses represent correlations; other numbers are causal paths.)

minute path coefficients might be found significant (Heise, 1975, p. 195; Kerlinger & Pedhazur, 1973, p. 318). One criterion recommended by Land (1969) is to delete all paths with coefficients (betas) less than .05. This is fairly common practice.

Of course, studies will differ greatly from each other in the size of their paths and in the usefulness of the results. If we could improve patient recovery time even 3% by making some easy change in our practice, we would surely want to do so. And we might wish to try it, even when we are not sure of the result, as long as it would do no harm. On the other hand, if the changes called for were very expensive and required nursing time needed for more urgent, life-and-death matters, we would be reluctant to accept uncertain, doubtful, or weak results as forcing such a change.

In other words, which paths to delete from a causal model must, in most research, be partly a subjective decision. What is required is that we always make clear what criteria we are using and why we choose to give more attention to some paths than to others.

One practice is to have a succession of path models representing the same analysis, in which we progressively delete paths as we use higher standards. Thus, we may first show a complete model (which may often be a rather bushy mess). Second, we may select only those paths with an absolute value (plus or minus) of .02 or larger and show the new diagram. This will usually reduce and clarify the model. Third, we may delete all paths except those with at least .05 or higher. And last, if the model has enough strong relationships, we may use a criterion still higher, such as .10 or more. It is remarkable how our understanding may be enriched by such a sequence. After all, no one path is the "true" representation, exactly, and all paths may help us study the causal system.

EXPERIMENTS IN PATH ANALYSIS

Such path models may help in identifying the nature of experiments and in understanding their results. In this section, two expansions of the former example of achievement in nursing school are presented. First, our subjects attend different types of nursing schools (*i.e.,* 2-year vs. 4-year), and we wish to add the variable, type of nursing school, to our model. Such a model may be drawn as in Figure 14-7.

Again, how we draw this model is very important and depends on our reasoning about the way education works. In the sense of "weak causal ordering," we are entitled to place the family influences prior to the school selection.

False "Experiments"

Too often, investigators regard just one relationship by itself, such as that between Nursing School Type and Achievement, and draw conclusions filled with errors and exaggerations. For example, let us suppose that the correlation between School Type and Achievement were .30. The implication might be that simply by changing School Type, we would increase Achievement nearly one third of a standard deviation, on the average. But suppose that the more complete, four-variable model had correlations as in Table 14-5.

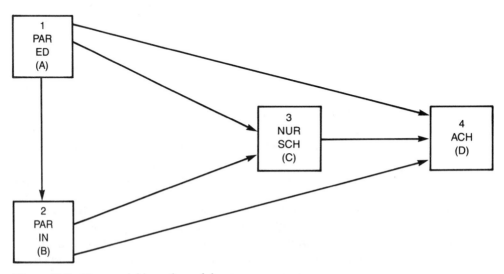

Figure 14-7   Four variable path model.

Table 14-5   Correlations of Hypothetical Data for Effects of Nursing School Type

Variables	A	B	C	D
A. Parent education	1.00	.50	.30	.50
B. Parent income		1.00	.40	.40
C. Nursing-school type			1.00	.30
D. Achievement test				1.00

Note that school type is correlated 0.30 with Achievement but that the prior variables are correlated with both School Type and with Achievement. So we may properly be inquisitive about the causal relations among these four variables.

An SAS Analysis of the Problem

Let us use the Statistical Analysis System (SAS) to give us the path analysis we seek. Since SAS is currently the most widely available and widely used such package in the world, we may gain some feel for recursive path models from such an example.

In the Nursing School model, we are mainly interested in the path coefficients, and these are produced by SAS in the form shown in Figure 14-8. In this example, a correlation matrix, already produced by previous analysis, was our input. More commonly, SAS works directly with individual data, but the use of the correlation matrix is easy, and the resulting analysis takes only a few seconds, thus saving expensive computer processing time.

The important path coefficients are all found under the heading of "parameter estimate." For the first model, regressing B on A (Parent Income on Parent Education), we find .500 to be the path. In the second model, Nursing School (C) is regressed on Parent Education (A) and Parent Income (B). The resulting paths are .133 for A (Parent Education) and .333 for B (Parent Income). These, then, are the causal forces bearing on selection into Nursing School Type. For the third model, we find the paths bearing on Achievement (D) are .384 from Parent Education (A); .160 from Parent Income (B); and .121 from Nursing School Type (C). We may draw these paths into a new diagram, as shown in Figure 14-9.

Of course, with all the causal variables having influences on each other, we expect to see the path coefficients considerably smaller than were the correlations. Such is the case in Figure 14-9. Note that no paths are eliminated from the model, because no paths fell below the arbitrary test of .05. Observe that the effect of School Type has shrunk to about one third of the power that we might, previously, have estimated. Even without eliminating such a path, then, we have greatly altered our theoretical understanding of it. Although these are fictitious data, this analysis illustrates a common finding in path models: that we must control for pre-existing causes and not be misled simply by those variables that might have caught our attention or that come under our own control.

Procedure Cards

PROC SYSREG;

    MODEL   B = A;
    MODEL   C = A B;
    MODEL   D = A B C;

Output

MODEL:	MODEL01			SSE	74.250000	F RATIO	32.67
				DFE	98	PROB > F	0.0001
DEP VAR:	B			MSE	0.757653	R-SQUARE	0.2500

VARIABLE	DF	PARAMETER ESTIMATE	STANDARD ERROR	T RATIO	PROB > |T|
INTERCEPT	1	0	0.087043		
A	1	0.500000	0.087482	5.7155	0.0001

MODEL:	MODEL02			SSE	81.840000	F RATIO	10.17
				DFE	97	PROB > F	0.0001
DEP VAR:	C			MSE	0.843711	R-SQUARE	0.1733

VARIABLE	DF	PARAMETER ESTIMATE	STANDARD ERROR	T RATIO	PROB > |T|
INTERCEPT	1	0	0.091854		
A	1	0.133333	0.106598	1.2508	0.2140
B	1	0.333333	0.106598	3.1270	0.0023

MODEL:	MODEL03			SSE	70.082419	F RATIO	13.20
				DFE	96	PROB > F	0.0001
DEP VAR:	D			MSE	0.730025	R-SQUARE	0.2921

VARIABLE	DF	PARAMETER ESTIMATE	STANDARD ERROR	T RATIO	PROB > |T|
INTERCEPT	1	0	0.085442		
A	1	0.383871	0.099953	3.8405	0.0002
B	1	0.159677	0.104034	1.5349	0.1281
C	1	0.120968	0.094447	1.2808	0.2033

Figure 14-8 Computer output from SAS for the nursing school problem.

A True Experiment

The above study of Nursing School Type may illustrate a common error in understanding: When seen in a path model, we observe that selection into nursing schools will not be random, but rather will be correlated with other variables of importance. Nursing-school selection, then, will seldom be a "true" experiment. Suppose, however, that there is some true experiment that we used, such as a film

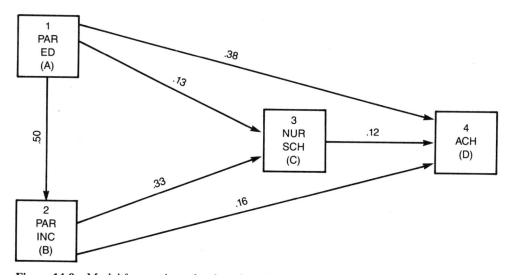

Figure 14-9   Model for nursing school study, with causal paths included.

aimed at improving the instruction of certain practices, and we wish to find out whether it improves the general Achievement tests scores for the field. When we say "true" experiment, we mean that every subject has an equal chance of being placed in a particular experimental group. A true experiment would be drawn as in Figure 14-10.

In Figure 14-10, note that Variable 4, our Experimental variable, has no lines connecting it with Parent Education, Parent Income, or Nursing School Type. Why not? Because, if the assignment is truly random, there will be no important correlations with any prior variables. In fact, one test of whether the treatments were assigned randomly is to inspect the correlations and the resulting paths. Indeed, after the analysis is completed, the correlation of EXP and ACH should be very close to the path coefficient for the same two variables.

If we should find that the effects of the Experiment were overlapping the background variables, we might wish to redraw the model, showing the apparent influences of the background variables on the experimental assignment. The fact is, in the real world of experimentation with human subjects, there are frequently compromises with availability, self-selection, and other soft influences, which may distort true randomness. In such cases, there is great power in including all the available variables that might influence the apparent outcomes.

MULTIPLE REGRESSION OR
ANALYSIS OF COVARIANCE

Note, the model in Figure 14-10 is quite similar to the basic situation of the analysis of covariance (ANCOVA; see Chapter 11); that is, we are mainly interested here in the relation between the experiment and student achievement after controlling for

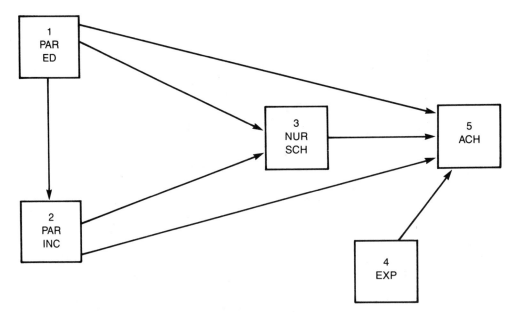

Figure 14-10   Inclusion of a "true" experiment in the nursing-school model.

the background variables that might otherwise muddy or distort the view. True, we could use either approach. For purposes of this chapter, however, and of general understanding of causal modeling, multiple regression might be more descriptive and useful.

"UNMEASURED" VARIABLES

One important possibility in path modeling is to work with what we call "unmeasured" variables. Yet the term may seem a contradiction: How can we possibly use something that is not measured in our data set? The answer is not really so strange. We may not have an item about being "chronically ill," yet we may easily make such a category from other questions. We may ask about recent complaints and absences from work for illness and follow some rule of our own to differentiate the "chronically ill" from the others in our data set. Or we may, in another data set, combine items about children and about marital status to infer information about "fatherless" families. In a sense, although we did not measure such a variable directly, we are able to quantify it and to investigate it.

A more common way of finding out about "unmeasured" variables is through the use of somewhat more advanced mathematical methods. Suppose that we have no direct "measure" of self-esteem but that we pose the following question:

How do you feel about each of the following statements?

1. At times I think that I am no good at all.
2. When I make plans, I am almost certain that I can make them work.
3. On the whole, I am satisfied with myself.

The subject responds by checking one of five choices, from Agree Strongly to Disagree Strongly. Looking over these statements, we might predict that they will be related—that if one agreed with the first statement, one would probably disagree with the second and third. (These items are from the Rosenberg Self-Esteem Scale, 1972.)

Now let us suppose that we seek not three related items, but rather, within the three responses to these items, we seek for a certain trait in the person, or disposition, that contributes something to each of the three responses. We may call this disposition "self-esteem" (*SE*), and we can explore *SE* in these three items and their intercorrelations. A path diagram as shown in Figure 14-11 can be used to test our assumptions. Note that the "unmeasured" variable is drawn as a circle, and the "measured" variables are drawn as squares.

We could find how strongly Self-Esteem is related to each item and then use the strength of the relationship as a way of calculating a Self-Esteem variable for each person in our data set. Algebra can be used to determine the appropriate weights. More often than not, however, researchers may solve for unmeasured variables through the use of factor analysis and factor scores, as described in Chapter 13. For working with the intricacies of unmeasured variables in path models, you are encouraged to study the texts by Duncan (1975), Heise (1975), Kenny (1979), Li (1975), and Pedhazur (1982).

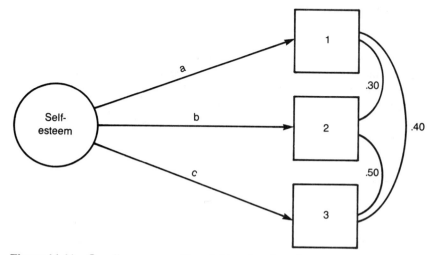

Figure 14-11   One "unmeasured" variable related to three measured variables.

MEASUREMENT MODELS AND STRUCTURAL MODELS

In our examples of "unmeasured" variables, we studied them only in relation to the "measured" variables they are presumed to cause. Such diagrams are often called "measurement models." On the other hand, when we study how different variables influence each other, our diagrams are often called "structural models." These structural models commonly consist of a mixture of causal influences. For further examples see the work of Jöreskog and Sörbom (1979).

Consider a very simple diagram of a structural model involving both "measured" and "unmeasured" variables. Suppose that we have information on patients in rehabilitation and are interested in the possible earlier return home caused by prescribed exercise. We therefore have gathered some data on prescribed exercise from the patients and nurses and on length of stay in the hospital. The correlation between those two variables is .30. The observed data may be represented as in Figure 14-12.

We recognize, of course, that there are many influences bearing on when patients leave the hospital and that neither measure is exactly what we wanted to test. For example, we took the patients' reports about how much they complied with the prescribed exercise regimen, and such reports will not be entirely reliable or valid. Also, when the patient is released partly depends on the physician's philosophy, how crowded the hospital is, the economic status of the patient, and a number of other factors in addition to patient fitness.

Reliability and Causal Paths

Thus, we redesign our model, reflecting our true research interest and trying to correct for some of the distractions in our data. The result is seen in Figure 14-13. Here we show some important changes in our thinking about the problem. Note that there is only a curved line, now, between the two observed variables, showing that this correlation is not considered to be causal in this new model. Rather, the causal influence we seek is now shown between the "unmeasured" variables of exercise, on the one hand, and of rehabilitation, on the other. These "unmeasured" variables are causal, as well, for their own observed variables. One possible question, then, is what are the paths from the "unmeasured" variables to the observed variables?

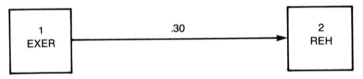

Figure 14-12   Observed data for exercise and rehabilitation.

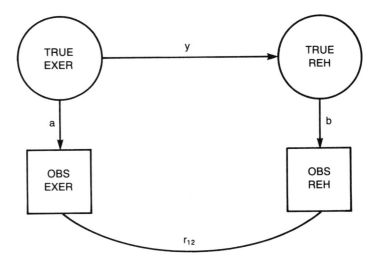

Figure 14-13 "Unmeasured" variables in the study of exercise and rehabilitation.

Calculating Validity

If we seek further information about Figure 14-13, we might collect other knowledge about the exercise of the patient, seeking some estimate of validity or reliability. One method is to take a sub-sample of patients and to explore the accuracy of their reports by checking for their own consistency, by observation, and by checking with the nurses. From such inquiry, we calculate that the validity of "Exercise" is .80 in the patient reports and that the validity of "Rehabilitation" is .70. Thus, a in Figure 14-13 = .80 and b = .70. We are now interested in the "true" path from "Exercise" to "Rehabilitation," after adjusting for the weaknesses of the observed measures.

Calculating "True" Paths

The tracing rule may be applied in this investigation. According to this rule, the one correlation between the observed measures is only a shadow, whereas the true path is between the "unmeasured" variables, which are hidden from view. But we do know that the correlation must result from the product of the paths between the two observed variables. Therefore, we may write that $r = a \times y \times b$, hence

$$.30 = (.80)\, y\, (.70),$$
$$.30 = .56y$$
$$y = .30/.56 = .536.$$

We observe that the "true," or theoretical, path from Exercise to Rehabilitation (.536) is a great deal larger than the observed path .30.

Importance of the Theoretical Paths

The result here is the usual case: The estimated theoretical influences are generally larger than the observed paths, because the errors in measurement will usually be in a random direction, weakening and attenuating the true effects.

There are two lessons to be learned from such examples. First, we should not be misled by the weakness of our observed relationships, and, second, we should always remember that, if our measurements were improved, the paths would almost surely be greater than what we see. Still, for some purposes, we would not wish merely to stress the higher, theoretical values, because this might set up expectations of results that we would never accomplish in the real world of health practice. In short, we shall often wish to look at the "true" paths of influence between the variables that interest us. But we should not expect the "real-world" data to confirm these predictions to the same extent as theory would suggest.

In ordinary research practice, we may often wish to use what data are available economically and report the outcomes, but include in our report whatever background information we can supply about the reliability and validity of our variables and the necessary adjustments in understanding of our observed results.

TIME-LAGGED MODELS

Usually, researchers will find it more profitable and productive to work with recursive models, in which one variable points clearly to others and there is an assumed hierarchy leading from the first variable to the last. Needless to say, life itself is not always so simple, and some pairs of variables are quite difficult to sort into cause and effect. Does depression lead to illness, or does illness lead to depression? Does self-esteem lead to achievement, or is it the other way around? We could name many such questions where, given our present knowledge, we might be doubtful about the cause–effect relationship or might argue that the causes work both ways. How may we handle such problems?

Where the Problem is Minor

In the first place, depending on where our doubtful path occurs, it may not make any important difference in our outcome whether A causes B, or B causes A. For example, if our main concern is on other relationships and the questionable path occurs earlier in a large model, the direction of such an early arrow may be trivial in its later effects. The doubtful path itself may be weak and, thus, unimportant. We should be aware that any importance of earlier paths is typically in estimating indirect effects, and these will usually be quite small later in the causal chain. In any case, we can often directly resolve the question of importance: The model can usually be run both ways, first with A influencing B, then with B influencing A. This will frequently show that the principal concerns are not importantly affected by the arrow. And the results of such trials may be briefly reported, to satisfy the critical reader, so that questioning of some disagreement about cause will not be a barrier to the acceptance of the research as a whole.

Cross-Lagged Designs

On the other hand, suppose that such a question of causal direction is close to the heart of our research. How may we seek out an answer? One type of solution has been used extensively and may, like a straight recursive model, be analyzed by rather simple methods. This type of model is often termed *cross-lagged panel correlation (CLPC)*. It is so-named because there is a "lag" of time between the two periods, and the interest is in the "cross" correlations, across both time and variable. Such a case is shown in Figure 14-14.

In Figure 14-14, note that there are two variables, *A* and *B*, measured on two occasions, 1 and 2. From the four measures, there are six correlations, and they may be separated into three different types:

1. $r_{A_1 B_1}$ and $r_{A_2 B_2}$ are synchronous correlations (with *A* and *B* measured at the same time)
2. $r_{A_1 A_2}$ and $r_{B_1 B_2}$ are autocorrelations (the same variables measured twice)
3. $r_{A_1 B_2}$ and $r_{B_1 A_2}$ are cross-lagged correlations (different variables at different times)

Figure 14-14 is drawn differently from the earlier diagrams, showing the model with some straight lines but without any arrows. The straight lines are shown because, in the logic of causality, we believe that the earlier events might cause the later events—at least, the reverse would not be defended. On the other hand, two curved lines are used for the synchronous correlations, because we are being agnostic about the direction of cause. But this notation is not "standard." There are various ways of drawing such CLPC designs and various ways of analyzing them.

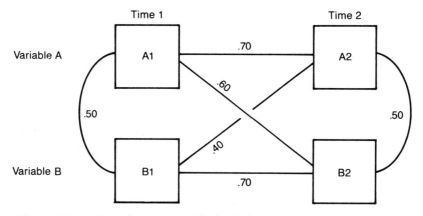

Figure 14-14   Cross-lagged panel design in its simplest form.

Method of Simple Difference

Such designs attracted much attention when explained in a classic early work on research design (Campbell & Stanley, 1963). In the earliest suggestion, a researcher was mainly interested in this question: Does A cause B more than B causes A?

This question was answered by a comparison of $r_{A_1 B_2}$ and $r_{B_1 A_2}$. If $r_{A_1 B_2}$ was greater than $r_{B_1 A_2}$ and this contrast was statistically significant, A (at Time 1) was possibly causing B (at Time 2) more than $B1$ was causing $A2$.

Doubts About the Simple Method

In the past decades, there have been increasing doubts about the simple comparison of the cross-lagged correlations. If the reliability of $B2$ is greater than that for $A2$, all correlations with $B2$ might be expected to be relatively higher, including $r_{A_1 B_2}$, but this would say little about causality. For the cross-lagged correlations to be a good index of relative causality, it is expected that the whole construct of relations remains stable from Time 1 to Time 2 (the principle of stationarity), and this condition is not easy to verify. Many researchers would now urge that such data be set forth in more of an explicit and defensible path model and be solved by the use of multiple regression and other methods (Cook & Campbell, 1979, Chapter 7; Kenny, 1979, Chapter 12).

For these reasons, we will not describe such cross-lagged designs further in this book. But you should be aware that this is one method of exploring the possible direction of influence between two variables, or their possible mutual influence. Even when you decide to use the straight recursive models, you should be aware of such alternatives and sometimes consider their use.

COMPLEX PACKAGES (LISREL)

When we try to model real and important causal networks, there is no limit to how complex these may become. They may involve hundreds of variables in the same model, and the model itself may have a number of "unmeasured" variables and feedback loops. Should we attempt realistic models of such complex situations? And if so, how should we proceed?

How Complex a Model?

Research inevitably involves some trade-off of realism and simplicity. The usual purpose is a many-to-few reduction, taking a mass of often indigestible data and finding some elementary regularities within it. After all, this is the usual goal of statistics: It is no accident that the most commonly used numbers, such as the mean or the standard deviation, may summarize many thousands of cases. And when more advanced statistics are used, as in multiple regression, where we may use 20 variables or many more to predict just one, we are summarizing an enormously complex situation with a few weightings.

The same search for simplicity, for parsimony, for elegance, motivates us in building path models. We are always doing violence to the "complete data" by our models. The question is, how may we best understand what the important causes are? And beyond understanding, what guides may there be in our models for our future practice? Very often, we can really use only a few central messages, so that our principal goal is to understand these few as well as we can. Starting with dozens, even hundreds of causal variables, we may wish to slash through most of these in our actual discussion, to concentrate on the most important findings and implications.

There are some packages available for very complex models, and these have found favor among a number of experts in research methodology. The most widely used among these complex packages is one called LISREL (for LInear Structural RELations), which is the work of Karl Jöreskog (1973) and others (Jörkeskog & Sörbom, 1979).

Here we will give one illustration to demonstrate the kind of analysis that LISREL makes possible. Let us suppose that we have three unmeasured variables of interest to us:

A = PATCARE—Patient Care, with 4 variables
B = PATSAT—Patient Satisfaction, with 3 variables
C = RECSPD—Recovery Speed, with 3 variables

We show this model in Figure 14-15. There we have taken PATCARE to be the principal causal variable, and we plan to estimate its workings through four accepted indices of the quality of patient care. Because these are the indicators of "cause" in our model, they are termed X_1 through X_4. We represent them all as indicators of the central factor of patient care.

In Figure 14-15, we also show two major outcome variables, patient satisfaction and recovery speed. These we attempt to quantify through five indicators, Y_1 through Y_5. We observe that one of these Y variables, Y_3, is a part of both outcome factors. Finally, we see that we are treating patient satisfaction and recovery speed as being mutually causal. We wish, if possible, to estimate what the flow is between these two variables.

As we have drawn this model, there are 14 unknowns for which we seek solutions: four paths from A to the X variables, six paths from B and C to the Y variables, and the four principal paths of our "unmeasured" variables A, B, and C. For input data, we have nine measured variables, with a resulting correlation matrix that will give us $9 \times 8/2 = 36$ correlation coefficients.

Supplying LISREL Input

In addition to the observed matrices, we will have many more numbers or constraints to supply to LISREL. There are, in fact, eight different matrices to be set up, the size of these depending on the numbers of variables, "measured" and

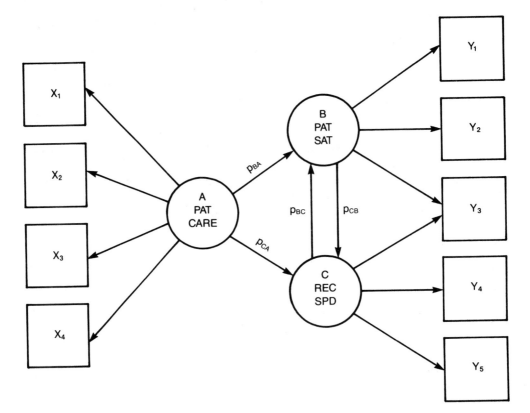

Figure 14-15   A complex model for analysis of covariance structures.

"unmeasured," in our model. In effect, these matrices are the equivalent of the arrows or curved lines that we draw in our model (or choose not to draw).

LISREL's Two Basic Components

For LISREL models such as Figure 14-15, there are two kinds of components present. One is the "measurement model," consisting of the relations of the "unmeasured" variables (A, B, and C) with their respective "measured" variables. (For example, the paths from A to X_1, X_2, X_3, and X_4.) The second component of LISREL is the "structural equation model," consisting of the relations among the unmeasured variables. In Figure 14-15, this structural equation model would seek the four paths among the circles: p_{BA}, p_{CA}, p_{BC}, and p_{CB}.

For our purposes now, we will not bother with actual numbers, neither the observed correlations among the X and Y variables, nor the eight input matrices required, nor the outcome data from LISREL, which may print out for many pages.

Our present purpose is to show that such complex models can, at least in principle, be analyzed by such available packages.

Difficulties of the LISREL Methods

Those of us who have worked with LISREL, or who have tried to help colleagues or graduate students work with LISREL, are bound to have mixed feelings about its general use, given the present state of the art. There have been many improvements in LISREL, over six different versions of the package, and there are now some competitors to LISREL that may promise a more understandable and workable tool for most researchers. Many able researchers have worked for months with LISREL without success or have produced outcomes that are not understandable or useful. Even David Kenny (1979), a noted causal researcher, warns that "one should take care not to fall into the many common traps. . . ." He confesses, "When I run LISREL I presume I have made an error. I check and recheck my results . . . with every error, we must surely be learning" (p. 183).

Furthermore, we recognize that none of the complex results of such programs have any magic in them: They produce only what we have, knowingly or not, permitted them to produce. For example, if we are able to show mutual causal paths (as in Fig. 14-15 for *A* and *B*), it is because we have supplied some apparent "instrumental variables." Such variables are difficult to locate. The fact that we do not really know how LISREL has done it should not inspire confidence in us. To the contrary, it should make us wary. Sometimes there may be a great problem in interpreting what is meant by the paths among the "unmeasured variables."

The above cautions might appear to be almost a condemnation of the LISREL approach. They are not that. Rather, they are intended to protect the optimistic worker from losing months of precious time in an often fruitless search for a solution that will either not appear or will not be understandable to the researcher or to those wishing to publish or use the research. Nonetheless, if the researcher has a particular interest in advanced methodology, such approaches may be worth the difficulty.

ANOTHER APPROACH TO
COMPLEX MODELS

Suppose that we do have an interest in the kinds of relations we have seen in Figure 14-15, but wish to avoid the difficulties of LISREL and related packages. Then how may we proceed?

First, we can resolve the "measurement model" by separate factor analyses run with the three "unmeasured" variables: PATCARE, PATSAT, and RECSPD. Such factor analysis, as we have already seen in Chapter 13, is fairly easy to run from widely available and reliable packages such as SAS, SPSS, or BMDP. Virtually every large computer system will have such packages, and many micro-computers have them in handy software, as well.

Second, we may assign factor scores to each of the cases in the data set. These will often be assigned within the available statistical packages, as well. Now each subject in the data set will have measured scores for PATCARE, PATSAT, and RECSPD. In effect, we have stripped away the formerly measured variables, X and Y, in Figure 14-15. We now have just three circles, with our three principal concerns, and the arrows between them. Or, since we may now term them "measured" variables, we might draw our three main variables as in Figure 14-15. Note that we still have the mutually causal paths between PATSAT and RECSPD. The actual solutions of such reciprocal causation cannot be treated here because of their many complications (*e.g.,* Blalock, 1971, Chapters 13–15; Heise, 1975, pp. 160–185; Kenny, 1979, Chapter 6).

For our purposes here, we would probably wish to simplify the model of Figure 14-16 to a recursive design. One way of doing this would be to take recovery speed as the final object, thus eliminating p_{BC} from the figure. Or, we might run the model both ways, first treating B as the object, then C. If this simplification proved to be too damaging to our research, it might well pay us to consult the more detailed references on mutual causes and try to fit some of these methods into our data. These remain issues that depend greatly on the judgments of the researcher.

When we do run these factor scores, as in Figure 14-16, instead of the "unmeasured" variables in Figure 14-15, what do we gain or lose? On the loss side, remember that with "unmeasured" variables, we typically obtain much stronger paths, because the unreliability of the actual measures is adjusted for. We can expect, therefore, that the paths in Figure 14-16 will be considerably weaker than those in the "structural equation model" of Figure 14-15. On the gain side, the factor scores are easier to understand. Also, they are usually closer to the data that we can actually predict.

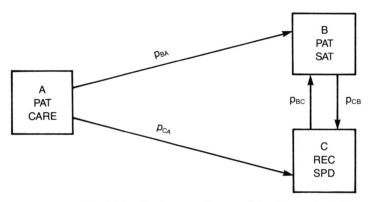

Figure 14-16 Variables in the complex model, after calculating factor scores.

PATH ANALYSIS AS A TOOL: A FINAL WORD

Obviously, path models can become very complex and can lead the researcher to almost endless questions of method and justification. But the last thing that we wish to do is to intimidate a researcher, who is seeking to understand and explain some of the interesting data in the health professions.

Rather, we offer path models as a way of placing a great deal of material into some meaningful pattern. Data are clearly useless unless we have some general organizing principle. Very often, quite simple diagrams can help us decide what it is that we are after, what data we need to collect or examine, and how we may present our case.

For most of your uses, you will probably be content with the completely recursive models, in which you are willing to draw causal arrows from some beginning variable to the intermediate variables, and on to the final variables. In such models, you will frequently want to set forth correlation matrices, then path coefficients for the diagrams, then tables of decomposition into direct causal relations, indirect causes, and noncausal covariation. Frequently, you may wish to combine a number of variables into single measures by the use of factor analysis or some other principle, so that you can see the important relations more clearly. And you will ordinarily wish to use some standard multiple regression packages, such as we find in SAS or SPSS.

Naturally, you will wish to be clear about your assumptions in the models, trying to justify your arrows and priorities. You may also wish to explore data several ways to be sure that any doubtful decisions are not too damaging to the conclusions. It is also important to be aware of what can conceivably be done through very advanced methods or through such packages as LISREL.

But you should recognize that there are countless important topics in the health professions—topics that require better understanding. You should not let "the best" so intimidate you that it becomes the "enemy of the good." The methods of path analysis, usually the straightforward methods of recursive models, will often illuminate the shadowy corners of both theory and practice.

EXERCISES FOR CHAPTER 14

1. What has been the role played by causes in scientific research?

2. What have been the two principal approaches to cause?

3. What are the advantages and disadvantages of path analysis for revealing causes, compared with "true" experiments?

4. Here are some possible questions you might have about health care. For each,

decide whether it seems suitable for causal modeling or for some noncausal approach.

a. In planning a hospital wing, you wish to know what the population will be in 10 years. Would this be a causal question?

b. Your hospital area does not presently offer a visit from a local minister. You are curious about certain possible advantages. How would you explore this?

c. You believe that certain information on the admissions form (*e.g.*, age, ethnic group, illness history, family status) might be related to patient satisfaction. How would you investigate this?

5. You are interested in understanding how long married nurses continue in the profession, and you have a big sample in one of the national data sets. Among the variables that interest you are the following (with a variable name):

Number of Children (NCH)
Level of husband's occupation (HOC)
Ethnic background of nurse (ETH)
Occupation of nurse's father (FOC)
College grade average (GRA)

Your target, persistence in nursing, you call PER.

Decide in what order these would normally occur. Assume a "weak causal ordering," and draw a path diagram as shown in this chapter, with the earliest variables on the left and later variables on the right.

Questions 6–14 refer to the following path model, where the numbers represent the path coefficients.

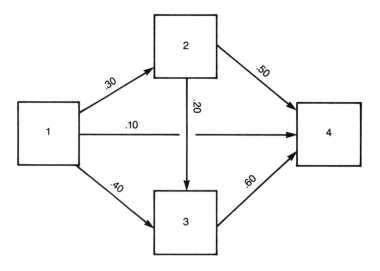

6. How may one describe this path model?

7. We observe that $p_{12} = 0.30$. What would be the correlation between variables 1 and 2?

8. What is the indirect causal influence of 1 on 3?

9. What is the indirect causal influence of 1 on 2?

10. What is the indirect causal influence of 2 on 3?

11. What is the indirect causal influence of 2 on 4?

12. What is the total causal influence of 4 on the other variables?

13. What is the correlation of 1 with 3?

14. What is the correlation of 2 with 3?

CHAPTER 15

Canonical Correlation and Discriminant Function Analysis

Barbara Hazard Munro

OBJECTIVES FOR CHAPTER 15

After reading this chapter and completing the exercises, you should be able to

1. Determine what types of questions may be answered using canonical correlation and discriminant function analysis.
2. Define the following terminology: canonical variate, canonical weights, structure coefficients, centroids, discriminant functions.
3. Describe significance testing, including the use of Wilks' lambda as a measure of variance accounted for.
4. Interpret the results section of research studies that report these techniques.

CANONICAL CORRELATION

When calculating a multiple correlation, you have more than one independent variable but only one dependent variable. Suppose, however, that you have more than one dependent variable. For example, in a study of post-myocardial infarction (MI) patients, we might wish to predict outcomes based on the patient's age, score on the Jenkins' Activity Survey, and type of MI. The outcomes (dependent variables) that we want to investigate are time to return to work and psychological adaptation. We could, of course, run two separate multiple regressions, with time to return to work as the dependent variable in one and psychological adaptation as the dependent variable in the other. That would not allow us to explore all the variation in the data, however. A method that takes all the information into account, thus giving a better understanding of all the relationships, is *canonical correlation*. This technique measures the relationship between a *set* of independent variables and a *set* of dependent variables. The method of least squares is used to give two composites, one for the independent variables, sometimes called the variables "on the left," and one for the dependent variables, or "variables on the right." Many authors reserve the term *multivariate analysis* for situations in which there is more than one dependent variable.

Although the variables are weighted through the procedure of canonical correlation, the main emphasis of this technique is on assessing relationships, rather than on prediction. More than one canonical correlation coefficient can be generated from a single analysis, because each coefficient represents the relationship between one factor in one of the groups of variables and a related factor in the other group. In that way, canonical correlation is like factor analysis. As we know, there may be several factors in a group of variables. If there are three factors in one set of variables and three related factors in the second group of variables, three canonical correlation coefficients might emerge, one for each pair of factors. There cannot be more canonical correlation coefficients (Rcs) than there are variables in the smaller set. For example, if you had four independent variables ($X1, X2, X3, X4$) and three dependent variables ($Y1, Y2, Y3$), the most Rcs that could be calculated would be three. The variance accounted for by each Rc is unique. The first canonical correlation accounts for the largest amount of variance, the second accounts for the second largest amount, and so on. The procedure ends when there are no significant Rcs left.

A *canonical variate* is a weighted composite of the variables in a set. It is a "new" variable or construct derived from the original variables. *Canonical weights*, which are in standard score form, are generated for each variable. Although like standardized regression coefficients (Betas), they are used more for explanation than for prediction. Because they are in standard score form, they indicate the relative importance of the variable with which they are associated. They must be interpreted with caution, however. Canonical weights, like the Betas in regression equations, may be quite unstable in that they may vary a great deal from one analysis to another. Because of that, many researchers prefer to interpret loadings called *structure coefficients*. Those loadings represent the correlation between the canonical variates and the real (or original) variables. If there is a high correlation between the new variable (canonical variate) and the original variables, the canonical variate is representing what the original variables were measuring. Loadings or structure coefficients of .30 or higher are treated as meaningful (Pedhazur, 1982, p. 732). They are interpreted like the loadings in factor analysis. The higher loadings give meaning to the canonical correlation and are used to name it. The square of a loading is the proportion of variance accounted for, so you can say how much of the variance is accounted for by an Rc.

Computation is done by computers. Once you go beyond two variables in each set, the calculations are overwhelming, even with a calculator. Because it is necessary to use a computer to calculate this statistic, there are not many examples in the nursing literature. Because the technique has great potential for use in research done by health professionals, we expect to see more reports of the use of canonical correlation in the future.

To test the significance of a canonical correlation, Bartlett's test of Wilks' lambda (Λ) is used. Lambda varies from 0 to 1 and stands for the error variance, that variance *not* accounted for by the independent variables. Thus, it is interpreted in an opposite way to the squared multiple correlation, R^2. A 1.0 means that the independent variables are *not* accounting for any of the variance in the dependent variable, and a 0 means that the independent variables are accounting for *all* of the variance. The *smaller* the lambda, the *greater* the variance accounted for. $1 - \Lambda$ would be equivalent to R^2. A chi-square statistic (called *Bartlett's test*) is used to test the significance of lambda.

The redundancy of the variables is often mentioned when canonical correlation results are presented. The higher the redundancy, or correlation among a group of variables, the better the ability to predict from one group to another.

Example of a Computer Printout

Figure 15-1 contains the printout generated by the SPSS CANCORR program. A much more sophisticated output can be produced by the SPSS MANOVA program or by SAS CANCORR. We use this one for demonstration because it is straightforward.

Data were collected from nurses and nurses' aides (working in home care agencies) about their demographic characteristics and their feelings about death. In the analysis presented here, three measures of feelings about death were correlated with seven demographic characteristics. The three measures included the desire to avoid dying people (AVOID), being fearful of death (SCARE), and being uncertain about what to say or do with dying people (UNCER). The seven demographic variables included level of education (EDUC); years of working experience in nursing (YEARS); whether or not they had been present when someone died (PRESENT); AGE; RACE (Caucasian or Black); birth order, that is, whether they were first-born, second-born, and so on (SIBPOS); and how religious they were (RELIGIOS).

Because there were three variables in the smaller set, three canonical correlations can be calculated (①). We see that the first $Rc = .63932$. Wilks' lambda $= .54734$ so this canonical correlation accounts for about 45% of the variance $(1 - .54734)$. The chi-square test of lambda is significant at the .002 level. Neither of the other RCs is significant. They account for only 7% and 2% of the variance, respectively.

This particular program generates only the standardized coefficients, which is unfortunate because the structure coefficients are more interpretable. We would advise using one of the more sophisticated programs in an actual analysis.

The coefficients are only produced for the significant Rc (②). Using the criterion that coefficients should be .30 or higher to be meaningful, we see that this Rc represents a cluster of variables. Those high on this factor have lower education (negative correlation), are older, tend to avoid dying people, and are afraid of death. Those low on this factor have the opposite characteristics.

Figure 15-1 SPSS CANCORR output.

Procedure Cards

```
1       16

CANCORR    VARIABLES = AVOID, SCARE, UNCER, EDUC, YEARS, PRESENT, AGE, RACE, SIBPOS,
           RELIGIOS/RELATE = AVOID TO UNCER WITH EDUC TO RELIGIOS/

OPTIONS    2
```

Output

---------------C A N O N I C A L   C O R R E L A T I O N---------------- RELATE LIST 1

NUMBER	EIGENVALUE	CANONICAL CORRELATION	WILKS LAMBDA	CHI-SQUARE	D.F.	SIGNIFICANCE
1	0.40872	0.63932	0.54734	44.29784	21	0.002
2	0.05812	0.24108	0.92569	5.67561	12	0.932
3	0.01719	0.13112	0.98281	1.27460	5	0.938

COEFFICIENTS FOR CANONICAL VARIABLES OF THE SECOND SET

                   CANVAR 1

```
EDUC       -0.72354
YEARS       0.15212
PRESENT    -0.16034
AGE         0.56064
RACE       -0.13832
SIBPOS      0.18263
RELIGIOS   -0.12117
```

COEFFICIENTS FOR CANONICAL VARIABLES OF THE FIRST SET

                   CANVAR 1

```
AVOID       0.52376
SCARE       0.61083
UNCER      -0.13436
```

323

EXAMPLES FROM PUBLISHED RESEARCH

Example 1

Research Question
Marriner and Craigie (1977) sought to determine nursing educators' perceptions of the general importance of given job characteristics to job satisfaction.

Data Gathered
A three-part questionnaire was sent to nurse educators in 13 western states. The three parts included demographics, rating of the importance of job factors to job satisfaction and own satisfaction, and open-ended questions. The sample included 822 respondents, of whom 477 gave complete data.

Tabular Presentation and Description of Results
Canonical correlation was used to examine the following three relationships: demographic variables with importance variables, demographic variables with satisfaction variables, and importance variables with satisfaction variables. Only the results of the first canonical correlation analysis (demographics with importance) will be presented here. Because this is one of the few examples of canonical correlation in the nursing literature, and because it is very well presented, you are encouraged to study the original article. The results are shown in Table 15-1. Note that the authors use the structure coefficients (or loadings) for interpretation.

Five significant canonical correlations were derived. The first ($Rc = .7226$) demonstrates a relationship between the demographic factor of seniority and the importance factor that ties together issues of importance to senior faculty such as retirement benefits, sabbatical leave policies, and so on. In the second Rc, the relationship was between young, well-educated male faculty (demographic variate) and the "ambition" factor, that is, those elements of importance that relate to opportunities for getting ahead, such as facilities and financial support for research. The third Rc demonstrates a relationship between those who support their families and interest in health insurance and vice versa.

The fourth Rc was significant, but it accounted for only a small amount of variance. The demographic factor was difficult to interpret, but the authors report that "it seems to indicate persons who have had many job opportunities from which to choose, are employed full-time, but have delivered few speeches. This group felt that consulting policies, professional travel, promotion policies, and administrative leadership style are important" (p. 357). A low factor score would imply the opposite characteristics.

The fifth Rc indicated a relationship between working full time in a large department and having written few articles with a feeling that tuition waivers and student advising load are important.

Table 15-1 Canonical Correlations between the Importance and Demographic Domains

	Factors			
Pairs of Factors	*Demographic*		*Importance*	
First	Salary	.82[b]	Retirement benefits	−.69[b]
$R_c = .7226$[a]	Age	.74	Sabbatical policies	−.51
$p = .0005$	Tenure	.68	Health insurance	−.45
	Years of employment	.67	Institutional governance	−.44
	Academic rank	.65	Office space	−.38
	Publications	.60	Financial support–	
	Educational preparation	.49	research	−.36
	Support of family	−.40	Secretarial services	−.35
	Full or part time	−.38	Tuition waiver	.34
	Books published	.35	Student assistants	−.32
	Speeches	.32	Quality of students	−.32
	Number of academic		Student advising load	−.32
	appointments	.31	Faculty club	−.32
			Departmental	
			governance	−.31
			Facilities for research	−.31
Second	Years of employment	.42	Facilities for research	.47
$R_c = .6145$	Support of family	.41	Financial support–	
$p = .0005$	Age	.40	research	.47
	Sex	−.34	Summer school	
	Educational preparation	−.32	teaching	.45
			Promotion policies	.36
			Student assistants	.31
			Tuition waiver	.30
			Reappointment policies	.30
Third	Support of family	−.70	Health insurance	−.59
$R_c = .5142$	Publications	−.38	Facilities for research	.35
$p = .0005$	Books published	−.38	Financial support–	
	Research under way	−.37	research	.35
	Speeches	−.32		
	Educational preparation	−.30		
Fourth	Job opportunities	−.40	Consulting policies	.48
$R_c = .5013$	Speeches	.33	Professional travel	
$p = .0005$	Full or part time	.32	policies	.37
			Administrative leadership	
			style	.34
			Promotion policies	.33
Fifth	Head count	−.51	Tuition waiver	.50
$R_c = .4933$	Publications	.33	Student advising load	.34
$p = .01$	Full or part time	.32		

[a] R_c = the canonical correlation coefficient or the maximal correlation that can be developed between two linear functions of variables

[b] This is the correlation of the factor with the individual variables listed (only correlations above .30 are reported)

From Marriner, A., & Craigie, D. (1977). Job satisfaction and mobility of nursing educators. *Nursing Research, 26* (5), 349–360.

Conclusions

"Several canonical correlations in the study indicated that nursing educators tended to be dissatisfied with what they felt was important and satisfied with what they did not feel was important. . . . The domains in the study were related to each other, but much of each domain was not predicted because of the relatively small amount of variance extracted by the correlated factors" (Marriner & Craigie, 1977, p. 360).

Example 2

Another example of a study using canonical correlation is one done by Speegle, Bayer, and Greene (1979). Their study was designed to quantify patients' expressions of discomfort about 1½ years after an acute coronary event and to examine associations between those scores and other variables. Eighty-three subjects were included in the study. Canonical correlation was used to measure the relationship between physical symptoms and measures of mood. The Rc was .67 ($p < .001$). "The significant associations suggest that expressions of discomfort as measured in these subjects 17 months after an acute coronary event might be predicted on the basis of some demographic, clinical, and emotional characteristics. Most impressive is the association between variables recognizable at the time of the acute event and discomfort scores generated 17 months later" (p. 137).

DISCRIMINANT FUNCTION ANALYSIS

In multiple regression, the dependent variable is continuous, but there may be occasions when we want to use a categorical variable as the dependent variable. If the categorical variable is dichotomous, we can simply code it as 1 or 0 and use multiple regression. If the dependent variable has more than two categories, however, we are no longer able to use multiple regression. *Discriminant function analysis* is a technique that allows us to distinguish among groups, based on some predictor variables. The mathematical function that combines information from predictor variables so as to obtain the maximum discrimination among groups is called the *discriminant function*. With two groups, the results are the same as using multiple regression with a dummy-coded dependent variable.

The question that we are trying to answer with this technique is: Which set of predictors will most clearly distinguish among these groups? Tripp and Duffey (1981) used this technique to predict graduation and two categories of nongraduation (dropouts and non-admitted applicants) in a master's degree program in nursing. We might want to know which information would most clearly differentiate college graduates, dropouts, and transfers or which factors differentiate the following groups of patients: cardiac, cancer, and arthritis.

We are interested in both explanation and prediction. We want to know which factors are most related to these groups and, also, how well we could predict group membership. This is a powerful statistical tool that was first used to aid in personnel selection and placement. The researchers looked for variables that would differentiate among those successful or not in various jobs; then, that information was used in the selection and placement of new personnel. It has also been used for predicting voting patterns of politicians.

The aim of the procedure is to find a way to maximize the discrimination among groups. As with canonical correlation, more than one statistic may be derived. The most discriminant functions that can be derived are one less than the number of categories in the dependent variable or the number of independent variables, whichever is smaller. The first discriminant function derived from the data is the one that explains most of the between group variance. The second discriminant function explains the next largest piece of variance, and so on. These functions are uncorrelated with each other. All the variables may be entered at once, or a stepwise procedure may be used to select the "most discriminating" variables. Eigenvalues and their associated canonical correlations are used to judge which are the "most discriminating" variables.

As with multiple regression, each variable is weighted, and those weights may be used to calculate a discriminant score for each subject. The mean of the discriminant scores for a given group, say the cancer group (when trying to discover factors that differentiate between cardiac, cancer, and arthritis patients), is called the *centroid*.

The discriminant functions are calculated by a method similar to factor analysis. Principal components analysis is done on a matrix of indices of discrimination between and within groups. This type of analysis discriminates among subjects, rather than among variables. Rotation may be used to increase the interpretability of the functions.

Wilks' lambda (Λ) is used to measure the association between the independent and dependent variables. Using the discriminant function scores, the members of the "known" groups are classified to see how well the system works. We want to know what percent are classified correctly and what percent are classified incorrectly.

The analysis produces *raw coefficients* (like bs in multiple regression), *standardized coefficients* (like betas), and *structure coefficients* (like those in canonical correlation). The raw coefficients are commonly used for calculating scores for each individual. The standardized coefficients represent the relative importance of the independent variables with which they are associated. Like betas, they should be interpreted with caution, however, because they tend to be unstable.

The correlations between the discriminant score for each individual and the scores on the original variables are called *structure coefficients*, or *loadings*. The square of that coefficient is the proportion of variance in a particular variable explained by the discriminant functions. Structure coefficients of 0.30 or greater are considered "meaningful" (Pedhazur, 1982, p. 704). These coefficients are used for "interpretation" of the discriminant functions.

Example of a Computer Printout

The example in Figure 15-2 was generated by the SPSS DISCRIMINANT program. Only selected parts of the output are included here. Using data gathered in a study of admission procedures at Yale School of Nursing and discriminant analysis, we seek to determine whether we could discriminate among those who chose the five specialty programs at Yale. The five nursing specialty programs (GROUPs 1–5) are Community Health, Midwifery, Medical-Surgical, Pediatric, and Psychiatric. The predictor variables are those measures gathered by the Admissions Committee, and they include sex, race, marital status (MS), years of experience in nursing or related field (EXPER), GRE-Verbal, GRE-Math, undergraduate GPA (BACH), admission's essay (AUTO), scores of references (REFTOT), and interview score (TOT).

Because there are five groups, four discriminant functions are possible. On the left side of the table with Canonical Discriminant Functions, we see the four functions with their associated eigenvalues and canonical correlations (①). These statistics "denote the relative ability of each function to separate the groups" (Nie, Hull, Jenkins, Steinbrenner & Bent, 1975, p. 440). We see that the first function accounts for 54% of the variance. The right side of the table (②) "shows the changes in Wilks' lambda (and their associated chi-square tests of statistical significance) as the information in successive discriminant functions is removed" (Nie et al., 1975, p. 440). Before any functions were removed, lambda was .4896974, which means that there is a considerable amount of discriminating power in the variables being used. When function one is created, lambda is .7063009, and the chi-square test indicates that there is no statistically significant amount of discriminating power left ($p = .3107$). Thus, function 1 is the only one contributing significantly to the variance accounted for.

Examining the coefficients (③), we see that race, marital status, experience, GRE-Math, essay, and interview are responsible for most of the variance accounted for by function 1. Sex, race, undergraduate GPA, and essay are the discriminating variables on function 2. Experience, GRE-Verbal, GRE-Math, essay, and interview are the important predictors for function 3. Sex, GRE-Math, and references are the most important for function 4.

Examining the centroids (④) shows us that the maximal discrimination of function 1 is between Group 2, the midwives (.975) and Group 5, the psychiatric nurses (−.866). Other functions are interpreted similarly. On function 4, the Community Health and Pediatric groups are most widely separated, with the other three groups clustering close to the middle of the range.

In the classification results (⑤), we see that prediction of the Community Health group was the poorest, only 17.6 percent of Group 1 were predicted to be members of Group 1. This may be due to the fact that Group 1 contains FNPs and Community Health Clinical Specialists and those groups are quite different. The best prediction was for the Psychiatric Group (#5), 60 percent of the group membership was accurately predicted. Overall, the correct classification equalled 50.53 percent, not bad for five groups.

Examples from Published Research

Smith and Shamansky (1983) investigated the relationship between consumer values and intentions to use Family Nurse Practitioner (FNP) services.

Research Questions

1. To what extent could consumers be categorized as potential users or non-users of FNP services?
2. What was the demographic profile of potential users of FNP services?
3. What was the buying behavior of potential users of FNP services?
4. What was the level of demand for FNP services? (p. 301)

Data Gathered

A telephone survey was used to collect data from a stratified random sample of Seattle residents. A 42-item instrument containing two subscales was used. On the first subscale, respondents were asked to rate various aspects of the FNP role on a four-point scale, from very important to not important. The second subscale measured respondents' reactions to innovations. The sample contained 239 respondents.

Tabular Presentation of Results

Tables 15-2 and 15-3 are from this study. Discriminant analysis was used to differentiate between subjects who would use FNP services and those who would not. Results of discriminant analysis of the FNP subscale indicated that seven of the variables correctly classified users vs. non-users of FNP services in 85% of the cases ($p = .00001$). This group of predictors was more accurate in predicting potential user status (85%) than of non-user status (55%). Wilks' lambda was .6884. Prior knowledge of the FNP role was the strongest predictor. Table 15-2 presents the order, in terms of predictive strength, of the seven variables.

Discriminant analysis was also performed on the innovation subscale. With eight optimum predictors, potential users were correctly classified 98.5% of the time, and potential non-users, 82.8% of the time. Table 15-3 lists the eight predictors.

Conclusions

"From interpretation of this study's data, a profile emerges of a potential group of users of FNP services: younger women, professionally employed or specializing in homemaking, middle or upper income, single or with small families" (p. 305).

SUMMARY

It is hoped that this overview of these two techniques will enable you to understand research reports that contain these techniques. We would hope that you would

(*Text continues on page 333*)

Figure 15-2 SPSS DISCRIMINANT output.

Procedure Cards

```
1          16
DISCRIMINANT  GROUPS = PREP(1,5)/
              VARIABLES = SEX,RACE,MS,PROG,EXPER,GREV,GREM,BACH,AUTO,REFTOT,TOT/
              ANALYSIS = SEX TO TOT/

OPTIONS    5,11
```

Output

CANONICAL DISCRIMINANT FUNCTIONS

②

FUNCTION	EIGENVALUE	PERCENT OF VARIANCE	CUMULATIVE PERCENT	CANONICAL CORRELATION	AFTER FUNCTION	WILKS' LAMBDA	CHI-SQUARED	D.F.	SIGNIFICANCE
①					0	0.4896974	61.758	40	0.0152
1*	0.44232	54.12	54.12	0.5537807	1	0.7063009	30.077	27	0.3107
2*	0.17681	21.63	75.76	0.3876166	2	0.8311833	15.994	16	0.4534
3*	0.16875	20.65	96.40	0.3799827	3	0.9714476	2.5057	7	0.9267
4*	0.02939	3.60	100.00	0.1689746					

*MARKS THE 4 CANONICAL DISCRIMINANT FUNCTION(S) TO BE USED IN THE REMAINING ANALYSIS.

STANDARDIZED CANONICAL DISCRIMINANT FUNCTION COEFFICIENTS

	FUNC 1	FUNC 2	FUNC 3	FUNC 4
③ SEX	0.11357	-0.51796	-0.27073	0.56383
RACE	-0.49523	0.41343	-0.17338	-0.14622
MS	0.44272	0.12553	-0.18964	-0.37427
EXPER	-0.67978	0.26169	0.53326	0.17706
GREV	0.11876	0.19794	-0.58150	0.31738
GREM	0.52314	0.28208	0.81741	0.56576
BACH	-0.11350	-0.72093	-0.04909	-0.02912
AUTO	0.62911	0.44701	-0.44724	0.10241
REFTOT	-0.03967	-0.11410	0.24333	-0.49438
TOT	0.45716	-0.21051	0.64027	-0.05028

CANONICAL DISCRIMINANT FUNCTIONS EVALUATED AT GROUP MEANS (GROUP CENTROIDS)

GROUP	FUNC 1	FUNC 2	FUNC 3	FUNC 4
④ 1	0.11712	-0.25409	-0.26399	0.32245
2	0.97544	0.63018	-0.28916	-0.06858
3	0.23046	-0.05090	0.73511	0.00624
4	0.37609	-0.80433	-0.30373	-0.22410
5	-0.86585	0.18626	-0.09892	-0.05516

CLASSIFICATION RESULTS –

		PREDICTED GROUP MEMBERSHIP				
ACTUAL GROUP	NO. OF CASES	1	2	3	4	5
GROUP 1	17	3	4	1	5	4
		17.6%	23.5%	5.9%	29.4%	23.5%
⑤ GROUP 2	15	4	8	1	1	1
		26.7%	53.3%	6.7%	6.7%	6.7%
GROUP 3	21	3	2	12	3	1
		14.3%	9.5%	57.1%	14.3%	4.8%
GROUP 4	12	2	1	1	7	1
		16.7%	8.3%	8.3%	58.3%	8.3%
GROUP 5	30	2	3	3	4	18
		6.7%	10.0%	10.0%	13.3%	60.0%

PERCENT OF "GROUPED" CASES CORRECTLY CLASSIFIED: 50.53%

Table 15-2   Seven Optimum Predictor Variables of the FNP Subset

Variable Statements	Wilk's Lambda	Significance
1. Do you know what a FNP is?	.8748	.0006
2. How important is it to know that the FNP can provide care for your whole family?	.8085	.0001
3. Have you ever received care from an FNP?	.7537	.0000
4. How important is it to know that the FNP may make a house call if you couldn't come to the office?	.7376	.0000
5. How important would it be to know about the difference between an FNP and other registered nurses?	.7169	.0000
6. How important is it to know that the FNP will take a history and do a physical exam?	.7030	.0000
7. How important is the amount of time you need to wait to see the FNP?	.6884	.0000

From Smith, D. W., Shamansky, S. L. (1983). Determining the market for family nurse practitioner services: the Seattle experience. *Nursing Research,* 32(5), 301–305.

Table 15-3   Eight Optimum Predictor Variables of the Innovation Subscale

Variable Statements	Wilk's Lambda	Significance
1. My family might favor my going to an FNP for health care.	.5653	.0000
2. If FNP and MD care costs are equal, then FNP care is worth the money it costs.	.3947	.0000
3. If I went to an FNP for health care, I would tell my friends about it.	.3488	.0000
4. FNP care is a service intended for a person like me.	.3262	.0000
5. I understand what services an FNP could provide for me.	.3132	.0000
6. I understand the difference between FNP and MD care.	.2992	.0000
7. I would gain a great deal if I did what the FNP told me and the treatment worked.	.2855	.0000
8. I might need to change the way I take care of myself if I went to an FNP.	.2813	.0000

From Smith, D. W., Shamansky, S. L. (1983). Determining the market for family nurse practitioner services: the Seattle experience. *Nursing Research,* 32(5), 301–305.

consider the use of these techniques when appropriate, because they are powerful statistical measures that could be very useful in studying problems related to the delivery of health-related care.

EXERCISES FOR CHAPTER 15

In items 1 to 3, select the appropriate technique from the list below:
   A. Multiple regression
   B. Canonical correlation
   C. Discriminant function analysis

1. _____You wish to measure the relationship between the predictor variables of level of stress, social supports, and job satisfaction, and the outcome variables: absentee rate and job performance.

2. _____You want to find out which variables are related to developing one of the following diseases: cancer, heart disease, arthritis.

3. _____You want to predict longevity given the stage of illness, age, and level of hope.

4. Match the term with the definition.

_____A. canonical variate	a. correlation between canonical variate and original variables.
_____B. canonical weight	b. indicates relative importance of variables.
_____C. structure coefficient	c. mathematical technique allowing maximal distancing of groups based on predictor variables.
_____D. centroid	d. weighted composite of variables in a set.
_____E. discriminant function	e. mean of discriminant scores for a group.

5. In canonical correlation, which of the following is usually interpreted?
   A. canonical weights
   B. structure coefficients

6. If lambda equals .48, how much variance has been accounted for?

Bibliography

Armstrong, G. D. (1981). Parametric statistics and ordinal data: A pervasive misconception. *Nursing Research, 30* (1), 60–62.

Asher, A. B. (1976). *Causal modeling.* Sage University Papers: Quantitative Applications in the Social Sciences Series. Beverly Hills: Sage Publications.

Atkins, A. C., & Munro, B. H. (1984). Attitudes of visiting nurses and home health aides toward death and dying. Unpublished manuscript.

Ballard, S., & McNamara, R. (1983). Quantifying nursing needs in home health care. *Nursing Research, 32* (4), 236–241.

Barsevick, A., & Llewellyn, J. (1982). A comparison of the anxiety-reducing potential of two techniques of bathing. *Nursing Research, 31* (1), 22–27.

Blalock, H. M., Jr. (Ed.) (1971). *Causal models in the social sciences.* Chicago: Aldine.

Blashfield, R. K. (1980). Proposition regarding use of cluster analysis in clinical research. *Journal of Consulting and Clinical Psychology, 48,* 456–459.

Bock, R. D. (1967). Multivariate analysis of variance of repeated measures. In C. W. Harris (Ed.). *Problems in measuring change* (pp 85–103). Madison, Wisconsin: The University of Wisconsin Press.

Bohachick, P. (1984). Progressive relaxation training in cardiac rehabilitation: Effect on psychologic variables. *Nursing Research, 33* (5), 283–287.

Campbell, D. T., & Stanley, J. C. (1963). *Experimental and quasi-experimental designs for research.* Chicago: Rand McNally.

Coffman, R. A. (1979). *Coping with stress: The graduate school experience.* Unpublished Master's Thesis, Yale University School of Nursing, New Haven, CT.

Cohen, J. (1977). *Statistical power analysis for the behavioral sciences.* (Rev. ed.) New York: Academic Press.

Cook, T. D., & Campbell, D. T. (1979). *Quasi-experimentation: Design and analysis issues for field settings.* Chicago: Rand McNally.

Dickoff, J., & James, P. (1968). A theory of theories: A position paper. *Nursing Research, 17,* 197–203.

Dickoff, J., James, P., & Wiedenbach, E. (1968). Theory in a practice discipline: Practice oriented theory. *Nursing Research, 17,* 415–435.

Diers, D. (1979). *Research in Nursing Practice.* Philadelphia: J. B. Lippincott.

Dixon, J. (1984). Effect of nursing interventions on nutritional and performance status in cancer patients. *Nursing Research, 33*(6), 330–335.

Dixon, J. K., & Koerner, B. (1976). Faculty and student perceptions of effective classroom teaching in nursing. *Nursing Research, 25,* 300–305.

Dixon, W. J. (Ed.) (1983). *BMDP Biomedical Computer Program.* Berkeley: University of California Press.

Duncan, O. D. (1975). *Introduction to structural equation models.* New York: Academic Press.

Fawcett, J. (1978). The "what" of theory development. In *Theory development: What, why, how?* New York: National League for Nursing (Pub. No. 15-1708).

Finn, J. D., & Mattsson, I. (1978). *Multivariate analysis in educational research—Applications of the multivariance program.* Chicago: National Educational Resources.

Fisher, R. A. (1935). *The design of experiments.* London: Oliver & Boyd.

Fisher, R. A. (1970). Statistical methods for research workers (14th ed.). Darien, CT: Hafner Publishing Co.

Greenhouse, S. W., & Geisser, S. (1959). On methods in the analysis of profile data. *Psychometrika, 24,* 95–112.

Hald, A. (1952). *Statistical tables and formulas.* New York: John Wiley & Sons.

Hays, W. (1973). *Statistics for the social sciences.* New York: Holt, Rinehart & Winston.

Heidt, P. (1981). Effect of therapeutic touch on anxiety level of hospitalized patients. *Nursing Research, 30*(1), 32–37.

Heise, D. R. (1975). *Causal analysis.* New York: Wiley-Interscience.

Helwig, J. T., & Council, K. A. (Eds.) (1979). *SAS user's guide.* Cary, North Carolina: SAS Institute, Inc.

Hinkle, D. E., Wiersma, W., & Jurs, S. G. (1982). *Basic behavioral statistics.* Boston: Houghton Mifflin.

Jöreskog, K. G. (1973). A general method for estimating a linear structural equation system. In A. S. Goldberger & O. D. Duncan (Eds.). *Latent models in the social sciences.* New York: Seminar.

Jöreskog, K. G., & Sörbom, D. (1979). *Advances in factor analysis and structural equation models.* Cambridge, Mass.: Clark Abt. Associates.

Kenny, D. (1979). *Correlation and causality.* New York: Wiley.

Keppel, G. (1973). *Design and analysis—A researcher's handbook.* Englewood Cliffs, N.J.: Prentice-Hall.

Kerlinger, F. N. (1973). *Foundations of behavioral research* (2nd ed.). New York: Holt, Rinehart & Winston.

Kerlinger, F. N., & Pedhazur, E. S. (1973). *Multiple regression in behavioral research.* New York: Holt, Rinehart & Winston.

Lamontagne, L. L. (1984). Children's locus of control beliefs as predictors of preoperative coping behavior. *Nursing Research, 33*(2), 76–79, 85.

Land, K. C. (1969). Principles of path analysis. In E. F. Borgatta (Ed.). *Sociological methodology: 1969.* San Francisco: Jossey-Bass.

Li, C. C. (1975). *Path Analysis: A primer.* Pacific Grove, Calif.: Boxwood.

Mahon, N. E. (1982). The relationship of self-disclosure, interpersonal dependency, and life changes to loneliness in young adults. *Nursing Research, 31*(6), 343–347.

Marriner, A., & Craigie, D. (1977). Job satisfaction and mobility of nursing educators. *Nursing Research, 26*(5), 349–360.

Matthews, K. A., Glass, D. C., Rosenman, R. H., & Bortner, R. W. (1977). Competitive drive, pattern A and coronary heart disease: A further analysis of some data from the western collaborative group study. *Journal of Chronic Diseases, 30,* 489–498.

Moses, E. B., Spencer, W. E., & Roman, R. (1982). *The registered nurse population—an overview.* (DHHS Publication No. HRS-P-OD-83-1). Washington, D.C.: U.S. Dept. of Health & Human Services.

Munro, B. H. (1983). Job satisfaction among recent graduates of schools of nursing. *Nursing Research, 32*(6), 350–355.

Munro, B. H. (1985). Predicting success in graduate clinical specialty programs. (Brief). *Nursing Research, 34*(1), 54–57.

Munro, B. H., & Krauss, J. B. (1985). The success of non-RNs in graduate nursing programs. *Journal of Nursing Education, 24*(5), 192–196.

Munro, B. H., & Sexton, D. L. (1984). Path analysis: A method for theory testing. *Western Journal of Nursing Research, 6*(1), 97–106.

Nie, N. H., Hull, C. H., Jenkins, J. G., Steinbrenner, K., & Bent, D. H. (1975). *Statistical package for the social sciences* (2nd ed.). New York: McGraw-Hill Book Co.

Norbeck, J. S., Lindsey, A. M., & Carrieri, V. L. (1983). Further development of the Norbeck social support questionnaire: Normative data and validity testing. *Nursing Research, 32*(1), 4–9.

Numan, I. M., Barklind, K. S., & Lubin, B. (1981). Correlates of depression in chronic dialysis patients: Morbidity and mortality. *Research in Nursing and Health, 4*(3), 295–297.

Nunnally, J. C. (1978). *Psychometric theory* (2nd ed.). New York: McGraw-Hill.

Pearson, E. S., & Hartley, H. O. (Eds.) (1966). *Biometrika tables for statisticians.* Vol. I (3rd ed.). Cambridge: University Press.

Pedhazur, E. J. (1982). *Multiple regression in behavioral research, explanation and prediction* (2nd ed.). New York: Holt, Rinehart & Winston.

Polit, D. F., & Hungler, B. P. (1983). Nursing research—principles and methods (2nd ed.). Philadelphia: J. B. Lippincott.

Popham, W. J., & Sirotnik, K. A. (1973). *Educational statistics: use and interpretation* (2nd ed.) New York: Harper & Row.

Rice, V. H., & Johnson, J. E. (1984). Preadmission self-instruction booklets, post admission exercise performance, and teaching time. *Nursing Research, 33*(3), 147–151.

Rosenberg, M. (1972). *Society and the adolescent self-image.* Princeton: Princeton University Press.

Rummel, R. J. (1970). *Applied factor analysis.* Evanston: Northwestern University Press.

Schmale, A. H. Jr., & Iker, H. P. (1964). The effect of hopelessness in the development of cancer. *Psychosomatic Medicine, 26,* 634–639.

Sexton, D. L., & Munro, B. H. (1985). Impact of a husband's chronic illness (COPD) on the spouse's life. *Research in Nursing & Health, 8*(1), 83–90.

Siegel, S. (1956). *Nonparametric statistics for the behavioral sciences.* New York: McGraw-Hill.

Smith, D. W., & Shamansky, S. L. (1983). Determining the market for family nurse practitioner services: The Seattle experience. *Nursing Research, 32*(5), 301–305.

Snedecor, G. W. (1938). *Statistical methods.* Ames, Iowa: Collegiate Press.

Speegle, E. K., Bayer, L. R., Greene, W. A. (1979). Convalescent discomfort following acute coronary events. *Nursing Research, 28*(3), 132–138.

Spence, J. T., Cotton, J. W., Underwood, B. H., & Duncan, C. P. (1976). *Elementary statistics.* New Jersey: Prentice-Hall, Inc.

Stevens, S. S. (1951). Mathematics, measurements, and psychophysics. In S. S. Stevens (Ed.). *Handbook of experimental psychology.* New York: John Wiley & Sons, pp. 1–49.

Stitt, F. W., Frane, M., & Frane, J. W. (1977). Mood change in rheumatoid arthritis: Factor analysis as a tool in clinical research. *Journal of Chronic Diseases, 30,* 135–145.

Thurstone, L. L. (1947). *Multiple-factor analysis.* Chicago: University of Chicago Press.

Tripp, A., & Duffy, M. (1981). Discriminant analysis to predict graduation–nongraduation in a master's degree program in nursing. *Research in Nursing & Health, 4*(4), 345–353.

Tryon, R. C., & Bailey, D. E. (1970). *Cluster analysis.* New York: McGraw-Hill.

Visintainer, M. A., & Wolfer, J. A. (1975). Psychological preparation for surgical pediatric patients: The effect on children's and parents' stress responses and adjustment. *Pediatrics, 56,* 187–202.

Volicer, B. J. (1981). *Advanced statistical methods with nursing research applications.* Bedford, MA: MERESTAT.

Williams, R. A., & Nicholaisen, S. M. (1982). Sudden infant death syndrome: Parents' perceptions and responses to the loss of their infant. *Research in Nursing and Health, 5*(2), 55–61.

Winer, B. J. (1962). *Statistical principles in experimental design.* New York: McGraw-Hill.

Wolfer, J. A., & Visintainer, M. A. (1975). Pediatric surgical patients' and mothers' distress and coping behavior as a function of psychological preparation and stress-point nursing care. *Nursing Research, 24,* 244–255.

Wright, S. (1921). Correlation and causation. *Journal of Agricultural Research, 20,* 557–585.

Ziemer, M. M. (1983). Effects of information on postsurgical coping. *Nursing Research, 32*(5), 282–287.

APPENDIX A
Answers to Exercises

Chapter 1

1. Variable   **Level of Measurement**

Variable	Level of Measurement
Sex	Nominal
Weight	Ratio
Rank in class	Ordinal
Temperature—Farenheit	Interval
Marital status	Nominal
Height	Ratio

2. FREQUENCY DISTRIBUTION

Scores	f	Relative Frequency	Cumulative Percent
1–7	2	7	7
8–14	4	13	20
15–21	7	23	43
22–28	9	30	73
29–35	5	17	90
36–42	2	7	97
43–49	1	3	100
	30	100%	

3. Histogram, frequency polygon, and cumulative percentage polygon:

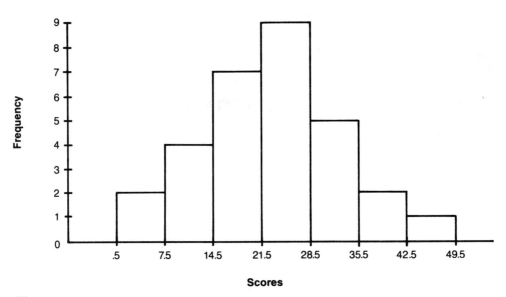

Histogram

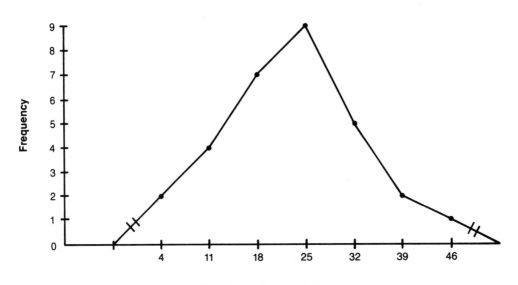

Frequency Polygon

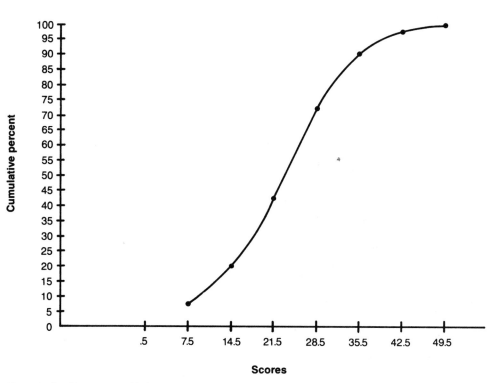

Cumulative Percentage Polygon

Chapter 2

Data Sets $X1$ and $X2$. First rearrange the sets from highest to lowest and calculate $\Sigma X1$ and $\Sigma X2$.

$X1$	$X2$
20	22
19	17
18	15
16	12
14	10
7	9
7	9
6	9
5	6
2	6
2	$\Sigma X2 = \overline{115}$
1	
$\Sigma X1 = \overline{117}$	

1. Mean for $X1 = \dfrac{117}{12} = 9.75$

Mean for $X2 = \dfrac{115}{10} = 11.5$

2. Median for $X1 = \dfrac{7+7}{2} = 7$

Median for $X2 = \dfrac{9+10}{2} = 9.5$

3. Mode for $X1 = 2$ and 7

Mode for $X2 = 9$

4. Range for $X1 = 20 - 1 = 19$

Range for $X2 = 22 - 6 = 16$

5. Interquartile range for $X1$:

$Q1 = \tfrac{12}{4} = $ 3rd score $= 2$
$Q3 = 12 \times \tfrac{3}{4} = $ 9th score $= 16$
$Q3 - Q1 = 16 - 2 = 14$

Interquartile range for $X2$:

$Q1 = \tfrac{10}{4} = $ 2.5th score $= \dfrac{9+6}{2} = 7.5$

$Q3 = 10 \times \tfrac{3}{4} = $ 7.5th score $= \dfrac{12+15}{2} = 13.5$

$Q3 - Q1 = 13.5 - 7.5 = 6$

6. Semi-interquartile range for $X1$:

$\dfrac{Q_3 - Q_1}{2} = \dfrac{16 - 2}{2} = \dfrac{14}{2} = 7$

Semi-interquartile range for $X2$:

$\dfrac{Q_3 - Q_1}{2} = \dfrac{13.5 - 7.5}{2} = \dfrac{6}{2} = 3$

For Variances and Standard deviations, you need to square the scores:

$X1$	$X1^2$	$X2$	$X2^2$
20	400	22	484
19	361	17	289
18	324	15	225
16	256	12	144
14	196	10	100
7	49	9	81
7	49	9	81
6	36	9	81
5	25	6	36
2	4	6	36
2	4	$\Sigma X2 = 115$	$\Sigma X2^2 = 1557$
1	1		
$\Sigma X1 = 117$	$\Sigma X1^2 = 1705$		

7. Variance for $X1$:   **Variance for $X2$:**

$$s^2 = \frac{1705 - \frac{(117)^2}{12}}{12 - 1}$$

$$s^2 = \frac{1705 - \frac{13689}{12}}{11}$$

$$s^2 = \frac{1705 - 1140.75}{11}$$

$$s^2 = \frac{564.25}{11}$$

$$s^2 = 51.295$$

$$s^2 = \frac{1557 - \frac{(115)^2}{10}}{10 - 1}$$

$$s^2 = \frac{1557 - \frac{13225}{10}}{9}$$

$$s^2 = \frac{1557 - 1322.25}{9}$$

$$s^2 = \frac{234.5}{9}$$

$$s^2 = 26.056$$

8. Standard deviation for $X1$:   **Standard deviation for $X2$:**

$$s = \sqrt{\frac{1705 - \frac{(117)^2}{12}}{12 - 1}}$$

$$s = \sqrt{51.295}$$

$$s = 7.162$$

$$s = \sqrt{\frac{1557 - \frac{(115)^2}{10}}{10 - 1}}$$

$$s = \sqrt{26.056}$$

$$s = 5.105$$

Chapter 3

1. a. $68\% = \pm 1z$
80 ± 20
68% fall between 60 and 100

b. $96\% = \pm 2z$
80 ± 40
96% fall between 40 and 120

2. left, lower   **3.** below   **4.** 0, 1

5. a. Standard scores and T-scores:

Raw Scores	Standard Scores $z = \frac{X = \overline{X}}{s}$	T-Scores $T = 10z + 50$
58	$z = \frac{58 - 70}{5} = -2.4$	$T = (10)(-2.4) + 50 = 26$
65	$z = \frac{65 - 70}{5} = -1.0$	$T = (10)(-1.0) + 50 = 40$
73	$z = \frac{73 - 70}{5} = 0.6$	$T = (10)(.6) + 50 = 56$
82	$z = \frac{80 - 70}{5} = 2.4$	$T = (10)(2.4) + 50 = 74$

b. Percentiles: Areas between mean and z-score (Appendix B)

Raw Score	z-Score	Tabled Values	Percentiles
58	-2.4	49.18	$50 - 49.18 = .82$
65	-1.0	34.13	$50 - 34.13 = 15.87$
73	.6	22.57	$50 + 22.57 = 72.57$
82	2.4	49.18	$50 + 49.18 = 99.18$

c. New Distribution:
Transformed z-scores $= (\text{new } s)(z) + (\text{new } \overline{X})$
$$= 25z + 100$$

z-Scores	Transformed Scores
-2.4	$25(-2.4) + 100 = 40$
-1.0	$25(-1.0) + 100 = 75$
.6	$25(.6) + 100 = 115$
2.4	$25(2.4) + 100 = 160$

6. $s_{\overline{x}} = \dfrac{s}{\sqrt{n}}$

a. $= \dfrac{6}{\sqrt{120}} = 0.55$

b. $95\% = \overline{X} \pm 1.96\, s_{\overline{x}}$
$$= 75 \pm (1.96)(0.55)$$
$$= 75 \pm 1.08$$
$$= 73.92 \text{ to } 76.08$$

c. $99\% = \overline{X} \pm 2.58\, s_{\overline{x}}$
$$= 75 \pm (2.58)(0.55)$$
$$= 75 \pm 1.42$$
$$= 73.58 \text{ to } 76.42$$

Chapter 4

1. reject

2. accept

3. a. reject
b. accept
c. reject
d. accept
[For a two-tailed test at the .05 level, the z-score must be at least 1.96 for it to be significant. If the result is significant, you *reject* the null hypothesis.)

4. a. accept
   b. reject
   c. reject
   d. reject
   [For a one-tailed test, the z-score must be $+2.33$ or higher at the .01 level. The directional hypothesis states that one group will be significantly higher, so, if the z-score is $+2.33$ or greater, you accept the directional hypothesis.]

5. one-tailed

6. one-tailed

7. a. Type II
   b. no error
   c. no error
   d. Type I

8. parametric

9. medium (.5)
   50

Chapter 5

	$p < .05$	$p < .01$
1. a.	accept	accept
b.	accept	accept
c.	reject	accept
d.	reject	reject
e.	reject	reject

[Should have used the two-tailed test. If significant, *reject* the null hypothesis.]

2. a.	accept	reject
b.	reject	reject
c.	accept	reject
d.	accept	accept
e.	reject	reject

[Should have used the one-tailed test. If positive and significant, *accept* the directional hypothesis. If negative, *reject* the hypothesis.]

3. Neither, they are both of equal strength.

4. Eta, also called the correlation ratio.

5. Multiple correlation

6. Partial correlation

7. Semi-partial correlation

8. $r = .81$ Yes, it is significant at $<.05$. It is also significant at $<.01$.

9. $z_r = .867$
standard error $= .07$
95%—$z_r s = .73$ and 1.004
            confidence interval is $.625$—$.765$
99%—$z_r s = 0.686$ and 1.048
            confidence interval is $.595$—$.780$

Chapter 6

1. Multiple regression   2. B

3. A $10 + (.8)(40) - (.4)(64) = 16.4$
   B $10 + (.8)(34) - (.4)(57) = 14.4$
   C $10 + (.8)(65) - (.4)(72) = 33.2$
   D $10 + (.8)(58) - (.4)(84) = 22.8$

4. B   5. b

6. $\Sigma X = 55$
   $\Sigma Y = 60$
   $\Sigma X^2 = 385$
   $\Sigma Y^2 = 464$
   $\Sigma XY = 403$
   $\overline{X} = 5.5$
   $\overline{Y} = 6$
   $\Sigma x^2 = 82.5$
   $\Sigma y^2 = 104$
   $\Sigma xy = 73$
   $Y' = 1.16 + 0.88X$
   standard error $= 2.22$

7. 95% $8 \pm (1.96)(2.2) = 3.688 - 12.312$
   99% $8 \pm (2.58)(2.2) = 2.324 - 13.676$

8. $p < .05$ $p < .01$

a.	ns	ns
b.	sig	ns
c.	sig	sig
d.	sig	ns

Chapter 7

1. Is participation in ITP related to a decrease in elopement?
   $X^2 = .065$ with 1 df not significant
   Individuals in the ITP program do not elope less often that those in the CTP program. Because the chi-square is not significant, it is inappropriate to calculate phi.

2. $X^2 = 2.46$ with 2 df not significant
   Although nurses chose plan c less frequently, the differences were not statistically significant.

3. $X^2 = 1348.439$, 1 df, $p < 0.001$
   This hospital, with an infection rate of 5.49%, has significantly less infections than the JAH estimate.

4. Someone might have been counted twice.

5. $X^2 = 121.028$, 4 df, $p < .001$
   Diploma and AD nurses select medical-surgical nursing more often than BSN students. BSN students select psychiatric nursing most often, pediatric nursing second, and medical-surgical nursing third. Pediatrics tends to be chosen about equally by the three groups. It is the second choice for all groups.

6. The phi coefficient is .232 and demonstrates the strength of the relationship between two variables in a 2 × 2 design.

Chapter 8

1. Variances of two groups are unequal; therefore, you must use the separate formula.

$$t = -2.795, df = 24$$

This value is significant at $< .01$; therefore, relaxation therapy significantly reduced diastolic blood pressure.

2. Case 1   1.771
      Case 2   2.160
      Case 3   2.479
      Case 4   2.779
      Case 5   2.617

3. Individuals who receive the experimental drug will work more days than those in the control group.
. Variances of two groups are equivalent. Pooled formula is used.

$$t = 1.996, 31 \text{ df}, p < .05.$$

4. Is there a difference between children raised in an orphanage and those raised in foster care in terms of the age at which they begin to interact with others? Variances are equivalent, use pooled formula.

$$t = .802, 8 \text{ df, not significant}$$

5. Hope to get a non-significant t, thus showing that groups did not differ on those variables. This would demonstrate that random assignment had worked.

6. The correlated t-test formula is used.

$$t = 40.82, 19 \text{ df}, p < .0005.$$

Your treatment has significantly increased hair growth.

Chapter 9

1. Variance for Group 1 = 1.6, for Group 2, 1.85. Not significantly different.

Source	SS	df	MS	F	p
Between	48.05	2	24.025	15.034	< .01
Within	47.95	30	1.598		
Total	96.00	32			

There is a significant difference among the three groups in hours of pain control.

2. Scheffé, $F_{cv} = 6.64$
   Groups 1 and 2, 3.6, ns
   Groups 1 and 3, 29, sig
   Groups 2 and 3, 12.35, sig

The laughter group (3) had significantly more pain free hours than either of the other two groups.

3. df

df	MS	F	p
2	248.02	4.83	< .05
42	51.31		

There is a significant difference in days to resumption of weight-bearing among participants in these three programs.

4. HSD = 6.364

Only the difference between II and III is significant. Group II, with a mean of 22, scored significantly higher than Group III ($\overline{X}$ = 14).

Chapter 10

1. Does adding the visual component to a taped lession enhance learning? Is there any difference in knowledge retention between those who discuss the tape with a nurse and those who discusss it with other patients and a nurse? Is there any interaction between type of teaching and type of follow-up discussion?

SUMMARY TABLE

Source	SS	df	MS	F	p
Between	88.475	3			
Teaching	70.225	1	70.225	38.021	<.01
Discussion	18.225	1	18.225	9.867	<.01
Teaching × Discussion	.025	1	.025	.014	ns
Within	66.5	36	1.847		
Total	154.975	39			

The homogeneity of variance assumption was met. The groups did not have significantly different variances. Those taught by audio-visual tape do significantly better than those taught by audio tape. Those with group discussion do significantly better than those in the one-to-one discussion condition. There is no interaction between type of teaching and type of discussion.

2. **THREE-WAY ANOVA SUMMARY TABLE**

Source	SS	df	MS	F	p
Between Groups		7			
Treatment		3			
Marital Status		2			
Race		2			
Interactions					
Treatment × Marital Status		6			
Treatment × Race		6			
Marital Status × Race		4			
Treatment × Marital Status × Race		12			
Within		764			
Total		799			

Chapter 11

1. To reduce the error variance and thus to increase the power of the test.

2. No, the use of ANCOVA supposes that the groups are basically similar, except for the covariate (in this case verbal ability). Because men and women are *not* similar in all aspects except verbal ability, this would be an incorrect use of ANCOVA.

3. It means that there is no interaction between the covariate and the levels of the independent variable(s); that is, the action of the covariate in relation to the dependent variable should be the same for all groups.

4. $F = .116/.0038 = 30.53$, 1,100 df, $p < .01$
   Cannot use ANCOVA for this analysis.

5. $\sum y_{tot}^2 = 546.2$
   $\sum y_{within}^2 = 193.4$
   $\sum x_{tot}^2 = 592$
   $\sum x_{within}^2 = 591.8$
   $\sum xy_{tot} = -319$
   $\sum xy_{within} = -327.4$

SUMMARY TABLE

Source	SS	df	MS	F	p
Between	362.04	1	362.04	502.83	<.01
Within	12.27	17	.72		
Total	374.31	18			

There is a significant difference between experimental and control group after controlling for covariate.

Groups	Original Means	Adjusted Means
Experimental	14.9	14.955
Control	6.5	6.445

The adjusted means are not very different from the original means.

Chapter 12

1. Correlations across repeated measures are equivalent. Variances across repeated measures are equivalent.

2.   SUMMARY TABLE

Source of Variation	SS	df	MS	F	p
Between Subjects		59			
Treatment	804.75	3	268.25	5.06	< .01
Within Group	2970.50	56	53.04		
Within Subjects					
Time	982.60	2	491.3	6.00	<.01
Treatment × Time	498.00	6	83.0	1.01	ns
Time × Within Group	9170.90	112	81.88		

There is a significant difference among the treatment groups, and there are significant changes over time. Post-hoc tests would be done on both of these factors. There is no treatment by time interaction.

3.   SUMMARY TABLE

Source of Variation	SS	df	MS	F	p
Between Subjects		19			
Within Subjects		40			
Treatments	106.8	2	53.4	1.85	ns
Residual	1094.4	38	28.8		
Total		59			

Treatments do not make a difference.

4. No

5. Multivariate Approach, Greenhouse-Geisser Procedure

6. Original   **After Procedure**

Original	After Procedure
3/27	1/9
6/81	2/27
9/300	3/100

Chapter 13

1. a. Factor analysis
   b. Neither
   c. Cluster analysis followed by subsequent analysis (probably analysis of variance)
   d. Factor analysis followed by analysis of variance. (Also, one may conduct a cluster analysis on a limited number of variables.)

2. a. With the exception of one item, "eating," all items have a high loading on one and only one factor. Simple structure is closely approached.

b.	I	II
Walking in the neighborhood	.81	
Walking from room to room	.75	
Climbing stairs	.72	
Shopping and marketing	.68	
Bathing		.87
Dressing		.82
Care of hair		.73

("Eating" may or may not be included in this table depending on one's choice of a criteria for factor loadings.)

c. One may name the factors *Mobility* and *Appearance Self-care*. A wide variety of other answers would also be "correct."

d. Eigenvalue is 2.3876, or 2.4. The factor accounts for 29.8% of variance.

e. .5850, or 59% of the variance in this item has been explained by the two factors.

3. a. Four factors should be rotated. It is standard to use 5% of variance accounted for as the cut-off, and that level corresponds to a breaking point in these results.

b. 48.0%

c. 38.4%

Chapter 14

1. The study of causes has stimulated much of our scientific research.

2. Experiments and causal modeling.

3. Path analysis can often be used when a "true" experiment is impossible or unfeasible. The reliance on correlations and the inability to control extraneous effects must be considered when drawing inferences from path analysis.

4. The three problems:

a. Probably not causal. You would wish to study much information, probably, but it is a predictive question as it is framed.

b. Assuming the availability of religious counselors, you migth wish to try an experiment, with patients randomly assigned to be offered such visits. You might judge its help by finding whether those offered these opportunities expressed satisfaction, compared with those who did not.

Note: You might be wise to study such an experimental effect *in context of* a path model with the background variables of the patient and the medical conditions of length of stay, severity of illness.
c. Such data would strongly imply a causal model of the kind discussed in this chapter.

5. You remember that the order should reflect a "weak causal ordering," and should not have any illogical arrow directions. One possible model is the following:

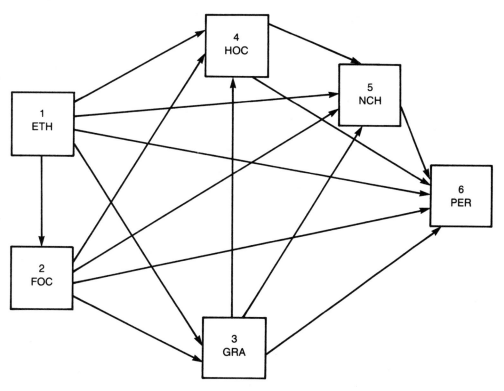

6. Complete recursive model.

7. Same, .30 (because there are no other influences on 2).

8. Multiply the paths on the indirect route: $(.30)(.20) = .06$.

9. There are no paths for indirect influence.

10. None.

11. Multiply: $(.20)(.60) = .12$.

12. None.

13. The correlation $= .40 + (.30)(.20) = .40 + .06 = .46$.

14. The correlation of 2 and 3 $= .20 + (.30)(.40) = .32$.

Chapter 15

  1. B

  2. C

  3. A

4A. d

4B. b

4C. a

4D. e

4E. c

  5. B

  6. 52%

APPENDIX B

Percent of Total Area of Normal Curve Between a *z*-Score and the Mean

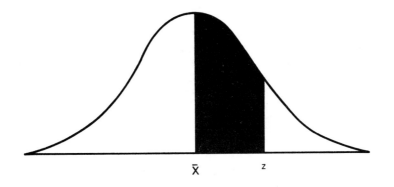

z	0.00	0.01	0.02	0.03	0.04	0.05	0.06	0.07	0.08	0.09
0.0	00.00	00.40	00.80	01.20	01.60	01.99	02.39	02.79	03.19	03.59
0.1	03.98	04.38	04.78	05.17	05.57	05.96	06.36	06.75	07.14	07.53
0.2	07.93	08.32	08.71	09.10	09.48	09.87	10.26	10.64	11.03	11.41
0.3	11.79	12.17	12.55	12.93	13.31	13.68	14.06	14.43	14.80	15.17
0.4	15.54	15.91	16.28	16.64	17.00	17.36	17.72	18.08	18.44	18.79
0.5	19.15	19.50	19.85	20.19	20.54	20.88	21.23	21.57	21.90	22.24
0.6	22.57	22.91	23.24	23.57	23.89	24.22	24.54	24.86	25.17	25.49
0.7	25.80	26.11	26.42	26.73	27.04	27.34	27.64	27.94	28.23	28.52
0.8	28.81	29.10	29.39	29.67	29.95	30.23	30.51	30.78	31.06	31.33
0.9	31.59	31.86	32.12	32.38	32.64	32.90	33.15	33.40	33.65	33.89

*% area
under norm.
curve below
X + 12*

z	0.00	0.01	0.02	0.03	0.04	0.05	0.06	0.07	0.08	0.09
1.0	34.13	34.38	34.61	34.85	35.08	35.31	35.54	35.77	35.99	36.21
1.1	36.43	36.65	36.86	37.08	37.29	37.49	37.70	37.90	38.10	38.30
1.2	38.49	38.69	38.88	39.07	39.25	39.44	39.62	39.80	39.97	40.15
1.3	40.32	40.49	40.66	40.82	40.99	41.15	41.31	41.47	41.62	41.77
1.4	41.92	42.07	42.22	42.36	42.51	42.65	42.79	42.92	43.06	43.19
1.5	43.32	43.45	43.57	43.70	43.83	43.94	44.06	44.18	44.29	44.41
1.6	44.52	44.63	44.74	44.84	44.95	45.05	45.15	45.25	45.35	45.45
1.7	45.54	45.64	45.73	45.82	45.91	45.99	46.08	46.16	46.25	46.33
1.8	46.41	46.49	46.56	46.64	46.71	46.78	46.86	46.93	46.99	47.06
1.9	47.13	47.19	47.26	47.32	47.38	47.44	47.50	47.56	47.61	47.67
2.0	47.72	47.78	47.83	47.88	47.93	47.98	48.03	48.08	48.12	48.17
2.1	48.21	48.26	48.30	48.34	48.38	48.42	48.46	48.50	48.54	48.57
2.2	48.61	48.64	48.68	48.71	48.75	48.78	48.81	48.84	48.87	48.90
2.3	48.93	48.96	48.98	49.01	49.04	49.06	49.09	49.11	49.13	49.16
2.4	49.18	49.20	49.22	49.25	49.27	49.29	49.31	49.32	49.34	49.36
2.5	49.38	49.40	49.41	49.43	49.45	49.46	49.48	49.49	49.51	49.52
2.6	49.53	49.55	49.56	49.57	49.59	49.60	49.61	49.62	49.63	49.64
2.7	49.65	49.66	49.67	49.68	49.69	49.70	49.71	49.72	49.73	49.74
2.8	49.74	49.75	49.76	49.77	49.77	49.78	49.79	49.79	49.80	49.81
2.9	49.81	49.82	49.82	49.83	49.84	49.84	49.85	49.85	49.86	49.86
3.0	49.87									
3.5	49.98									
4.0	49.997									
5.0	49.99997									

*Below
X x*

From: Hald, A. (1952). Statistical tables and formulas. New York: John Wiley & Sons. (Table 1).

APPENDIX C

Critical Values of the Correlation Coefficient

	Level of Significance for One-Tailed Test			
	.05	.025	.01	.005
	Level of Significance for Two-Tailed Test			
df	.10	.05	.02	.01
1	.988	.997	.9995	.9999
2	.900	.950	.980	.990
3	.805	.878	.934	.959
4	.729	.811	.882	.917
5	.669	.754	.833	.874
6	.622	.707	.789	.834
7	.582	.666	.750	.798
8	.549	.632	.716	.765
9	.521	.602	.685	.735
10	.497	.576	.658	.708
11	.476	.553	.634	.684
12	.458	.532	.612	.661
13	.441	.514	.592	.641
14	.426	.497	.574	.623
15	.412	.482	.558	.606
16	.400	.468	.542	.590
17	.389	.456	.528	.575
18	.378	.444	.516	.561
19	.369	.433	.503	.549
20	.360	.423	.492	.537
21	.352	.413	.482	.526
22	.344	.404	.472	.515

df	Level of Significance for One-Tailed Test			
	.05	.025	.01	.005
	Level of Significance for Two-Tailed Test			
	.10	.05	.02	.01
23	.337	.396	.462	.505
24	.330	.388	.453	.496
25	.323	.381	.445	.487
26	.317	.374	.437	.479
27	.311	.367	.430	.471
28	.306	.361	.423	.463
29	.301	.355	.416	.456
30	.296	.349	.409	.449
35	.275	.325	.381	.418
40	.257	.304	.358	.393
45	.243	.288	.338	.372
50	.231	.273	.322	.354
60	.211	.250	.295	.325
70	.195	.232	.274	.303
80	.183	.217	.256	.283
90	.173	.205	.242	.267
100	.164	.195	.230	.254
125		.174		.228
150		.159		.208
200		.138		.181
300		.113		.148
400		.098		.128
500		.088		.115
1000		.062		.081

From: Fisher, R. A. (1970). *Statistical methods for research workers*. (14th ed.). Darien, CT: Hafner Publishing Co. (Table V.A., p. 211)

APPENDIX D

Transformation of r to z_r

r	z_r	r	z_r	r	z_r	r	z_r	r	z_r
.000	.000	.200	.203	.400	.424	.600	.693	.800	1.099
.005	.005	.205	.208	.405	.430	.605	.701	.805	1.113
.010	.010	.210	.213	.410	.436	.610	.709	.810	1.127
.015	.015	.215	.218	.415	.442	.615	.717	.815	1.142
.020	.020	.220	.224	.420	.448	.620	.725	.820	1.157
.025	.025	.225	.229	.425	.454	.625	.733	.825	1.172
.030	.030	.230	.234	.430	.460	.630	.741	.830	1.188
.035	.035	.235	.239	.435	.466	.635	.750	.835	1.204
.040	.040	.240	.245	.440	.472	.640	.758	.840	1.221
.045	.045	.245	.250	.445	.478	.645	.767	.845	1.238
.050	.050	.250	.255	.450	.485	.650	.775	.850	1.256
.055	.055	.255	.261	.455	.491	.655	.784	.855	1.274
.060	.060	.260	.266	.460	.497	.660	.793	.860	1.293
.065	.065	.265	.271	.465	.504	.665	.802	.865	1.313
.070	.070	.270	.277	.470	.510	.670	.811	.870	1.333
.075	.075	.275	.282	.475	.517	.675	.820	.875	1.354
.080	.080	.280	.288	.480	.523	.680	.829	.880	1.376
.085	.085	.285	.293	.485	.530	.685	.838	.885	1.398
.090	.090	.290	.299	.490	.536	.690	.848	.890	1.422
.095	.095	.295	.304	.495	.543	.695	.858	.895	1.447
.100	.100	.300	.310	.500	.549	.700	.867	.900	1.472
.105	.105	.305	.315	.505	.556	.705	.877	.905	1.499
.110	.110	.310	.321	.510	.563	.710	.887	.910	1.528
.115	.116	.315	.326	.515	.570	.715	.897	.915	1.557
.120	.121	.320	.332	.520	.576	.720	.908	.920	1.589

r	z_r	r	z_r	r	z_r	r	z_r	r	z_r
.125	.126	.325	.337	.525	.583	.725	.918	.925	1.623
.130	.131	.330	.343	.530	.590	.730	.929	.930	1.658
.135	.136	.335	.348	.535	.597	.735	.940	.935	1.697
.140	.141	.340	.354	.540	.604	.740	.950	.940	1.738
.145	.146	.345	.360	.545	.611	.745	.962	.945	1.783
.150	.151	.350	.365	.550	.618	.750	.973	.950	1.832
.155	.156	.355	.371	.555	.626	.755	.984	.955	1.886
.160	.161	.360	.377	.560	.633	.760	.996	.960	1.946
.165	.167	.365	.383	.565	.640	.765	1.008	.965	2.014
.170	.172	.370	.388	.570	.648	.770	1.020	.970	2.092
.175	.177	.375	.394	.575	.655	.775	1.033	.975	2.185
.180	.182	.380	.400	.580	.662	.780	1.045	.980	2.298
.185	.187	.385	.406	.585	.670	.785	1.058	.985	2.443
.190	.192	.390	.412	.590	.678	.790	1.071	.990	2.647
.195	.198	.395	.418	.595	.685	.795	.1085	.995	2.994

From Hinkle, D. E., Wiersma, W., & Jurs, S. G. (1982). *Basic behavioral statistics* (Appendix E.6, p. 372). Boston: Houghton Mifflin. Copyright © 1982 by Houghton Mifflin Company. Used by permission.

APPENDIX E

The 5% and 1% Points for the Distribution of *F*

(Table begins on page 362)

5% = roman type; 1% = boldface type

n_1 degrees of freedom (for greater mean square)*

n_2		1	2	3	4	5	6	7	8	9	10	11	12	14	16	20	24	30	40	50	75	100	200	500	∞
1	.05	161	200	216	225	230	234	237	239	241	242	243	244	245	246	248	249	250	251	252	253	253	254	254	254
	.01	**4,052**	**4,999**	**5,403**	**5,625**	**5,764**	**5,859**	**5,928**	**5,981**	**6,022**	**6,056**	**6,082**	**6,106**	**6,142**	**6,169**	**6,208**	**6,234**	**6,258**	**6,286**	**6,302**	**6,323**	**6,334**	**6,352**	**6,361**	**6,366**
2	.05	18.51	19.00	19.16	19.25	19.30	19.33	19.36	19.37	19.38	19.39	19.40	19.41	19.42	19.43	19.44	19.45	19.46	19.47	19.47	19.48	19.49	19.49	19.50	19.50
	.01	**98.49**	**99.00**	**99.17**	**99.25**	**99.30**	**99.33**	**99.34**	**99.36**	**99.38**	**99.40**	**99.41**	**99.42**	**99.43**	**99.44**	**99.45**	**99.46**	**99.47**	**99.48**	**99.48**	**99.49**	**99.49**	**99.49**	**99.50**	**99.50**
3	.05	10.13	9.55	9.28	9.12	9.01	8.94	8.88	8.84	8.81	8.78	8.76	8.74	8.71	8.69	8.66	8.64	8.62	8.60	8.58	8.57	8.56	8.54	8.54	8.53
	.01	**34.12**	**30.82**	**29.46**	**28.71**	**28.24**	**27.91**	**27.67**	**27.49**	**27.34**	**27.23**	**27.13**	**27.05**	**26.92**	**26.83**	**26.69**	**26.60**	**26.50**	**26.41**	**26.35**	**26.27**	**26.23**	**26.18**	**26.14**	**26.12**
4	.05	7.71	6.94	6.59	6.39	6.26	6.16	6.09	6.04	6.00	5.96	5.93	5.91	5.87	5.84	5.80	5.77	5.74	5.71	5.70	5.68	5.66	5.65	5.64	5.63
	.01	**21.20**	**18.00**	**16.69**	**15.98**	**15.52**	**15.21**	**14.98**	**14.80**	**14.66**	**14.54**	**14.45**	**14.37**	**14.24**	**14.15**	**14.02**	**13.93**	**13.83**	**13.74**	**13.69**	**13.61**	**13.57**	**13.52**	**13.48**	**13.46**
5	.05	6.61	5.79	5.41	5.19	5.05	4.95	4.88	4.82	4.78	4.74	4.70	4.68	4.64	4.60	4.56	4.53	4.50	4.46	4.44	4.42	4.40	4.38	4.37	4.36
	.01	**16.26**	**13.27**	**12.06**	**11.39**	**10.97**	**10.67**	**10.45**	**10.27**	**10.15**	**10.05**	**9.96**	**9.89**	**9.77**	**9.68**	**9.55**	**9.47**	**9.38**	**9.29**	**9.24**	**9.17**	**9.13**	**9.07**	**9.04**	**9.02**
6	.05	5.99	5.14	4.76	4.53	4.39	4.28	4.21	4.15	4.10	4.06	4.03	4.00	3.96	3.92	3.87	3.84	3.81	3.77	3.75	3.72	3.71	3.69	3.68	3.67
	.01	**13.74**	**10.92**	**9.78**	**9.15**	**8.75**	**8.47**	**8.26**	**8.10**	**7.98**	**7.87**	**7.79**	**7.72**	**7.60**	**7.52**	**7.39**	**7.31**	**7.23**	**7.14**	**7.09**	**7.02**	**6.99**	**6.94**	**6.90**	**6.88**
7	.05	5.59	4.74	4.35	4.12	3.97	3.87	3.79	3.73	3.68	3.63	3.60	3.57	3.52	3.49	3.44	3.41	3.38	3.34	3.32	3.29	3.28	3.25	3.24	3.23
	.01	**12.25**	**9.55**	**8.45**	**7.85**	**7.46**	**7.19**	**7.00**	**6.84**	**6.71**	**6.62**	**6.54**	**6.47**	**6.35**	**6.27**	**6.15**	**6.07**	**5.98**	**5.90**	**5.85**	**5.78**	**5.75**	**5.70**	**5.67**	**5.65**
8	.05	5.32	4.46	4.07	3.84	3.69	3.58	3.50	3.44	3.39	3.34	3.31	3.28	3.23	3.20	3.15	3.12	3.08	3.05	3.03	3.00	2.98	2.96	2.94	2.93
	.01	**11.26**	**8.65**	**7.59**	**7.01**	**6.63**	**6.37**	**6.19**	**6.03**	**5.91**	**5.82**	**5.74**	**5.67**	**5.56**	**5.48**	**5.36**	**5.28**	**5.20**	**5.11**	**5.06**	**5.00**	**4.96**	**4.91**	**4.88**	**4.86**
9	.05	5.12	4.26	3.86	3.63	3.48	3.37	3.29	3.23	3.18	3.13	3.10	3.07	3.02	2.98	2.93	2.90	2.86	2.82	2.80	2.77	2.76	2.73	2.72	2.71
	.01	**10.56**	**8.02**	**6.99**	**6.42**	**6.06**	**5.80**	**5.62**	**5.47**	**5.35**	**5.26**	**5.18**	**5.11**	**5.00**	**4.92**	**4.80**	**4.73**	**4.64**	**4.56**	**4.51**	**4.45**	**4.41**	**4.36**	**4.33**	**4.31**
10	.05	4.96	4.10	3.71	3.48	3.33	3.22	3.14	3.07	3.02	2.97	2.94	2.91	2.86	2.82	2.77	2.74	2.70	2.67	2.64	2.61	2.59	2.56	2.55	2.54
	.01	**10.04**	**7.56**	**6.55**	**5.99**	**5.64**	**5.39**	**5.21**	**5.06**	**4.95**	**4.85**	**4.78**	**4.71**	**4.60**	**4.52**	**4.41**	**4.33**	**4.25**	**4.17**	**4.12**	**4.05**	**4.01**	**3.96**	**3.93**	**3.91**
11	.05	4.84	3.98	3.59	3.36	3.20	3.09	3.01	2.95	2.90	2.86	2.82	2.79	2.74	2.70	2.65	2.61	2.57	2.53	2.50	2.47	2.45	2.42	2.41	2.40
	.01	**9.65**	**7.20**	**6.22**	**5.67**	**5.32**	**5.07**	**4.88**	**4.74**	**4.63**	**4.54**	**4.46**	**4.40**	**4.29**	**4.21**	**4.10**	**4.02**	**3.94**	**3.86**	**3.80**	**3.74**	**3.70**	**3.66**	**3.62**	**3.60**
12	.05	4.75	3.88	3.49	3.26	3.11	3.00	2.92	2.85	2.80	2.76	2.72	2.69	2.64	2.60	2.54	2.50	2.46	2.42	2.40	2.36	2.35	2.32	2.31	2.30
	.01	**9.33**	**6.93**	**5.95**	**5.41**	**5.06**	**4.82**	**4.65**	**4.50**	**4.39**	**4.30**	**4.22**	**4.16**	**4.05**	**3.98**	**3.86**	**3.78**	**3.70**	**3.61**	**3.56**	**3.49**	**3.46**	**3.41**	**3.38**	**3.36**

13	4.67	3.80	3.41	3.18	3.02	2.92	2.84	2.77	2.72	2.67	2.63	2.60	2.55	2.51	2.46	2.42	2.38	2.34	2.32	2.28	2.26	2.24	2.22	2.21
	9.07	**6.70**	**5.74**	**5.20**	**4.86**	**4.62**	**4.44**	**4.30**	**4.19**	**4.10**	**4.02**	**3.96**	**3.85**	**3.78**	**3.67**	**3.59**	**3.51**	**3.42**	**3.37**	**3.30**	**3.27**	**3.21**	**3.18**	**3.16**
14	4.60	3.74	3.34	3.11	2.96	2.85	2.77	2.70	2.65	2.60	2.56	2.53	2.48	2.44	2.39	2.35	2.31	2.27	2.24	2.21	2.19	2.16	2.14	2.13
	8.86	**6.51**	**5.56**	**5.03**	**4.69**	**4.46**	**4.28**	**4.14**	**4.03**	**3.94**	**3.86**	**3.80**	**3.70**	**3.62**	**3.51**	**3.43**	**3.34**	**3.26**	**3.21**	**3.14**	**3.11**	**3.06**	**3.02**	**3.00**
15	4.54	3.68	3.29	3.06	2.90	2.79	2.70	2.64	2.59	2.55	2.51	2.48	2.43	2.39	2.33	2.29	2.25	2.21	2.18	2.15	2.12	2.10	2.08	2.07
	8.68	**6.36**	**5.42**	**4.89**	**4.56**	**4.32**	**4.14**	**4.00**	**3.89**	**3.80**	**3.73**	**3.67**	**3.56**	**3.48**	**3.36**	**3.29**	**3.20**	**3.12**	**3.07**	**3.00**	**2.97**	**2.92**	**2.89**	**2.87**
16	4.49	3.63	3.24	3.01	2.85	2.74	2.66	2.59	2.54	2.49	2.45	2.42	2.37	2.33	2.28	2.24	2.20	2.16	2.13	2.09	2.07	2.04	2.02	2.01
	8.53	**6.23**	**5.29**	**4.77**	**4.44**	**4.20**	**4.03**	**3.89**	**3.78**	**3.69**	**3.61**	**3.55**	**3.45**	**3.37**	**3.25**	**3.18**	**3.10**	**3.01**	**2.96**	**2.89**	**2.86**	**2.80**	**2.77**	**2.75**
17	4.45	3.59	3.20	2.96	2.81	2.70	2.62	2.55	2.50	2.45	2.41	2.38	2.33	2.29	2.23	2.19	2.15	2.11	2.08	2.04	2.02	1.99	1.97	1.96
	8.40	**6.11**	**5.18**	**4.67**	**4.34**	**4.10**	**3.93**	**3.79**	**3.68**	**3.59**	**3.52**	**3.45**	**3.35**	**3.27**	**3.16**	**3.08**	**3.00**	**2.92**	**2.86**	**2.79**	**2.76**	**2.70**	**2.67**	**2.65**
18	4.41	3.55	3.16	2.93	2.77	2.66	2.58	2.51	2.46	2.41	2.37	2.34	2.29	2.25	2.19	2.15	2.11	2.07	2.04	2.00	1.98	1.95	1.93	1.92
	8.28	**6.01**	**5.09**	**4.58**	**4.25**	**4.01**	**3.85**	**3.71**	**3.60**	**3.51**	**3.44**	**3.37**	**3.27**	**3.19**	**3.07**	**3.00**	**2.91**	**2.83**	**2.78**	**2.71**	**2.68**	**2.62**	**2.59**	**2.57**
19	4.38	3.52	3.13	2.90	2.74	2.63	2.55	2.48	2.43	2.38	2.34	2.31	2.26	2.21	2.15	2.11	2.07	2.02	2.00	1.96	1.94	1.91	1.90	1.88
	8.18	**5.93**	**5.01**	**4.50**	**4.17**	**3.94**	**3.77**	**3.63**	**3.52**	**3.43**	**3.36**	**3.30**	**3.19**	**3.12**	**3.00**	**2.92**	**2.84**	**2.76**	**2.70**	**2.63**	**2.60**	**2.54**	**2.51**	**2.49**
20	4.35	3.49	3.10	2.87	2.71	2.60	2.52	2.45	2.40	2.35	2.31	2.28	2.23	2.18	2.12	2.08	2.04	1.99	1.96	1.92	1.90	1.87	1.85	1.84
	8.10	**5.85**	**4.94**	**4.43**	**4.10**	**3.87**	**3.71**	**3.56**	**3.45**	**3.37**	**3.30**	**3.23**	**3.13**	**3.05**	**2.94**	**2.86**	**2.77**	**2.69**	**2.63**	**2.56**	**2.53**	**2.47**	**2.44**	**2.42**
21	4.32	3.47	3.07	2.84	2.68	2.57	2.49	2.42	2.37	2.32	2.28	2.25	2.20	2.15	2.09	2.05	2.00	1.96	1.93	1.89	1.87	1.84	1.82	1.81
	8.02	**5.78**	**4.87**	**4.37**	**4.04**	**3.81**	**3.65**	**3.51**	**3.40**	**3.31**	**3.24**	**3.17**	**3.07**	**2.99**	**2.88**	**2.80**	**2.72**	**2.63**	**2.58**	**2.51**	**2.47**	**2.42**	**2.38**	**2.36**
22	4.30	3.44	3.05	2.82	2.66	2.55	2.47	2.40	2.35	2.30	2.26	2.23	2.18	2.13	2.07	2.03	1.98	1.93	1.91	1.87	1.84	1.81	1.80	1.78
	7.94	**5.72**	**4.82**	**4.31**	**3.99**	**3.76**	**3.59**	**3.45**	**3.35**	**3.26**	**3.18**	**3.12**	**3.02**	**2.94**	**2.83**	**2.75**	**2.67**	**2.58**	**2.53**	**2.46**	**2.42**	**2.37**	**2.33**	**2.31**
23	4.28	3.42	3.03	2.80	2.64	2.53	2.45	2.38	2.32	2.28	2.24	2.20	2.14	2.10	2.04	2.00	1.96	1.91	1.88	1.84	1.82	1.79	1.77	1.76
	7.88	**5.66**	**4.76**	**4.26**	**3.94**	**3.71**	**3.54**	**3.41**	**3.30**	**3.21**	**3.14**	**3.07**	**2.97**	**2.89**	**2.78**	**2.70**	**2.62**	**2.53**	**2.48**	**2.41**	**2.37**	**2.32**	**2.28**	**2.26**
24	4.26	3.40	3.01	2.78	2.62	2.51	2.43	2.36	2.30	2.26	2.22	2.18	2.13	2.09	2.02	1.98	1.94	1.89	1.86	1.82	1.80	1.76	1.74	1.73
	7.82	**5.61**	**4.72**	**4.22**	**3.90**	**3.67**	**3.50**	**3.36**	**3.25**	**3.17**	**3.09**	**3.03**	**2.93**	**2.85**	**2.74**	**2.66**	**2.58**	**2.49**	**2.44**	**2.36**	**2.33**	**2.27**	**2.23**	**2.21**
25	4.24	3.38	2.99	2.76	2.60	2.49	2.41	2.34	2.28	2.24	2.20	2.16	2.11	2.06	2.00	1.96	1.92	1.87	1.84	1.80	1.77	1.74	1.72	1.71
	7.77	**5.57**	**4.68**	**4.18**	**3.86**	**3.63**	**3.46**	**3.32**	**3.21**	**3.13**	**3.05**	**2.99**	**2.89**	**2.81**	**2.70**	**2.62**	**2.54**	**2.45**	**2.40**	**2.32**	**2.29**	**2.23**	**2.19**	**2.17**
26	4.22	3.37	2.98	2.74	2.59	2.47	2.39	2.32	2.27	2.22	2.18	2.15	2.10	2.05	1.99	1.95	1.90	1.85	1.82	1.78	1.76	1.72	1.70	1.69
	7.72	**5.53**	**4.64**	**4.14**	**3.82**	**3.59**	**3.42**	**3.29**	**3.17**	**3.09**	**3.02**	**2.96**	**2.86**	**2.77**	**2.66**	**2.58**	**2.50**	**2.41**	**2.36**	**2.28**	**2.25**	**2.19**	**2.15**	**2.13**
27	4.21	3.35	2.96	2.73	2.57	2.46	2.37	2.30	2.25	2.20	2.16	2.13	2.08	2.03	1.97	1.93	1.88	1.84	1.80	1.76	1.74	1.71	1.68	1.67
	7.68	**5.49**	**4.60**	**4.11**	**3.79**	**3.56**	**3.39**	**3.26**	**3.14**	**3.06**	**2.98**	**2.93**	**2.83**	**2.74**	**2.63**	**2.55**	**2.47**	**2.38**	**2.33**	**2.25**	**2.21**	**2.16**	**2.12**	**2.10**

5% = roman type; 1% = boldface type

n_1 degrees of freedom (for greater mean square)*

n_2	1	2	3	4	5	6	7	8	9	10	11	12	14	16	20	24	30	40	50	75	100	200	500	∞
28	4.20	3.34	2.95	2.71	2.56	2.44	2.36	2.29	2.24	2.19	2.15	2.12	2.06	2.02	1.96	1.91	1.87	1.81	1.78	1.75	1.72	1.69	1.67	1.65
	7.64	**5.45**	**4.57**	**4.07**	**3.76**	**3.53**	**3.36**	**3.23**	**3.11**	**3.03**	**2.95**	**2.90**	**2.80**	**2.71**	**2.60**	**2.52**	**2.44**	**2.35**	**2.30**	**2.22**	**2.18**	**2.13**	**2.09**	**2.06**
29	4.18	3.33	2.93	2.70	2.54	2.43	2.35	2.28	2.22	2.18	2.14	2.10	2.05	2.00	1.94	1.90	1.85	1.80	1.77	1.73	1.71	1.68	1.65	1.64
	7.60	**5.42**	**4.54**	**4.04**	**3.73**	**3.50**	**3.33**	**3.20**	**3.08**	**3.00**	**2.92**	**2.87**	**2.77**	**2.68**	**2.57**	**2.49**	**2.41**	**2.32**	**2.27**	**2.19**	**2.15**	**2.10**	**2.06**	**2.03**
30	4.17	3.32	2.92	2.69	2.53	2.42	2.34	2.27	2.21	2.16	2.12	2.09	2.04	1.99	1.93	1.89	1.84	1.79	1.76	1.72	1.69	1.66	1.64	1.62
	7.56	**5.39**	**4.51**	**4.02**	**3.70**	**3.47**	**3.30**	**3.17**	**3.06**	**2.98**	**2.90**	**2.84**	**2.74**	**2.66**	**2.55**	**2.47**	**2.38**	**2.29**	**2.24**	**2.16**	**2.13**	**2.07**	**2.03**	**2.01**
32	4.15	3.30	2.90	2.67	2.51	2.40	2.32	2.25	2.19	2.14	2.10	2.07	2.02	1.97	1.91	1.86	1.82	1.76	1.74	1.69	1.67	1.64	1.61	1.59
	7.50	**5.34**	**4.46**	**3.97**	**3.66**	**3.42**	**3.25**	**3.12**	**3.01**	**2.94**	**2.86**	**2.80**	**2.70**	**2.62**	**2.51**	**2.42**	**2.34**	**2.25**	**2.20**	**2.12**	**2.08**	**2.02**	**1.98**	**1.96**
34	4.13	3.28	2.88	2.65	2.49	2.38	2.30	2.23	2.17	2.12	2.08	2.05	2.00	1.95	1.89	1.84	1.80	1.74	1.71	1.67	1.64	1.61	1.59	1.57
	7.44	**5.29**	**4.42**	**3.93**	**3.61**	**3.38**	**3.21**	**3.08**	**2.97**	**2.89**	**2.82**	**2.76**	**2.66**	**2.58**	**2.47**	**2.38**	**2.30**	**2.21**	**2.15**	**2.08**	**2.04**	**1.98**	**1.94**	**1.91**
36	4.11	3.26	2.86	2.63	2.48	2.36	2.28	2.21	2.15	2.10	2.06	2.03	1.98	1.93	1.87	1.82	1.78	1.72	1.69	1.65	1.62	1.59	1.56	1.55
	7.39	**5.25**	**4.38**	**3.89**	**3.58**	**3.35**	**3.18**	**3.04**	**2.94**	**2.86**	**2.78**	**2.72**	**2.62**	**2.54**	**2.43**	**2.35**	**2.26**	**2.17**	**2.12**	**2.04**	**2.00**	**1.94**	**1.90**	**1.87**
38	4.10	3.25	2.85	2.62	2.46	2.35	2.26	2.19	2.14	2.09	2.05	2.02	1.96	1.92	1.85	1.80	1.76	1.71	1.67	1.63	1.60	1.57	1.54	1.53
	7.35	**5.21**	**4.34**	**3.86**	**3.54**	**3.32**	**3.15**	**3.02**	**2.91**	**2.82**	**2.75**	**2.69**	**2.59**	**2.51**	**2.40**	**2.32**	**2.22**	**2.14**	**2.08**	**2.00**	**1.97**	**1.90**	**1.86**	**1.84**
40	4.08	3.23	2.84	2.61	2.45	2.34	2.25	2.18	2.12	2.07	2.04	2.00	1.95	1.90	1.84	1.79	1.74	1.69	1.66	1.61	1.59	1.55	1.53	1.51
	7.31	**5.18**	**4.31**	**3.83**	**3.51**	**3.29**	**3.12**	**2.99**	**2.88**	**2.80**	**2.73**	**2.66**	**2.56**	**2.49**	**2.37**	**2.29**	**2.20**	**2.11**	**2.05**	**1.97**	**1.94**	**1.88**	**1.84**	**1.81**
42	4.07	3.22	2.83	2.59	2.44	2.32	2.24	2.17	2.11	2.06	2.02	1.99	1.94	1.89	1.82	1.78	1.73	1.68	1.64	1.60	1.57	1.54	1.51	1.49
	7.27	**5.15**	**4.29**	**3.80**	**3.49**	**3.26**	**3.10**	**2.96**	**2.86**	**2.77**	**2.70**	**2.64**	**2.54**	**2.46**	**2.35**	**2.26**	**2.17**	**2.08**	**2.02**	**1.94**	**1.91**	**1.85**	**1.80**	**1.78**
44	4.06	3.21	2.82	2.58	2.43	2.31	2.23	2.16	2.10	2.05	2.01	1.98	1.92	1.88	1.81	1.76	1.72	1.66	1.63	1.58	1.56	1.52	1.50	1.48
	7.24	**5.12**	**4.26**	**3.78**	**3.46**	**3.24**	**3.07**	**2.94**	**2.84**	**2.75**	**2.68**	**2.62**	**2.52**	**2.44**	**2.32**	**2.24**	**2.15**	**2.06**	**2.00**	**1.92**	**1.88**	**1.82**	**1.78**	**1.75**
46	4.05	3.20	2.81	2.57	2.42	2.30	2.22	2.14	2.09	2.04	2.00	1.97	1.91	1.87	1.80	1.75	1.71	1.65	1.62	1.57	1.54	1.51	1.48	1.46
	7.21	**5.10**	**4.24**	**3.76**	**3.44**	**3.22**	**3.05**	**2.92**	**2.82**	**2.73**	**2.66**	**2.60**	**2.50**	**2.42**	**2.30**	**2.22**	**2.13**	**2.04**	**1.98**	**1.90**	**1.86**	**1.80**	**1.76**	**1.72**
48	4.04	3.19	2.80	2.56	2.41	2.30	2.21	2.14	2.08	2.03	1.99	1.96	1.90	1.86	1.79	1.74	1.70	1.64	1.61	1.56	1.53	1.50	1.47	1.45
	7.19	**5.08**	**4.22**	**3.74**	**3.42**	**3.20**	**3.04**	**2.90**	**2.80**	**2.71**	**2.64**	**2.58**	**2.48**	**2.40**	**2.28**	**2.20**	**2.11**	**2.02**	**1.96**	**1.88**	**1.84**	**1.78**	**1.73**	**1.70**
50	4.03	3.18	2.79	2.56	2.40	2.29	2.20	2.13	2.07	2.02	1.98	1.95	1.90	1.85	1.78	1.74	1.69	1.63	1.60	1.55	1.52	1.48	1.46	1.44
	7.17	**5.06**	**4.20**	**3.72**	**3.41**	**3.18**	**3.02**	**2.88**	**2.78**	**2.70**	**2.62**	**2.56**	**2.46**	**2.39**	**2.26**	**2.18**	**2.10**	**2.00**	**1.94**	**1.86**	**1.82**	**1.76**	**1.71**	**1.68**

df																								
55	4.02	3.17	2.78	2.54	2.38	2.27	2.18	2.11	2.05	2.00	1.97	1.93	1.88	1.83	1.76	1.72	1.67	1.61	1.58	1.52	1.50	1.46	1.43	1.41
	7.12	**5.01**	**4.16**	**3.68**	**3.37**	**3.15**	**2.98**	**2.85**	**2.75**	**2.66**	**2.59**	**2.53**	**2.43**	**2.35**	**2.23**	**2.15**	**2.06**	**1.96**	**1.90**	**1.82**	**1.78**	**1.71**	**1.66**	**1.64**
60	4.00	3.15	2.76	2.52	2.37	2.25	2.17	2.10	2.04	1.99	1.95	1.92	1.86	1.81	1.75	1.70	1.65	1.59	1.56	1.50	1.48	1.44	1.41	1.39
	7.08	**4.98**	**4.13**	**3.65**	**3.34**	**3.12**	**2.95**	**2.82**	**2.72**	**2.63**	**2.56**	**2.50**	**2.40**	**2.32**	**2.20**	**2.12**	**2.03**	**1.93**	**1.87**	**1.79**	**1.74**	**1.68**	**1.63**	**1.60**
65	3.99	3.14	2.75	2.51	2.36	2.24	2.15	2.08	2.02	1.98	1.94	1.90	1.85	1.80	1.73	1.68	1.63	1.57	1.54	1.49	1.46	1.42	1.39	1.37
	7.04	**4.95**	**4.10**	**3.62**	**3.31**	**3.09**	**2.93**	**2.79**	**2.70**	**2.61**	**2.54**	**2.47**	**2.37**	**2.30**	**2.18**	**2.09**	**2.00**	**1.90**	**1.84**	**1.76**	**1.71**	**1.64**	**1.60**	**1.56**
70	3.98	3.13	2.74	2.50	2.35	2.23	2.14	2.07	2.01	1.97	1.93	1.89	1.84	1.79	1.72	1.67	1.62	1.56	1.53	1.47	1.45	1.40	1.37	1.35
	7.01	**4.92**	**4.08**	**3.60**	**3.29**	**3.07**	**2.91**	**2.77**	**2.67**	**2.59**	**2.51**	**2.45**	**2.35**	**2.28**	**2.15**	**2.07**	**1.98**	**1.88**	**1.82**	**1.74**	**1.69**	**1.62**	**1.56**	**1.53**
80	3.96	3.11	2.72	2.48	2.33	2.21	2.12	2.05	1.99	1.95	1.91	1.88	1.82	1.77	1.70	1.65	1.60	1.54	1.51	1.45	1.42	1.38	1.35	1.32
	6.96	**4.88**	**4.04**	**3.56**	**3.25**	**3.04**	**2.87**	**2.74**	**2.64**	**2.55**	**2.48**	**2.41**	**2.32**	**2.24**	**2.11**	**2.03**	**1.94**	**1.84**	**1.78**	**1.70**	**1.65**	**1.57**	**1.52**	**1.49**
100	3.94	3.09	2.70	2.46	2.30	2.19	2.10	2.03	1.97	1.92	1.88	1.85	1.79	1.75	1.68	1.63	1.57	1.51	1.48	1.42	1.39	1.34	1.30	1.28
	6.90	**4.82**	**3.98**	**3.51**	**3.20**	**2.99**	**2.82**	**2.69**	**2.59**	**2.51**	**2.43**	**2.36**	**2.26**	**2.19**	**2.06**	**1.98**	**1.89**	**1.79**	**1.73**	**1.64**	**1.59**	**1.51**	**1.46**	**1.43**
125	3.92	3.07	2.68	2.44	2.29	2.17	2.08	2.01	1.95	1.90	1.86	1.83	1.77	1.72	1.65	1.60	1.55	1.49	1.45	1.39	1.36	1.31	1.27	1.25
	6.84	**4.78**	**3.94**	**3.47**	**3.17**	**2.95**	**2.79**	**2.65**	**2.56**	**2.47**	**2.40**	**2.33**	**2.23**	**2.15**	**2.03**	**1.94**	**1.85**	**1.75**	**1.68**	**1.59**	**1.54**	**1.46**	**1.40**	**1.37**
150	3.91	3.06	2.67	2.43	2.27	2.16	2.07	2.00	1.94	1.89	1.85	1.82	1.76	1.71	1.64	1.59	1.54	1.47	1.44	1.37	1.34	1.29	1.25	1.22
	6.81	**4.75**	**3.91**	**3.44**	**3.14**	**2.92**	**2.76**	**2.62**	**2.53**	**2.44**	**2.37**	**2.30**	**2.20**	**2.12**	**2.00**	**1.91**	**1.83**	**1.72**	**1.66**	**1.56**	**1.51**	**1.43**	**1.37**	**1.33**
200	3.89	3.04	2.65	2.41	2.26	2.14	2.05	1.98	1.92	1.87	1.83	1.80	1.74	1.69	1.62	1.57	1.52	1.45	1.42	1.35	1.32	1.26	1.22	1.19
	6.76	**4.71**	**3.88**	**3.41**	**3.11**	**2.90**	**2.73**	**2.60**	**2.50**	**2.41**	**2.34**	**2.28**	**2.17**	**2.09**	**1.97**	**1.88**	**1.79**	**1.69**	**1.62**	**1.53**	**1.48**	**1.39**	**1.33**	**1.28**
400	3.86	3.02	2.62	2.39	2.23	2.12	2.03	1.96	1.90	1.85	1.81	1.78	1.72	1.67	1.60	1.54	1.49	1.42	1.38	1.32	1.28	1.22	1.16	1.13
	6.70	**4.66**	**3.83**	**3.36**	**3.06**	**2.85**	**2.69**	**2.55**	**2.46**	**2.37**	**2.29**	**2.23**	**2.12**	**2.04**	**1.92**	**1.84**	**1.74**	**1.64**	**1.57**	**1.47**	**1.42**	**1.32**	**1.24**	**1.19**
1000	3.85	3.00	2.61	2.38	2.22	2.10	2.02	1.95	1.89	1.84	1.80	1.76	1.70	1.65	1.58	1.53	1.47	1.41	1.36	1.30	1.26	1.19	1.13	1.08
	6.66	**4.62**	**3.80**	**3.34**	**3.04**	**2.82**	**2.66**	**2.53**	**2.43**	**2.34**	**2.26**	**2.20**	**2.09**	**2.01**	**1.89**	**1.81**	**1.71**	**1.61**	**1.54**	**1.44**	**1.38**	**1.28**	**1.19**	**1.11**
∞	3.84	2.99	2.60	2.37	2.21	2.09	2.01	1.94	1.88	1.83	1.79	1.75	1.69	1.64	1.57	1.52	1.46	1.40	1.35	1.28	1.24	1.17	1.13	1.00
	6.64	**4.60**	**3.78**	**3.32**	**3.02**	**2.80**	**2.64**	**2.51**	**2.41**	**2.32**	**2.24**	**2.18**	**2.07**	**1.99**	**1.87**	**1.79**	**1.69**	**1.59**	**1.52**	**1.41**	**1.36**	**1.25**	**1.15**	**1.00**

* numerator
+ denominator
From: Snedecor, G. W. (1938). *Statistical methods*. Ames, Iowa: Collegiate Press. (Table 10-3, pp. 184–187).

APPENDIX F

Distribution of X^2 Probability

df	.20	.10	.05	.02	.01	.001
1	1.642	2.706	3.841	5.412	6.635	10.827
2	3.219	4.605	5.991	7.824	9.210	13.815
3	4.642	6.251	7.815	9.837	11.345	16.266
4	5.989	7.779	9.488	11.668	13.277	18.467
5	7.289	9.236	11.070	13.388	15.086	20.515
6	8.558	10.645	12.592	15.033	16.812	22.457
7	9.803	12.017	14.067	16.622	18.475	24.322
8	11.030	13.362	15.507	18.168	20.090	26.125
9	12.242	14.684	16.919	19.679	21.666	27.877
10	13.442	15.987	18.307	21.161	23.209	29.588
11	14.631	17.275	19.675	22.618	24.725	31.264
12	15.812	18.549	21.026	24.054	26.217	32.909
13	16.985	19.812	22.362	25.472	27.688	34.528
14	18.151	21.064	23.685	26.873	29.141	36.123
15	19.311	22.307	24.996	28.259	30.578	37.697
16	20.465	23.542	26.296	29.633	32.000	39.252
17	21.615	24.769	27.587	30.995	33.409	40.790
18	22.760	25.989	28.869	32.346	34.805	42.312
19	23.900	27.204	30.144	33.687	36.191	43.820
20	25.038	28.412	31.410	35.020	37.566	45.315
21	26.171	29.615	32.671	36.343	38.932	46.797
22	27.301	30.813	33.924	37.659	40.289	48.268
23	28.429	32.007	35.172	38.968	41.638	49.728
24	29.553	33.196	36.415	40.270	42.980	51.179
25	30.675	34.382	37.652	41.566	44.314	52.620
26	31.795	35.563	38.885	42.856	45.642	54.052
27	32.912	36.741	40.113	44.140	46.963	55.476
28	34.027	37.916	41.337	45.419	48.278	56.893
29	35.139	39.087	42.557	46.693	49.588	58.302
30	36.250	40.256	43.773	47.962	50.892	59.703

From: Fisher, R. A. (1970). *Statistical methods for research workers* (14th ed.). Darien, CT: Hafner Publishing. (Taken from Table III, pp. 112–113).

APPENDIX G

Distribution of *t*

	Level of significance for one-tailed test					
	.10	*.05*	*.025*	*.01*	*.005*	*.0005*
	Level of significance for two-tailed test					
df	*.20*	*.10*	*.05*	*.02*	*.01*	*.001*
1	3.078	6.314	12.706	31.821	63.657	636.619
2	1.886	2.920	4.303	6.965	9.925	31.598
3	1.638	2.353	3.182	4.541	5.841	12.941
4	1.533	2.132	2.776	3.747	4.604	8.610
5	1.476	2.015	2.571	3.365	4.032	6.859
6	1.440	1.943	2.447	3.143	3.707	5.959
7	1.415	1.895	2.365	2.998	3.499	5.405
8	1.397	1.860	2.306	2.896	3.355	5.041
9	1.383	1.833	2.262	2.821	3.250	4.781
10	1.372	1.812	2.228	2.764	3.169	4.587
11	1.363	1.796	2.201	2.718	3.106	4.437
12	1.356	1.782	2.179	2.681	3.055	4.318
13	1.350	1.771	2.160	2.650	3.012	4.221
14	1.345	1.761	2.145	2.624	2.977	4.140
15	1.341	1.753	2.131	2.602	2.947	4.073
16	1.337	1.746	2.120	2.583	2.921	4.015
17	1.333	1.740	2.110	2.567	2.898	3.965
18	1.330	1.734	2.101	2.552	2.878	3.922
19	1.328	1.729	2.093	2.539	2.861	3.883
20	1.325	1.725	2.086	2.528	2.845	3.850

	Level of significance for one-tailed test					
	.10	.05	.025	.01	.005	.0005
	Level of significance for two-tailed test					
df	.20	.10	.05	.02	.01	.001
21	1.323	1.721	2.080	2.518	2.831	3.819
22	1.321	1.717	2.074	2.508	2.819	3.792
23	1.319	1.714	2.069	2.500	2.807	3.767
24	1.318	1.711	2.064	2.492	2.797	3.745
25	1.316	1.708	2.060	2.485	2.787	3.725
26	1.315	1.706	2.056	2.479	2.779	3.707
27	1.314	1.703	2.052	2.473	2.771	3.690
28	1.313	1.701	2.048	2.467	2.763	3.674
29	1.311	1.699	2.045	2.462	2.756	3.659
30	1.310	1.697	2.042	2.457	2.750	3.646
40	1.303	1.684	2.021	2.423	2.704	3.551
60	1.296	1.671	2.000	2.390	2.660	3.460
120	1.289	1.658	1.980	2.358	2.617	3.373
∞	1.282	1.645	1.960	2.326	2.576	3.291

From Fisher, R. A. (1970). *Statistical methods for research workers* (14th ed.). Darien, CT: Hafner Publishing (Table IV, p. 176).

APPENDIX H

Values of q_α (the Studentized Range Statistic) at the 5% and 1% Levels of Significance

					k = Number of Means					
df_{wg}	α	2	3	4	5	6	7	8	9	10
1	.05	17.97	26.98	32.82	37.08	40.41	43.12	45.40	47.36	49.07
	.01	90.03	135.00	164.30	185.60	202.20	215.80	227.20	237.00	245.60
2	.05	6.08	8.33	9.80	10.88	11.74	12.44	13.03	13.54	13.99
	.01	14.04	19.02	22.29	24.72	26.63	28.20	29.53	30.68	31.69
3	.05	4.50	5.91	6.82	7.50	8.04	8.48	8.85	9.18	9.46
	.01	8.26	10.62	12.17	13.33	14.24	15.00	15.64	16.20	16.69
4	.05	3.93	5.04	5.76	6.29	6.71	7.05	7.35	7.60	7.83
	.01	6.51	8.12	9.17	9.96	10.58	11.10	11.55	11.93	12.27
5	.05	3.64	4.60	5.22	5.67	6.03	6.33	6.58	6.80	6.99
	.01	5.70	6.98	7.80	8.42	8.91	9.32	9.67	9.97	10.24
6	.05	3.46	4.34	4.90	5.30	5.63	5.90	6.12	6.32	6.49
	.01	5.24	6.33	7.03	7.56	7.97	8.32	8.61	8.87	9.10
7	.05	3.34	4.16	4.68	5.06	5.36	5.61	5.82	6.00	6.16
	.01	4.95	5.92	6.54	7.01	7.37	7.68	7.94	8.17	8.37
8	.05	3.26	4.04	4.53	4.89	5.17	5.40	5.60	5.77	5.92
	.01	4.75	5.64	6.20	6.62	6.96	7.24	7.47	7.68	7.86
9	.05	3.20	3.95	4.41	4.76	5.02	5.24	5.43	5.59	5.74
	.01	4.60	5.43	5.96	6.35	6.66	6.91	7.13	7.33	7.49
10	.05	3.15	3.88	4.33	4.65	4.91	5.12	5.30	5.46	5.60
	.01	4.48	5.27	5.77	6.14	6.43	6.67	6.87	7.05	7.21
11	.05	3.11	3.82	4.26	4.57	4.82	5.03	5.20	5.35	5.49
	.01	4.39	5.15	5.62	5.97	6.25	6.48	6.67	6.84	6.99
12	.05	3.08	3.77	4.20	4.51	4.75	4.95	5.12	5.27	5.39
	.01	4.32	5.05	5.50	5.84	6.10	6.32	6.51	6.67	6.81

| df_{wg} | α | \multicolumn{9}{c}{k = Number of Means} |
		2	3	4	5	6	7	8	9	10
13	.05	3.06	3.73	4.15	4.45	4.69	4.88	5.05	5.19	5.32
	.01	4.26	4.96	5.40	5.73	5.98	6.19	6.37	6.53	6.67
14	.05	3.03	3.70	4.11	4.41	4.64	4.83	4.99	5.13	5.25
	.01	4.21	4.89	5.32	5.63	5.88	6.08	6.26	6.41	6.54
15	.05	3.01	3.67	4.08	4.37	4.59	4.78	4.94	5.08	5.20
	.01	4.17	4.84	5.25	5.56	5.80	5.99	6.16	6.31	6.44
16	.05	3.00	3.65	4.05	4.33	4.56	4.74	4.90	5.03	5.15
	.01	4.13	4.79	5.19	5.49	5.72	5.92	6.08	6.22	6.35
17	.05	2.98	3.63	4.02	4.30	4.52	4.70	4.86	4.99	5.11
	.01	4.10	4.74	5.14	5.43	5.66	5.85	6.01	6.15	6.27
18	.05	2.97	3.61	4.00	4.28	4.49	4.67	4.82	4.96	5.07
	.01	4.07	4.70	5.09	5.38	5.60	5.79	5.94	6.08	6.20
19	.05	2.96	3.59	3.98	4.25	4.47	4.65	4.79	4.92	5.04
	.01	4.05	4.67	5.05	5.33	5.55	5.73	5.89	6.02	6.14
20	.05	2.95	3.58	3.96	4.23	4.45	4.62	4.77	4.90	5.01
	.01	4.02	4.64	5.02	5.29	5.51	5.69	5.84	5.97	6.09
24	.05	2.92	3.53	3.90	4.17	4.37	4.54	4.68	4.81	4.92
	.01	3.96	4.55	4.91	5.17	5.37	5.54	5.69	5.81	5.92
30	.05	2.89	3.49	3.85	4.10	4.30	4.46	4.60	4.72	4.82
	.01	3.89	4.45	4.80	5.05	5.24	5.40	5.54	5.65	5.76
40	.05	2.86	3.44	3.79	4.04	4.23	4.39	4.52	4.63	4.73
	.01	3.82	4.37	4.70	4.93	5.11	5.26	5.39	5.50	5.60
60	.05	2.83	3.40	3.74	3.98	4.16	4.31	4.44	4.55	4.65
	.01	3.76	4.28	4.59	4.82	4.99	5.13	5.25	5.36	5.45
120	.05	2.80	3.36	3.68	3.92	4.10	4.24	4.36	4.47	4.56
	.01	3.70	4.20	4.50	4.71	4.87	5.01	5.12	5.21	5.30
∞	.05	2.77	3.31	3.63	3.86	4.03	4.17	4.29	4.39	4.47
	.01	3.64	4.12	4.40	4.60	4.76	4.88	4.99	5.08	5.16

From: Pearson, E. S., & Hartley, H. O. (Eds.) (1966). Biometrika tables for statisticians. Vol. I. (3rd ed.). Cambridge: University Press (Table 29).

Index